T0259111

Pediatric Emergencies

Editors

RICHARD LICHENSTEIN
GETACHEW TESHOME

PEDIATRIC CLINICS
OF NORTH AMERICA

www.pediatric.theclinics.com

October 2013 • Volume 60 • Number 5

ELSEVIER

1600 John F. Kennedy Boulevard ● Suite 1800 ● Philadelphia, Pennsylvania, 19103-2899

http://www.theclinics.com

THE PEDIATRIC CLINICS OF NORTH AMERICA Volume 60, Number 5
October 2013 ISSN 0031-3955, ISBN-13: 978-0-323-22733-9

Editor: Kerry Holland
Developmental Editor: Donald Mumford

The Pediatric Clinics of North America (ISSN 0031-3955) is published bimonthly by Elsevier Inc., 360 Park Avenue South, New York, NY 10010-1710. Months of issue are February, April, June, August, October, and December. Periodicals postage paid at New York, NY and additional mailing offices. Subscription prices are $191.00 per year (US individuals), $462.00 per year (US institutions), $259.00 per year (Canadian individuals), $614.00 per year (Canadian institutions), $308.00 per year (international individuals), $614.00 per year (international institutions), $93.00 per year (US students and residents), and $159.00 per year (international and Canadian residents and students). To receive students/resident rare, orders must be accompanied by name of affiliated institution, date of term, and the signature of program/residency coordinator on institution letterhead. Orders will be billed at individual rate until proof of status is received. Foreign air speed delivery is included in all *Clinics* subscription prices. All prices are subject to change without notice. **POSTMASTER:** Send address changes to *The Pediatric Clinics of North America*, Elsevier Health Sciences Division, Subscription Customer Service, 3251 Riverport Lane, Maryland Heights, MO 63043. **Customer Service: 1-800-654-2452 (US and Canada). From outside of the US and Canada: 1-314-447-8871. Fax: 1-314-447-8029. For print support, E-mail: JournalsCustomerService-usa@elsevier.com. For online support, E-mail: JournalsOnlineSupport-usa@elsevier.com.**

Reprints. For copies of 100 or more, of articles in this publication, please contact the Commercial Reprints Department, Elsevier Inc., 360 Park Avenue South, New York, NY 10010-1710. Tel.: 212-633-3874; Fax: 212-633-3820; E-mail: reprints@elsevier.com.

The Pediatric Clinics of North America is also published in Spanish by McGraw-Hill Inter-americana Editores S.A., Mexico City, Mexico; in Portuguese by Riechmann and Affonso Editores, Rua Comandante Coelho 1085, CEP 21250, Rio de Janeiro, Brazil; and in Greek by Althayia SA, Athens, Greece.

The Pediatric Clinics of North America is covered in *MEDLINE/PubMed (Index Medicus)*, *Excerpta Medica*, *Current Contents*, *Current Contents/Clinical Medicine*, *Science Citation Index*, *ASCA*, *ISI/BIOMED*, and *BIOSIS*.

Printed and bound by CPI Group (UK) Ltd, Croydon, CR0 4YY

Transferred to digital print 2012

PROGRAM OBJECTIVE

The goal of the *Pediatric Clinics of North America* is to keep practicing physicians and residents up to date with current clinical practice in pediatrics by providing timely articles reviewing the state-of-the-art in patient care.

TARGET AUDIENCE

All practicing pediatricians, physicians and healthcare professionals who provide patient care to pediatric patients.

LEARNING OBJECTIVES

Upon completion of this activity, participants will be able to:
1. Review emerging concepts in pediatric emergency radiology.
2. Discuss common office procedures and analgesia considerations.
3. Recognize skin and soft tissue infections.

ACCREDITATION

The Elsevier Office of Continuing Medical Education (EOCME) is accredited by the Accreditation Council for Continuing Medical Education (ACCME) to provide continuing medical education for physicians.

The EOCME designates this enduringmaterial for a maximum of 15 *AMA PRA Category 1 Credit*(s)™. Physicians should claim only the credit commensurate with the extent of their participation in the activity.

All other health care professionals requesting continuing education credit for this enduring material will be issued a certificate of participation.

DISCLOSURE OF CONFLICTS OF INTEREST

The EOCME assesses conflict of interest with its instructors, faculty, planners, and other individuals who are in a position to control the content of CME activities. All relevant conflicts of interest that are identified are thoroughly vetted by EOCME for fair balance, scientific objectivity, and patient care recommendations. EOCME is committed to providing its learners with CME activities that promote improvements or quality in healthcare and not a specific proprietary business or a commercial interest.

The planning committee, staff, authors and editors listed below have identified no financial relationships or relationships to products or devices they or their spouse/life partner have with commercial interest related to the content of this CME activity:
Rajan Arora, MD; Shireen Atabaki, MD, MPH; Nicola Baker, MD; Fermin Barrueto Jr, MD; Reginald Brown, MD; Thomas Chun, MD; Forrest Closson, MD; Nicole Congleton; Susan J. Duffy, MD, MPH; Rajender K. Gattu, MD, FAAP, MRCP; Mike Gittelman, MD; Brynne Hunter; Kerry Holland; Emily R. Katz, MD; Indu Kumari; Sandy Lavery; Julie Leonard, MD, MPH; Richard Lichenstein, MD; Emily C. MacNeill, MD; Prashant Mahajan, MD, MPH, MBA; Maryann Mazer-Amirishani, PharmD, MD; Jill McNair; Marlene Melzer-Lange, MD; Rakesh Mistry, MD, MS; Getachew Teshome, MD, MPH; Sudhir Vashist, MD; Dale Woolridge, MD, PhD, FAAEM, FAACP, FACEP; Christian Wright, MD; Mark R. Zonfrillo, MD, MSCE; Joseph Zorc, MD, MSCEMD, MSCE.

The planning committee, staff, authors and editors listed below have identified financial relationships or relationships to products or devices they or their spouse/life partner have with commercial interest related to the content of this CME activity:
Amy Baxter, MD, FAAP, FACEP has an employment relationship and receives royalties/patents from MMJ Labs, LLC.
Susan Fuchs, MD has a research grant from UpToDate.
Kyle Nelson, MD's spouse has stock ownership and employment affiliation with Vertex Pharmaceuticals Incorporated.

UNAPPROVED/OFF-LABEL USE DISCLOSURE

The EOCME requires CME faculty to disclose to the participants:
1. When products or procedures being discussed are off-label, unlabelled, experimental, and/or investigational (not US Food and Drug Administration (FDA) approved); and
2. Any limitations on the information presented, such as data that are preliminary or that represent ongoing research, interim analyses, and/or unsupported opinions. Faculty may discuss information about pharmaceutical agents that is outside of FDA-approved labelling. This information is intended solely for CME and is not intended to promote off-label use of these medications. If you have any questions, contact the medical affairs department of the manufacturer for the most recent prescribing information.

TO ENROLL

To enroll in the *Pediatric Clinics of North America* Continuing Medical Education program, call customer service at 1-800-654-2452 or sign up online at http://www.theclinics.com/home/cme. The CME program is available to subscribers for an additional annual fee of USD 261.

METHOD OF PARTICIPATION

In order to claim credit, participants must complete the following:
1. Complete enrolment as indicated above.
2. Read the activity.
3. Complete the CME Test and Evaluation. Participants must achieve a score of 70% on the test. All CME Tests and Evaluations must be completed online.

CME INQUIRIES/SPECIAL NEEDS

For all CME inquiries or special needs, please contact elsevierCME@elsevier.com.

Contributors

EDITORS

RICHARD LICHENSTEIN
Professor and Director, Pediatric Emergency Medicine Research, Division of Emergency Medicine, Department of Pediatrics, University of Maryland School of Medicine, Baltimore, Maryland

GETACHEW TESHOME, MD, MPH
Assistant Professor and Medical Director, Division of Emergency Medicine, Department of Pediatrics, University of Maryland School of Medicine, Baltimore, Maryland

AUTHORS

RAJAN ARORA, MD
Division of Emergency Medicine, Pediatric Emergency Medicine Fellow, Carman and Ann Adam Department of Pediatrics, Children's Hospital of Michigan, Wayne State University School of Medicine, Detroit, Michigan

SHIREEN M. ATABAKI, MD, MPH
Associate Professor, Division of Emergency Medicine, Department of Pediatrics and Emergency Medicine, Children's National Medical Center, and The George Washington University School of Medicine, Washington, DC

NICOLA BAKER, MD
Department of Emergency Medicine, University of Arizona, Tucson, Arizona

FERMIN BARRUETO Jr, MD, FACEP, FAAEM, FACMT
Clinical Associate Professor, Department of Emergency Medicine, University of Maryland School of Medicine, Baltimore; Chairman, Department of Emergency Medicine, Upper Chesapeake Health Systems, Bel Air, Maryland

AMY BAXTER, MD
Director of Research, Pediatric Emergency Medicine Associates, Children's Healthcare of Atlanta Scottish Rite, Atlanta; Clinical Associate Professor, Department of Emergency Medicine, Medical College of Georgia at Georgia Regents University, Augusta, Georgia

REGINALD BROWN, MD
Instructor, Department of Emergency Medicine, University of Maryland School of Medicine, Baltimore, Maryland

THOMAS H. CHUN, MD, MPH
Associate Professor, Departments of Emergency Medicine and Pediatrics, Rhode Island Hospital, Providence, Rhode Island

FORREST T. CLOSSON, MD
Instructor of Pediatrics, Division of Emergency Medicine, Department of Pediatrics, University of Maryland School of Medicine, University of Maryland Children's Hospital, Baltimore, Maryland

SUSAN J. DUFFY, MD, MPH
Associate Professor, Departments of Emergency Medicine and Pediatrics, Rhode Island Hospital, Providence, Rhode Island

SUSAN FUCHS, MD, FAAP, FACEP
Associate Division Head, Division of Emergency Medicine, Ann & Robert H. Lurie Children's Hospital of Chicago; Professor of Pediatrics, Feinberg School of Medicine, Northwestern University, Chicago, Illinois

RAJENDER GATTU, MD
Assistant Professor of Pediatrics, Division of Emergency Medicine, Department of Pediatrics, University of Maryland School of Medicine, Baltimore, Maryland

MICHAEL A. GITTELMAN, MD
Professor, Clinical Pediatrics, University of Cincinnati School of Medicine; Division of Emergency Medicine, Co-Director, Comprehensive Children's Injury Center, Emergency Medicine Physician, Cincinnati Children's Hospital Medical Center, Cincinnati, Ohio

EMILY R. KATZ, MD
Clinical Assistant Professor, Department of Child and Family Psychiatry, Rhode Island Hospital, Providence, Rhode Island

JULIE C. LEONARD, MD, MPH
Division of Emergency Medicine, Department of Pediatrics, School of Medicine, Washington University in St. Louis, St Louis, Missouri

EMILY C. MACNEILL, MD
Assistant Professor, Department of Emergency Medicine, Carolinas Medical Center, Carolinas Healthcare System, Charlotte, North Carolina

PRASHANT MAHAJAN, MD, MPH, MBA
Division of Emergency Medicine, Division Chief and Research Director, Professor of Pediatrics & Emergency Medicine, Carman and Ann Adam Department of Pediatrics, Director, Center for Quality and Innovation, Children's Hospital of Michigan, Wayne State University School of Medicine, Detroit, Michigan

MARYANN MAZER-AMIRSHAHI, PharmD, MD
Clinical Assistant Professor, Department of Emergency Medicine, George Washington University; Instructor, Department of Clinical Pharmacology, Children's National Medical Center, Washington, DC

MARLENE D. MELZER-LANGE, MD
Medical Director, Emergency Department Trauma Center, Children's Hospital of Wisconsin; Professor, Department of Pediatrics, Section of Emergency Medicine, Medical College of Wisconsin, Milwaukee, Wisconsin

RAKESH D. MISTRY, MD, MS
Attending Physician, Section of Pediatric Emergency Medicine, Children's Hospital Colorado; Associate Professor of Pediatrics, University of Colorado School of Medicine, Aurora, Colorado

KYLE A. NELSON, MD, MPH
Attending Physician, Emergency Medicine, Boston Children's Hospital; Assistant Professor, Pediatrics, Harvard Medical School, Boston, Massachusetts

GETACHEW TESHOME, MD, MPH
Assistant Professor and Medical Director, Division of Emergency Medicine, Department of Pediatrics, University of Maryland School of Medicine, Baltimore, Maryland

SUDHIR VASHIST, MBBS, MD
Assistant Professor, Department of Pediatrics, Pediatric Cardiologist, Children's Heart Program, University of Maryland School of Medicine, Baltimore, Maryland

DALE WOOLRIDGE, MD, PhD
Department of Emergency Medicine, University of Arizona, Tucson, Arizona

CHRISTIAN C. WRIGHT, MD
Assistant Professor, Division of Emergency Medicine, Department of Pediatrics, University of Maryland School of Medicine, University of Maryland Children's Hospital, Baltimore, Maryland

MARK R. ZONFRILLO, MD, MSCE
Associate Director of Research, Division of Emergency Medicine, Director of Child Road Traffic Safety Research, Center for Injury Research and Prevention, Children's Hospital of Philadelphia; Assistant Professor of Pediatrics, Perelman School of Medicine, University of Pennsylvania, Philadelphia, Pennsylvania

JOSEPH J. ZORC, MD, MSCE
Attending Physician, Emergency Medicine, and Director, Emergency Information System, The Children's Hospital of Philadelphia; Associate Professor, Pediatrics, Perelman School of Medicine, University of Pennsylvania, Philadelphia, Pennsylvania

Contents

and medical toxicologists can be consulted to assist with the diagnosis of medicinal/drug overdoses, for advice about the pitfalls inherent in stabilizing children who have been exposed to toxic compounds, and for treatment recommendations based on the latest research.

Although most ingested foreign bodies in children pass spontaneously, certain foreign bodies can be harmful and they require special attention and emergent medical intervention to prevent significant morbidity and mortality. This article presents an overview of the epidemiology, diagnosis, management, and complications of foreign body ingestions in children. Particular attention is paid to coins, sharp objects, long objects, food bolus, caustic liquids, batteries, and magnets.

Because injury is the leading cause of morbidity and mortality in young patients, emergency departments have a significant opportunity to provide injury-prevention interventions at a teachable moment. The emergency department has the ability to survey injuries in the community, use the hospital setting to screen patients, provide products, offer resources to assist families within this setting to change their risky behaviors, and connect families to community resources. With a thoughtful, collaborative approach, emergency departments are an excellent setting within which to promote injury prevention among patients and families.

PEDIATRIC CLINICS OF NORTH AMERICA

FORTHCOMING ISSUES

December 2013
Pediatric Hematology
Catherine Manno, MD, *Editor*

February 2014
Adolescent Cardiac Issues
Richard Humes, MD, and
Pooja Gupta, MD, *Editors*

April 2014
Pediatric Dermatology
Kara Shah, MD, *Editor*

RECENT ISSUES

August 2013
Pediatric Otolaryngology
Harold S. Pine, MD, *Editor*

June 2013
Critical Care of the Pediatric Patient
Derek S. Wheeler, MD, *Editor*

April 2013
**Advances in the Diagnosis and Treatment
of Pediatric Infectious Diseases**
Chandy C. John, MD, *Editor*

RELATED INTEREST

Emergency Medicine Clinics of North America August 2013 (Volume 31:3)
Pediatric Emergency Medicine
Mimi Lu, MD, Dale Woolridge, MD, PhD, and Ann Dietrich, MD, *Editors*

Preface

Pediatric Emergencies

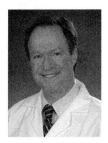 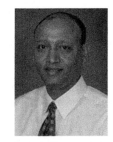

Richard Lichenstein, MD   Getachew Teshome, MD, MPH
Editors

Pediatric medicine continues to evolve along its complex path. As research deepens our understanding of injury and illness, clinicians are challenged to use the latest technology and rely on the new best evidence to optimize our care of patients. This is as true for conditions that are seemingly unchanging (head trauma and bronchiolitis) as it is for emerging conditions brought to our attention by the keen observations of clinicians in the field (magnet ingestions). We need to understand how to use technology judiciously and how to apply new knowledge that will provide meaningful solutions to the clinical scenarios we encounter every day.

These issues are amplified in the hotbed of the emergency department. Emergency physicians face the dilemma of being expected to apply practices based on best evidence, with access to all manner of laboratory and radiologic resources, and to do it as efficiently as possible for all types of medical and traumatic conditions. Emergency physicians must juggle the clinical needs of patients and parents as well as the administrative issues of time and cost. Practicing pediatricians are challenged even more so by the same problems and demands.

This issue of *Pediatric Clinics of North America* highlights diseases, injuries, populations, and emerging conditions in pediatric emergency medicine. Bronchiolitis, asthma, and fever will always be pediatricians' bread and butter. The latest developments in these illnesses are reviewed in this issue, with implications for their assessment and management. Skin infections and abscesses are likewise common, but our knowledge of resistance patterns and the new best practices for treatment is changing. Appropriate use of antibiotics and judicious use of incision and drainage are discussed. The evaluation of altered mental status is always challenging. We present a framework for a rational approach to evaluation and management of these patients. Concussion and head injury are frequent presentations for the practicing pediatrician. We now better understand how to evaluate and manage children

Pediatr Clin N Am 60 (2013) xv–xvii
http://dx.doi.org/10.1016/j.pcl.2013.08.001   **pediatric.theclinics.com**

with these injuries, and we know how to use CT scans more appropriately. New research has shed light on the risk of cervical spine injury after trauma, helping us understand the common practice of clearing the c-spine better. Moreover, the practical use of all types of radiologic examinations is reviewed as they pertain to acute pediatric illness and injury. Pediatric offices have evolved with a greater scope of practice and extended hours of availability, to the point that they can be seen as mini emergency departments. These clinical care sites need to be ready to assess and manage acute emergencies and common injuries by knowing simple procedures as well as lifesaving skills, because these sites will surely be incorporated in community emergency plans.

At every site of care, children need to be made comfortable when they are ill or injured. Analgesia and procedural sedation must always be considered to provide comfort for children. A child's first experience in a medical setting can leave lasting physical and psychological impressions. A comprehensive approach to pain relief and anxiolysis is the first step toward ensuring a rewarding medical encounter for patient and practitioner. Children assisted by technologic devices and others with acute psychiatric and behavioral problems are coming to emergency departments and office settings in increasing numbers. The practicing pediatrician needs to have a true appreciation of these patient groups and a clear plan for interacting with them and providing appropriate management and referral.

New drugs of abuse and foreign body ingestions pose unique diagnostic and treatment challenges. Clinicians are on the forefront for uncovering patterns of injury, ingestion, and illness that are likely to be encountered in any office setting. The magnet and bath salt ingestion stories told in this issue are the types of encounters that lead to research and innovation and ultimately improved children's health.

Finally, prevention efforts initiated and encouraged by pediatric office practitioners and emergency medicine physicians are critical for the safety and wellness of children. Injury prevention efforts are one of the true success stories in pediatrics. This issue reviews some evidence-based interventions that have been used successfully in emergency departments.

We would like to thank all our authors for their time and effort in preparing the manuscripts. Their expertise and enthusiasm were very much appreciated in this undertaking.

Our experience with the Pediatric Emergency Care Applied Research Network was integral for the planning and compilation of this *Pediatric Clinics of North America* issue. From this interaction, we have developed an intense respect for the process of research and evidenced-based medicine. Moreover, we have benefited from collaboration with members of the Section of Pediatric Emergency Medicine, Council on Injury, Violence, and Poison Prevention of the American Academy of Pediatrics, and at the University of Maryland School of Medicine. We are privileged to consider these people as colleagues, mentors, and friends.

We are forever grateful for our family and friends, but are especially thankful to our wives, Maura and Tsigie, and our children, Sarah, Mike, Eden, and Daniel. These are the people who inspire us daily to tackle challenges thoughtfully and with empathy and compassion.

Richard Lichenstein, MD
Pediatric Emergency Medicine Research
University of Maryland School of Medicine
110 South Paca Street, 8-S-139
Baltimore, MD 21201, USA

Getachew Teshome, MD, MPH
Division of Emergency Medicine
Department of Pediatrics
University of Maryland School of Medicine
22 South Greene Street–WGL-266
Baltimore, MD 21201, USA

E-mail addresses:
RLichenstein@peds.umaryland.edu (R. Lichenstein)
Gteshome@peds.umaryland.edu (G. Teshome)

Acute Bronchiolitis

Getachew Teshome, MD, MPH[a],*, Rajender Gattu, MD[a],
Reginald Brown, MD[b]

KEYWORDS

- Acute bronchiolitis • Wheezing • Respiratory syncytial virus

KEY POINTS

- Acute bronchiolitis is a clinical diagnosis based on history and physical examination. Clinicians should not routinely order laboratory and radiologic studies for diagnosis.
- Assess risk factors for severe disease such as age less than 12 weeks, a history of prematurity, hemodynamically significant cardiovascular disease, or immunodeficiency when making decisions about management of children with bronchiolitis.
- Respiratory syncytial virus accounts for an overwhelming majority of bronchiolitis infections followed by rhinovirus, parainfluenza, adenovirus, and *Mycoplasma*.
- A carefully monitored trial of α-adrenergic or β-adrenergic agents is an option. Inhaled bronchodilators should be continued only if there is a documented positive clinical response. Corticosteroids should not be used routinely in the management of bronchiolitis.
- Antibacterial medications should only be used in children with bronchiolitis who have specific evidence for the coexistence of a bacterial infection. When present, bacterial infection should be treated in the same manner as in the absence of bronchiolitis.

INTRODUCTION

Bronchiolitis is the most common lower respiratory tract infection to affect infants and toddlers. Bronchiolitis was originally described in 1901 by Wilhelm Lange, and is familiar to nearly every pediatrician and emergency physician. An abundance of new research has emerged over the last decade, changing some existing knowledge regarding bronchiolitis. Most of the research is stimulated by the increasing number of bronchiolitis-related primary care, Emergency Department (ED) visits, and hospital admissions in the United States. Physician, nursing, and financial resources used annually are higher than previously assumed, and rival those of influenza epidemics. A vast majority of bronchiolitis illness is attributed to respiratory syncytial virus (RSV),

Disclosures: None.
[a] Division of Emergency Medicine, Department of Pediatrics, University of Maryland School of Medicine, 22 South Greene Street, WGL 266, Baltimore, MD 21201, USA; [b] Department of Emergency Medicine, University of Maryland School of Medicine, 110 Paca Street, 6th Floor, Suite 200, Baltimore, MD 21201, USA
* Corresponding author.
E-mail address: gteshome@peds.umaryland.edu

Pediatr Clin N Am 60 (2013) 1019–1034
http://dx.doi.org/10.1016/j.pcl.2013.06.005
0031-3955/13/$ – see front matter © 2013 Elsevier Inc. All rights reserved.

although new knowledge has highlighted 2 additional viral agents. The paradigm of treatment with bronchodilators and steroids has drastically changed.[1] Novel therapies such as hypertonic saline nebulized therapy, helium/oxygen mixtures (heliox), and high-flow nasal cannula (HFNC) therapies are currently being investigated.

PUBLIC HEALTH BURDEN

Bronchiolitis hospitalizations have been increasing over the last 20 years. An estimated 132,000 to 172,000 RSV-associated hospitalizations occur annually in children younger than 5 years.[2] Hospital costs are estimated at US$700 million annually.[3] Experts have postulated that the increase in hospitalization is multifactorial, and includes increased survival of preterm infants, increased use of pulse oximetry, changes in admission criteria, and even increased attendance in day care. Fortunately, the number of deaths from bronchiolitis has decreased significantly to fewer than 500 annually in the United States, partially attributable to effective use of RSV immune globulin and RSV monoclonal antibody for high-risk infants.[3,4]

Hall and colleagues[5] demonstrated an expanded burden of RSV bronchiolitis by examining a cohort of children up to 5 years of age. The extrapolated data suggest that 2.1 million children under the age of 5 would require treatment each year, 25% or 500,000 of whom would seek treatment in the ED, with 57,000 hospitalizations each year. This burden equals that of influenza for ages 2 to 5 years. For infants aged less than 6 months, the burden of bronchiolitis exceeds that of influenza. Risk factors for RSV bronchiolitis requiring hospitalization were similar to those previously reported, and include male sex, chronic illness, lower socioeconomic status, smoke exposure, and contact with other children. Independent risks factors for severe illness were young age and prematurity.[6]

PATHOGENESIS

Bronchiolitis is characterized by bronchiole obstruction with edema, cellular debris, and mucus, resulting in symptoms of wheezing. Bronchiolitis takes place in the small thin-walled conducting passages of the lung of less than 2 mm in diameter. In addition to size, bronchioles differ from the larger bronchi in that they are absent of cartilage, goblet cells, or glands.

Small-bronchiole epithelium is circumferentially infected, but basal cells are spared. Both type 1 and 2 alveolar pneumocytes are also infected. Inflammatory infiltrates are centered on bronchial and pulmonary arterioles and consist of primarily CD69+ monocytes, CD3+ double-negative T cells, CD8+ T cells, and neutrophils. The neutrophil distribution is predominantly between arterioles and airways, whereas the mononuclear cell distributions are in both airways and lung parenchyma. Most inflammatory cells are concentrated submuscular to the airway, but many cells traverse the smooth muscle into the airway epithelium and lumen. Airway obstruction is a prominent feature attributed to epithelial and inflammatory cell debris mixed with fibrin, mucus, and edema, and compounded by compression from hyperplasic lymphoid follicles. These findings are important to our understanding of RSV pathogenesis, and may facilitate the development of new approaches to prevention and treatment.[7]

There are 2 main patterns of disease: acute bronchiolitis and interstitial pneumonia. In acute bronchiolitis, the main lesion is epithelial necrosis, which occurs when a dense plug is formed in the bronchiolar lumen, leading to air trapping air and other mechanical interference with ventilation. In interstitial pneumonia, there is widespread inflammation and necrosis of lung parenchyma with severe lesions of the bronchial and bronchiolar mucosa.[8]

Bronchioles make little contribution to airflow resistance in the healthy lung. However, in the setting of inflammation or obstruction, the bronchioles can produce significant impairment of lung function. In the pediatric population, bronchiolitis is nearly exclusively the result of viral infection, specifically RSV. Similar abnormality is also seen in adults with inhalation injury, postinfectious conditions, complications of lung or stem cell transplant, collagen vascular disease, and idiopathic causes.[9]

ETIOLOGY

The proportion of disease caused by specific viruses varies depending on the season and the year; RSV is the most common, followed by rhinovirus. Parainfluenza, adenovirus, and *Mycoplasma* also produce similar bronchiolitis illness. Recent evidence has also shown that metapneumovirus and human bocavirus have also caused bronchiolitis alone or as a coinfection with RSV.[10]

RSV is an enveloped, nonsegmented, negative-strand RNA virus of the family Paramyxoviridae. Humans are the only source of infection. Infection is via close or direct contact with contaminated secretions. RSV can persist on hands and surfaces for 30 minutes or more. RSV typically is seen in epidemics in North America between November and March. The incubation period is between 2 and 8 days. Infected hosts can shed the disease typically from 3 to 8 days, but immune-compromised hosts or infants can shed for as long as 4 weeks.[10]

Rhinovirus has long been known as an etiologic agent of the common cold; it can also cause bronchiolitis and infects the lower respiratory tract, and triggers asthma exacerbations in children, highlighting that this viral pathogen causes greater morbidity than previously recognized.[10]

Metapneumovirus was discovered in 2001 and is also of the Paramyxoviridae family. It causes upper respiratory infections in children of all ages and adults. In addition, it can cause asthma exacerbations, pneumonia, croup, and otitis media as well as bronchiolitis. Infections are generally from November to March, as for RSV. Recent studies link metapneumovirus with approximately 7% of bronchiolitis infections. Likewise, Human bocavirus, of the family Parvoviridae, was recently identified in 2005 as a source of upper respiratory infection in children. Bocavirus is identified as a coinfection in bronchiolitis 80% of the time. The pathogenesis of bocavirus is still being investigated.[11]

CLINICAL FEATURES

Bronchiolitis generally is a self-limited illness resulting in cough, fever, and rhinorrhea and lasting between 7 and 10 days. RSV is ubiquitous, with estimates of 90% of children infected with RSV in the first 2 years of life.[12] Nevertheless, RSV and non-RSV bronchiolitis can produce severe respiratory symptoms resulting in respiratory failure and even death.

Bronchiolitis is typically preceded by a 1- to 3-day history of upper respiratory tract symptoms, such as nasal congestion and/or discharge, cough, and low-grade fever followed by wheezing, and symptoms of respiratory distress including increased work of breathing with retractions.

Compared with other viruses that cause bronchiolitis, fever tends to be lower with RSV and higher with adenovirus.

Characteristic findings include tachypnea, mild intercostal and subcostal retractions, and expiratory wheezing. Additional auscultatory findings may include prolonged expiratory phase and coarse or fine crackles (rales). The chest may appear hyperexpanded with increased anteroposterior diameter, and may be hyperresonant to percussion. Hypoxemia (oxygen saturation <93%) commonly is detected by pulse oximetry.

Severity of illness and/or the need for hospitalization is determined by assessment of hydration status (eg, fluid intake, urine output), symptoms of respiratory distress (tachypnea, nasal flaring, retractions, grunting), presence of cyanosis, episodes of restlessness or lethargy, and history of apnea.

Children with severe illness have increased work of breathing (subcostal, intercostal, and supraclavicular retractions; nasal flaring; and expiratory grunting); they may appear cyanotic and have poor peripheral perfusion. Wheezing may not be audible if the airways are profoundly narrowed or when increased work of breathing results in exhaustion or respiratory failure.

Bronchiolitis usually is self-limited. Most children do not require hospitalization and recover within 28 days. In a cohort of 181 children, the median duration of illness (calculated as the reported duration of symptoms before initial hospital visit plus the time from first consultation to recovery) was 12 days. After 21 days, 18% were still ill and after 28 days, 9% were still ill. There was no association of duration of illness with age, sex, weight, age, or respiratory rate.[13]

In previously healthy infants older than 6 months who require hospitalization, the average length of hospitalization is 3 to 4 days, although it may be longer in children with bronchiolitis resulting from rhinovirus.[10]

DIFFERENTIAL DIAGNOSIS

Bronchiolitis should be differentiated form other causes of wheezing in children, such as viral-induced wheezing and asthma exacerbation, foreign-body aspiration, pneumonia, and congestive heart failure. Most can be distinguished by a through history and physical examination. Few might require radiologic studies.

Viral-Triggered Wheezing or Asthma

Asthma is a chronic airway hyperresponsiveness resulting in airway edema, hypersecretion of mucus, and smooth-muscle hypertrophy, and is difficult to distinguish from the initial exacerbation of bronchiolitis. A history of recurrent wheezing with response to bronchodilators supports the diagnosis of asthma.

Pediatricians and emergency physicians should use caution in definitely linking bronchiolitis with a diagnosis of asthma. These 2 entities are different in that bronchiolitis is an acute process, whereas asthma is a chronic condition characterized by acute exacerbations. Paradoxically, asthma generally presents as an acute illness, whereas bronchiolitis symptoms are more insidious. In addition, common asthma therapies such as bronchodilators and steroids do not have a consistent benefit in the treatment of bronchiolitis. Younger children are more at risk for bronchiolitis because airway edema, mucosal secretion, and debris have a more pronounced effect on the smaller airways. Thus bronchiolitis is not necessarily linked to the causative agent of asthma, airway hyperresponsiveness. Nevertheless, studies have shown that approximately 50% of infants who experience severe bronchiolitis are diagnosed with asthma by age 7 years.[14] Some evidence suggests that a genetic predisposition produces this high correlation between asthma and bronchiolitis. Other evidence leans toward airway injury from bronchiolitis as the causal link to asthma.

Gastroesophageal Reflux and Aspiration Pneumonia

Children with a history of gastroesophageal reflux disease can present with difficulty of breathing and persistent wheezing. In the presence of an upper respiratory tract infection, this can be difficult to distinguish from bronchiolitis. History of reflux associated with cough and chocking, recurrent stridor, chronic cough, and recurrent pneumonia are clinical characteristics that may help in distinguishing aspiration pneumonia from acute bronchiolitis.

Foreign-Body Aspiration

Foreign-body aspiration is a common cause of mortality and morbidity in children, especially in those younger than 2 years. Bronchial foreign body commonly presents with a history of choking followed by a focal area of wheezing or decreased air entry.

Pneumonia

Signs and symptoms may be similar in viral pneumonia and bronchiolitis, but children with bacterial pneumonia tend to appear more ill with higher fever.

Congestive Heart Failure

Infants with congestive heart failure often present with tachypnea and signs of respiratory distress, but a through history and physical examination reveals failure to thrive, excessive sweating, and interruption during feeding, accompanied by findings of a heart murmur or gallop rhythm and poor peripheral perfusion.

ASSESSMENT AND RISK STRATIFICATION

In the ED, evaluation of infants with symptoms concerning for bronchiolitis relies mainly on determining the risk of severe disease. High-risk populations include infants younger than 3 months; premature infants; and children with immunodeficiency, cystic fibrosis, cardiopulmonary, or neuromuscular disease. High-risk infants are susceptible to apneic episodes, severe respiratory distress, and respiratory failure (**Table 1**). Holman and colleagues[6] found that from 1996 to 1998, 55% of infant deaths from bronchiolitis were between the ages of 1 and 3 months. Very low body weight in premature infants was also an independent risk factor, with 30% mortality. The introduction of palivizumab has likely reduced the overall mortality. As a general consensus, RSV-positive infants younger than 2 months should be admitted for observation.[3,4]

Apnea

Preterm infants and infants younger than 2 months are at risk for apnea. Some even present with apnea in the absence of wheezing. The mechanism is unknown, but it is postulated that RSV can alter the sensitivity of laryngeal chemoreceptors and reinforce reflex apnea.[15]

Table 1 Risk factors for severe disease in children with acute bronchiolitis	
Risk Factor	**Complications**
Infants <3 mo	Apnea
Premature infants <34 wk gestation	Apnea, respiratory failure
Children with immunodeficiency	Respiratory failure
Hemodynamically significant congenital heart disease	Respiratory failure
Children with neuromuscular disorders	Respiratory failure
Cystic fibrosis	Respiratory failure

Respiratory Failure

Respiratory failure is one of the most serious complications of bronchiolitis, and commonly occurs in children with bronchopulmonary dysplasia, hemodynamically significant congenital heart disease, or immunosuppression, and in infants younger than 6 weeks in comparison with infants with no known risk factors.[16–18]

Risk stratification and disposition is derived by history and physical findings. Prolonged periods of increased work of breathing can result in significant dehydration from insensible losses, and intolerance of oral hydration. Infants with respiratory rates greater than 60 breaths/min are unlikely to tolerate oral hydration and thus should be admitted for parenteral hydration. Infants who are well appearing with mild hypoxemia (90%–95%), may be observed in the ED and discharged to home with reliable parents. Persistent hypoxemia oxygen saturation less than 93% requires hospital admission for oxygen therapy. Mucus plugging and nasal obstruction may produce transient hypoxemia, often complicating the evaluation and disposition of infants with bronchiolitis, and most infants oxygenate well after the plug or obstruction is cleared. Infants on oxygen therapy have a 4-fold increase in length of hospital stay.[12]

DIAGNOSIS

The diagnosis of bronchiolitis should be assessed based on the clinical presentation, including history, physical findings, and season. Severity should be likewise assessed by these clinical characteristics and age at presentation. The American Academy of Pediatrics (AAP) defines severe disease by persistent increased respiratory effort, apnea, or the need for intravenous hydration, supplemental oxygen, or mechanical ventilation. Patients at increased risk for a severe illness include infants of premature birth (<37 weeks' gestation) and young age (<12 weeks)[19,20]; and patients with underlying medical conditions such as chronic lung disease (bronchopulmonary dysplasia, cystic fibrosis, congenital anomaly),[16] hemodynamically significant congenital heart disease,[21–24] and the presence of an immunocompromised state.[19–22]

Several scoring instruments have been developed to assess the clinical severity of bronchiolitis. The lack of uniformity of clinical scoring systems in severity assessment of bronchiolitis, even among observers, makes its application limited in clinical practice.[23] The most widely used clinical score, the Respiratory Distress Assessment Instrument,[24] is reliable with respect to scoring but has not been validated for clinical predictive value in bronchiolitis. Few studies have shown the effectiveness of pulse oximetry in predicting clinical outcomes. Among hospitalized patients, the need for supplemental oxygen based on pulse oximetry has been associated with higher risk of prolonged hospitalizations, admission to the intensive care unit (ICU), and mechanical ventilation.[16,25,26] The concentration of lactate dehydrogenase (LDH), a marker of cell damage and inflammation in nasal-wash fluid, may provide an objective measure of disease severity in children with bronchiolitis. In one study, increased nasal-wash LDH was suggestive of robust antiviral response and was associated with decreased hospitalizations.[27]

Diagnostic laboratory tests are not routinely indicated in the evaluation of infants and children with bronchiolitis.[20] The complete blood count is sometimes used to evaluate for the possibility of coexistent bacterial infection in children with suspected bronchiolitis and fever. However, the risk of serious bacterial infection is low except for urinary tract infection (UTI) in infants older than 1 month.[28,29] Infants younger than 28 days with fever and symptoms/signs of bronchiolitis have the same risk for serious bacterial infection (SBI) as infants without bronchiolitis. Levine and colleagues[26,28,29] found the rate of SBI in febrile infants younger than 60 days with confirmed RSV to be 7.0%, compared with 12.5% for infants without RSV. Although the risk is less, it is not negligible.

Current evidence also does not support routine chest radiography in children with bronchiolitis. Chest radiography often does not change clinical decisions or predict disease progression. Radiographs may be useful when hospitalized children do not improve at the expected rate, if the severity of disease requires further evaluation, or if another diagnosis is suspected.[30]

Routine testing for specific viral agents do not alter the management or outcome of the illness and is not needed, especially in outpatient setting.[31–33] However, the identification of a viral etiologic agent during ED evaluation or in hospitalized patients has been associated with a decreased use of antibiotic treatment.[34–36]

In hospitalized patients, determination of a responsible virus may help to avoid nosocomial transmission by permitting isolation of patients. Identifying an etiologic agent may also be useful, if specific antiviral therapy is considered.[37]

When the etiologic diagnosis is necessary, nasal aspirates can be used to diagnose RSV infection. Rapid antigen tests are available for RSV, parainfluenza, adenovirus, and influenza virus. Immunofluorescence tests are also available for these viruses that cause bronchiolitis. Viral culture and polymerase chain reaction (PCR) are additional methods that can be used in identifying an etiologic agent. Antigen-detection tests and culture are generally reliable in younger children. The rapid tests vary in terms of sensitivity and specificity when compared with viral culture or PCR.[37]

The sensitivity for RSV rapid tests generally ranges from 80% to 90%. The sensitivity is approximately 50% to 70%, and the specificity is 90% to 95% for influenza. The interpretation of positive results should take into account the clinical characteristics of the case. If an important clinical decision is affected by the test result, the rapid test result should be confirmed by another test, such as viral culture or PCR.

TREATMENT

Bronchiolitis is a self-limited disease in healthy infants and children. The treatment is usually symptomatic, and the goal of therapy is to maintain adequate oxygenation and hydration. Infants with respiratory distress who have difficulty feeding safely should be given intravenous fluids. On the other hand, the possibility of fluid retention secondary to production of antidiuretic hormone has been reported in patients with bronchiolitis.[38,39] Clinicians should manage fluid balance accordingly. Bronchiolitis is associated with airway edema and sloughing of respiratory epithelium. Nasal suctioning may provide temporary relief, but there is no evidence to support routine deep suctioning of the pharynx or larynx. Supplemental oxygen is indicated if oxygen saturation falls persistently below 90% in previously healthy infants.

Several studies have shown that wide variation exists in the treatment of bronchiolitis (**Fig. 1**).[40–42] The difference in practice pattern suggests a lack of consensus among clinicians as to best practices. The AAP subcommittee on diagnosis and management of bronchiolitis has developed national guidelines for the treatment of bronchiolitis, based on systematic grading of the quality of evidence and strength of recommendation.[32] Various nonpharmacologic and pharmacologic therapies, controversies in its use, and recommendations are described here.

Pharmacologic Therapy

Bronchodilators

Use of bronchodilators (α- and β-adrenergic agents) for the treatment of bronchiolitis is controversial. Several studies consistently failed to show clinically significant

Exclude high-risk children with

- Cystic fibrosis, bronchopulmonary dysplasia, immunodeficiencies
- Hemodynamically significant congenital heart disease
- 2 months of age or less with apnea or cyanosis
- Severe respiratory distress requiring intubation or intensive care admission

Classify Severity

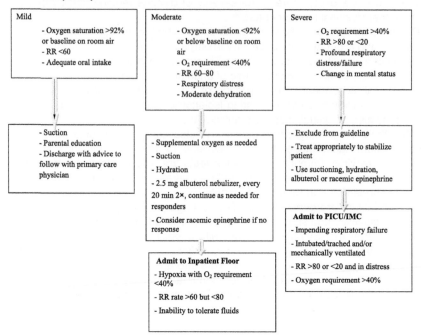

Fig. 1. Suggested treatment algorithm for children with acute bronchiolitis. IMC, intermediate care unit; PICU, pediatric intensive care unit; RR, respiratory rate (breaths/min).

improvement from the use of β2-agonists.[24,43–48] Bronchodilator use is controversial, with some studies showing a positive effect and others no effect.[49,50] Overall results of meta-analysis indicated that one-quarter of all children treated with bronchodilators have a transient improvement in clinical score of unclear clinical significance. Albuterol/salbutamol is the most widely used β2-agonist. Studies in an outpatient setting have shown a modest improvement in O_2 saturation or/and clinical score after albuterol treatment.[49,50] Studies with hospitalized patients have not demonstrated any clinical benefit for routine care.[51,52]

Nebulized epinephrine is another adrenergic agent that has demonstrated positive clinical effects when compared with albuterol nebulizer treatment in an outpatient setting,[53] possibly because of its additional vasoconstrictor effects in reducing microvascular leakage and mucosal edema. However, there is insufficient evidence to support the routine use of nebulized epinephrine for bronchiolitis especially in the home care setting, because of its short duration of action and potential adverse effects.

Other bronchodilators such as ipratropium, an anticholinergic, have not been shown to alter the course of viral bronchiolitis.

Corticosteroids/anti-inflammatory agents

Steroids have anti-inflammatory effects and, theoretically, are thought to reduce airway inflammation and edema. Several reports indicate that up to 60% of infants admitted to hospital for bronchiolitis receive corticosteroid therapy.[40,54,55] A meta-analysis evaluating the use of systemic glucocorticoids and inhaled glucocorticoids for acute bronchiolitis in children younger than 2 years included 17 trials and 2596 patients. No benefits were found in hospital-admission rate, length of stay, clinical score after 12 hours, or hospital revisit or readmission rates.[1,56]

The meta-analysis of 3 studies evaluating the efficacy of glucocorticoids in children with bronchiolitis who required mechanical ventilation also demonstrated no effect on mechanical ventilation or length of hospitalization.[57]

Antibiotics

Antibiotics should not be routinely used in the treatment of bronchiolitis. Children with bronchiolitis frequently receive antibacterial therapy because of fever or young age,[58,59] or concerns over secondary bacterial infection.[60] The rates of SBI range from 0% to 3.7% in patients with bronchiolitis and/or infections with RSV.[28,29,61] Febrile infants younger than 28 days with RSV bronchiolitis infections demonstrated that the overall risk of SBI, although significant, was not different between RSV-positive and RSV-negative infants.[33] When SBI was present, it was more likely to be a UTI than bacteremia or meningitis. In a study of 2396 infants with RSV bronchiolitis, 69% of the 39 patients with SBI had a UTI.[62] In children with bronchiolitis, antibiotics are warranted only when there is evidence of a coexisting bacterial infection such as positive urine or blood culture, pneumonia documented by consolidation on chest radiograph, or acute otitis media. Coexisting bacterial infections should be treated in a manner similar to that used in the absence of bronchiolitis.

Antiviral/ribavirin

The indication for specific antiviral therapy for bronchiolitis is controversial. Studies have shown mixed results. Although ribavirin has the potential to reduce number of days of mechanical ventilation and hospitalization, the data are insufficient to support its routine use to treat RSV bronchiolitis.[63–66] Cumbersome drug-delivery requirements,[67] potential health risks to care givers,[68] high cost,[69] and marginal benefit restrict this therapy to highly selected situations involving documented RSV bronchiolitis with severe disease, or those who are at risk for severe disease (immunocompromised or hemodynamically significant cardiopulmonary disease).

Other therapies

Heliox A meta-analysis of 4 randomized trials of heliox for the treatment of moderate to severe bronchiolitis has shown that heliox may improve the clinical score in the first hour, but did not reduce the rate of intubation, need for mechanical ventilation, or length of stay in the ICU.[70–74]

High-dose systemic steroids The anti-inflammatory properties of glucocorticoids are thought to reduce airway obstruction by decreasing bronchiolar swelling. There are a few small studies suggesting that high-dose systemic steroids early in the course of bronchiolitis may be effective in preventing the progression of inflammation or, at least, in modifying its course.[75]

Inhaled glucocorticoids In randomized controlled trials and meta-analysis, inhaled corticosteroids (budesonide, fluticasone, dexamethasone), have not been beneficial in reducing symptom duration, readmission rates, or subsequent wheezing episodes.[56,76–78]

Surfactant Evidence suggests that severe bronchiolitis may result in surfactant deficiency, and that therapy with surfactant on mechanically ventilated patients may shorten the duration of ventilation and ICU stay.[79–81]

Combination therapies

Multiple studies involving combination therapies including albuterol plus ipratropium,[82] albuterol plus oral prednisolone,[83] heliox with nebulized epinephrine, or HFNC oxygen[84] have not shown clinically significant improvement. Racemic epinephrine with steroids has shown short-term benefit in one study by decreasing the rate of hospitalization within 1 week of the ED visit.[85]

Nonpharmacologic Treatment

Chest physiotherapy

No differences were reported with different types of chest physiotherapy in infants with bronchiolitis, including vibration and percussion techniques, with respect to length of hospital stay, oxygen requirements, or severity score.[86]

Hypertonic saline

A few studies have shown that nebulized 3% or even 5% hypertonic saline is safe and effective for ambulatory treatment of bronchiolitis, and was associated with decreased mean length of hospital stay and improved clinical score.[39,87]

High-flow nasal cannula

This treatment is becoming more common for children with severe bronchiolitis. In contrast to the use of a nasal cannula for low-flow oxygen delivery in patients with mild respiratory distress, HFNC therapy involves delivery of heated and humidified oxygen via special devices at rates starting from 8 L/min to 40 L/min. In patients with respiratory distress or failure, humidified HFNC may be better tolerated than oxygen by face-mask in terms of comfort, and has been associated with better oxygenation. In an observational study, HFNC was associated with decreased rates of intubation in children younger than 24 months who were admitted to a pediatric intensive care unit (PICU) with bronchiolitis, in comparison with historical controls.[88]

Indications for hospitalization and admission to the PICU are described in **Table 2**.

Prophylaxis

Palivizumab is a monoclonal antibody that reduces hospitalizations due to RSV infection among children at high risk for severe disease (**Box 1**).[18] It is given in monthly injections during the RSV season (November through March in the United States).

Table 2
Indications for hospitalization

Inpatient Unit	Pediatric Intensive Care Unit (PICU)
Respiratory rate >60 breaths/min	Worsening respiratory distress
Increased work of breathing with retractions	Toxic appearance
Oxygen saturations <92% in room air	Lethargy
Cyanosis	Hypoxemia with oxygen requirements >40%
Apnea	Hypercapnia
Underlying chronic lung disease especially when the patient is on supplemental oxygen	
Hemodynamically significant congenital heart disease or pulmonary hypertension	
Poor oral intake	
Parent unable to care for the child at home	

Box 1
AAP recommendation: palivizumab prophylaxis may be considered for the following infants and children

Infants born at 28 weeks' of gestation or earlier during RSV season, whenever that occurs during the first 12 months of life

Infants born 32 to 35 weeks' gestation who are younger than 3 months at the start of the RSV season or who are born during RSV season if they have at least 1 of 2 risk factors: (1) infant attends child care; (2) infant has a sibling younger than 5 years

Infants born 29 to 32 weeks' gestation if they are younger than 6 months at the start of the RSV season

Infants and children younger than 2 years with cyanotic or complicated congenital heart disease

Infants and children younger than 2 years who have been treated for chronic lung disease within 6 months of the start of RSV season

Infants born before 35 weeks' gestation who have either congenital abnormalities of the airway or neuromuscular disease that compromises handling of the respiratory secretions

---

SUMMARY

RSV is common, and most patients do well with supportive care. Patients of premature birth or younger than 12 weeks, with underlying conditions such as bronchopulmonary dysplasia, cystic fibrosis, and hemodynamically significant congenital heart disease, are at risk for complications. Bronchiolitis is a self-limited disease in healthy infants and children. The treatment is usually symptomatic, and the goal of therapy is to maintain adequate oxygenation and hydration. Use of HFNC in the ED and ICU for severe cases is showing promise.

REFERENCES

1. Corneli HM, Zorc JJ, Majahan P, et al. Bronchiolitis Study Group of the Pediatric Emergency Care Applied Research Network (PECARN). A multicenter, randomized, controlled trial of dexamethasone for bronchiolitis. N Engl J Med 2007; 357(4):331–9.
2. Stockman LJ, Curns AT, Anderson LJ, et al. Respiratory syncytial virus-associated hospitalizations among infants and young children in the United States, 1997-2006. Pediatr Infect Dis J 2012;31(1):5.
3. Groothuis J, Simoes E, Hemming V. Respiratory syncytial virus (RSV) infection in preterm infants and the protective effects of RSV immune globulin (RSVIG). Pediatrics 1995;95(4):463–7.
4. The IMpact-RSV Study Group. Palivizumab, a humanized respiratory syncytial virus monoclonal antibody, reduces hospitalization from respiratory syncytial virus infection in high-risk infants. Pediatrics 1998;102(3):531–7.
5. Hall CB, Weinberg GA, Iwane MK, et al. The burden of respiratory syncytial virus infection in young children. N Engl J Med 2009;360(6):588.
6. Holman R, Shay D, Curns A, et al. Risk factors for bronchiolitis-associated deaths among infants in the United States. Pediatr Infect Dis J 2003;22(6): 483–90.
7. Johnson JE, Gonzales RA, Olson SJ, et al. The histopathology of fatal untreated human respiratory syncytial virus infection. Mod Pathol 2007;20(1):108.

8. Aherne W, Bird T, Court SD, et al. Pathological changes in virus infections of the lower respiratory tract in children. J Clin Pathol 1970;23(1):7.

9. Alverson B, Ralston S. Management of bronchiolitis: focus on hypertonic saline. Contemp Pediatr 2011;28(2):30–8.

10. Mansbach JM, Piedra PA, Teach SJ, et al. MARC-30 Investigators. Prospective multicenter study of viral etiology and hospital length of stay in children with severe bronchiolitis. Arch Pediatr Adolesc Med 2012;166(8):700.

11. American Academy of Pediatrics. Red book. Report of the Committee on Infectious Diseases. Respiratory syncytial virus. Elk Grove Village (IL): American Academy of Pediatrics; 2012. p. 609–18.

12. Zorc J, Phelan K. What's new for seasonal wheezing: an update on the AAP's bronchiolitis guidelines and the latest evidence on assessment and treatment. Contemp Pediatr 2008;25(2):54–62.

13. Swingler GH, Hussey GD, Zwarenstein M. Duration of illness in ambulatory children diagnosed with bronchiolitis. Arch Pediatr Adolesc Med 2000;154(10):997.

14. Bacharier L, Cohen R, Schweiger T, et al. Determinants of asthma after severe respiratory syncytial virus bronchiolitis. J Allergy Clin Immunol 2012;131(1): 91–100.e3.

15. Uren EC, Williams AL, Jack I, et al. Association of respiratory virus infections with sudden infant death syndrome. Med J Aust 1980;1(9):417.

16. Wang EE, Law BJ, Stephens D. Pediatric Investigators Collaborative Network on Infections in Canada (PICNIC) prospective study of risk factors and outcomes in patients hospitalized with respiratory syncytial viral lower respiratory tract infection. J Pediatr 1995;126(2):212.

17. Willson DF, Landrigan CP, Horn SD, et al. Complications in infants hospitalized for bronchiolitis or respiratory syncytial virus pneumonia. J Pediatr 2003; 143(Suppl 5):S142.

18. Committee on Infectious Diseases. From the American Academy of Pediatrics: policy statements—modified recommendations for use of palivizumab for prevention of respiratory syncytial virus infections. Pediatrics 2009;124(6): 1694–701.

19. Shaw KN, Bell LM, Sherman NH. Outpatient assessment of infants with bronchiolitis. Am J Dis Child 1991;145(2):151–5.

20. Chan PW, Lok FY, Khatijah SB. Risk factors for hypoxemia and respiratory failure in respiratory syncytial virus bronchiolitis. Southeast Asian J Trop Med Public Health 2002;33(4):806–10.

21. MacDonald NE, Hall CB, Suffin SC, et al. Respiratory syncytial viral infection in infants with congenital heart disease. N Engl J Med 1982;307(7):397–400.

22. Hall CB, Powel KR, MacDonald NE, et al. Respiratory syncytial viral infection in children with compromised immune function. N Engl J Med 1986;315(2): 77–81.

23. Viswanathan M, King VJ, Bordley C, et al. Management of bronchiolitis in infants and children. Evid Rep Technol Assess (Summ) 2003;(69):1–5.

24. Lowell DI, Lister G, Von Koss H, et al. Wheezing in infants: the response to epinephrine. Pediatrics 1987;79(6):939–45.

25. Brooks AM, McBride JT, McConnochie KM, et al. Predicting deterioration in previously healthy infants hospitalized with respiratory syncytial virus infection. Pediatrics 1999;104(3 Pt 1):463–7.

26. Schroeder AR, Marmor AK, Pantell RH, et al. Impact of pulse oximetry and oxygen therapy on length of stay in bronchiolitis hospitalizations. Arch Pediatr Adolesc Med 2004;158(6):527–30.

27. Laham FR, Troll AA, Bennett BL, et al. LDH concentration in nasal-wash fluid as a biochemical predictor of bronchiolitis severity. Pediatrics 2010;125(2): e225–33.
28. Kuppermann N, Bank DE, Walton EA, et al. Risks for bacteremia and urinary tract infections in young febrile children with bronchiolitis. Arch Pediatr Adolesc Med 1997;151(12):1207–14.
29. Levine DA, Platt SL, Dayan PS, et al. Risk of serious bacterial infection in young febrile infants with respiratory syncytial virus infections. Pediatrics 2004;113(6): 1728–34.
30. Carsin A, Gorincour G, Bresson V, et al. Chest radiographs in infants hospitalized for acute bronchiolitis: real information or just irradiation? Arch Pediatr 2012; 19(12):1308–15. http://dx.doi.org/10.1016/j.arcped.2012.09.019 [in French].
31. Bordley WC, Viswanthan M, King VJ, et al. Diagnosis and testing in bronchiolitis: a systematic review. Arch Pediatr Adolesc Med 2004;158(2):119–26.
32. American Academy of Pediatrics Subcommittee on Diagnosis and Management of Bronchiolitis. Diagnosis and management of bronchiolitis. Pediatrics 2006; 118(4):1774–93.
33. Harris JA, Huskins WC, Langley JM, et al, Pediatric Special Interest Group of the Society for Healthcare Epidemiology of America. Health care epidemiology perspective on the October 2006 recommendations of the Subcommittee on Diagnosis and Management of Bronchiolitis. Pediatrics 2007;120(4):890–2.
34. Smyth RL, Openshaw PJ. Bronchiolitis. Lancet 2006;368:312.
35. Vogel AM, Lennon DR, Harding JE, et al. Variations in bronchiolitis management between five New Zealand hospitals: can we do better? J Paediatr Child Health 2003;39:40.
36. Adcock PM, Stout GG, Hauck MA, et al. Effect of rapid viral diagnosis on the management of children hospitalized with lower respiratory tract infection. Pediatr Infect Dis J 1997;16:842.
37. Krilov LR, Lipson SM, Barone SR, et al. Evaluation of a rapid diagnostic test for respiratory syncytial virus (RSV): potential for bedside diagnosis. Pediatrics 1994;93(6 Pt 1):903–6.
38. Van Steensel-Moll HA, Hazelzet JA, van der Voort E, et al. Excessive secretion of antidiuretic hormone in infections with respiratory syncytial virus. Arch Dis Child 1990;65(11):1237–9.
39. Kuzik BA, Al-Qadhi SA, Kent S, et al. Nebulized hypertonic saline in the treatment of viral bronchiolitis in infants. J Pediatr 2007;151(3):266–70, 270.e1.
40. Willson DF, Horn SD, Hendley JO, et al. Effect of practice variation on resource utilization in infants for viral lower respiratory illness. Pediatrics 2001;108: 851–5.
41. Wang EE, Law BJ, Boucher FD, et al. Pediatric Investigators Collaborative Network on Infections in Canada (PICNIC) study of admission and management variation in patients hospitalized with respiratory syncytial viral lower respiratory tract infection. J Pediatr 1996;129:390–5.
42. Brand PL, Vaessen-Verberne AA. Differences in management of bronchiolitis between hospitals in the Netherlands. Eur J Pediatr 2000;159:343–7.
43. Alario AJ, Lewander WJ, Dennehy P, et al. The efficacy of nebulized metaproterenol in wheezing infants and young children. Am J Dis Child 1992;146:412–8.
44. Henry RL, Milner AD, Stokes GM. Ineffectiveness of ipratropium bromide in acute bronchiolitis. Arch Dis Child 1983;58:925–6.
45. Klassen TP, Rowe PC, Sutcliffe T, et al. Randomized trial of salbutamol in acute bronchiolitis. J Pediatr 1991;118:807–11.

46. Lines DR, Kattampallil JS, Liston P. Efficacy of nebulized salbutamol in bronchiolitis. Pediatr Rev Commun 1990;5:121–9.
47. Mallol J, Barrueo L, Girardi G, et al. Use of nebulized bronchodilators in infants under 1 year of age: analysis of four forms of therapy. Pediatr Pulmonol 1987;3: 298–303.
48. Tal A, Bavilski C, Yohai D, et al. Dexamethasone and salbutamol in the treatment of acute wheezing in infants. Pediatrics 1983;71:13–8.
49. Schweich PJ, Hurt TL, Walkley EI, et al. The use of nebulized albuterol in wheezing infants. Pediatr Emerg Care 1992;8:184–8.
50. Schuh S, Canny G, Reisman JJ, et al. Nebulized albuterol in acute bronchiolitis. J Pediatr 1990;117:633–7.
51. Dobson JV, Stephens-Groff SM, McMahon SR, et al. The use of albuterol in hospitalized infants with bronchiolitis. Pediatrics 1998;101:361–8.
52. Flores G, Horwitz RI. Efficacy of beta2-agonists in bronchiolitis: a reappraisal and meta-analysis. Pediatrics 1997;100:233–9.
53. Kristjansson S, Lodrup Carlsen KC, Wennergren G, et al. Nebulised racemic adrenaline in the treatment of acute bronchiolitis in infants and toddlers. Arch Dis Child 1993;69:650–4.
54. Behrendt CE, Decker MD, Burch DJ, et al. International variation in the management of infants hospitalized with respiratory syncytial virus. International RSV Study Group. Eur J Pediatr 1998;157:215–20.
55. Shay DK, Holman RC, Newman RD, et al. Bronchiolitis associated hospitalizations among US children, 1980-1996. JAMA 1999;282:1440–6.
56. Fernandes RM, Bialy LM, Vandermeer B, et al. Glucocorticoids for acute viral bronchiolitis in infants and young children. Cochrane Database Syst Rev 2010;(10):CD004878.
57. Davison C, Ventre KM, Luchetti M, et al. Efficacy of interventions for bronchiolitis in critically ill infants: a systematic review and meta-analysis. Pediatr Crit Care Med 2004;5(5):482–9.
58. Putto A, Ruuskanen O, Meruman O. Fever in respiratory virus infections. Am J Dis Child 1986;140:1159–63.
59. LaVia W, Marks MI, Stutman HR. Respiratory syncytial virus puzzle: clinical features, pathophysiology, treatment, and prevention. J Pediatr 1992;121:503–10.
60. Nichol KP, Cherry JD. Bacterial-viral interrelations in respiratory infections in children. N Engl J Med 1967;277:667–72.
61. Hall CB, Powell KR, Schnabel KC, et al. Risk of serious bacterial infection in infants hospitalized with respiratory syncytial viral infection. J Pediatr 1988; 113:266–71.
62. Purcell K, Fergie J. Concurrent serious bacterial infections in 2396 infants and children hospitalized with respiratory syncytial virus lower respiratory tract infections. Arch Pediatr Adolesc Med 2002;156:322–4.
63. Krilov LR, Mandel FS, Baron SR, et al. Follow-up of children with respiratory syncytial virus bronchiolitis in 1986 and 1987: potential effect of ribavirin on long term pulmonary function. Pediatr Infect Dis J 1997;16(3):273–6.
64. Reassessment of the indications for ribavirin therapy in respiratory syncytial virus infections. American Academy of Pediatrics Committee on Infectious Diseases. Pediatrics 1996;97(1):137–40.
65. Ventre K, Randolph AG. Ribavirin for respiratory syncytial virus infection of the lower respiratory tract in infants and young children. Cochrane Database Syst Rev 2007;(1):CD000181.

66. Randolph AG, Wang EE. Ribavirin for respiratory syncytial virus infection of the lower respiratory tract. Cochrane Database Syst Rev 2000;(2):CD000181.
67. Bradley JS, Conner JD, Compagiannis LS, et al. Exposure of health care workers to ribavirin during therapy for respiratory syncytial virus infections. Antimicrobial Agents Chemother 1990;34:668–70.
68. Rodriguez WJ, Bui RHD, Conner JD, et al. Environmental exposure of primary care personnel to ribavirin aerosol when supervising treatment of infants with respiratory syncytial virus infections. Antimicrobial Agents Chemother 1987; 31:1143–6.
69. Feldstein TJ, Swegarden JL, Atwood GF, et al. Ribavirin therapy: implementation of hospital guidelines and effect on usage and cost of therapy. Pediatrics 1995; 96:14–7.
70. Liet JM, Millotte B, Tucci M, et al. Canadian Critical Care Trials Group. Noninvasive therapy with helium-oxygen for severe bronchiolitis. J Pediatr 2005;147(6): 812–7.
71. Martinón-Torres F, Rodríguez-Núñez A, Martinón-Sánchez JM. Heliox therapy in infants with acute bronchiolitis. Pediatrics 2002;109(1):68–73.
72. Hollman G, Shen G, Zeng L, et al. Helium-oxygen improves clinical asthma scores in children with acute bronchiolitis. Crit Care Med 1998;26(10):1731–6.
73. Cambonie G, Milési C, Fournier-Favre S, et al. Clinical effects of heliox administration for acute bronchiolitis in young infants. Chest 2006;129(3):676–82.
74. Liet JM, Ducruet T, Gupta V, et al. Heliox inhalation therapy for bronchiolitis in infants. Cochrane Database Syst Rev 2010;(4):CD006915.
75. Weinberger MM. High-dose systemic corticosteroids may be effective early in the course of bronchiolitis. Pediatrics 2007;119(4):864–5 [discussion: 865–6].
76. King VJ, Viswanathan M, Bordley WC, et al. Pharmacologic treatment of bronchiolitis in infants and children: a systematic review. Arch Pediatr Adolesc Med 2004;158(2):127–37.
77. Cade A, Brownlee KG, Conway SP, et al. Randomised placebo controlled trial of nebulised corticosteroids in acute respiratory syncytial viral bronchiolitis. Arch Dis Child 2000;82(2):126–30.
78. Blom D, Ermers M, Bont L, et al. Inhaled corticosteroids during acute bronchiolitis in the prevention of post-bronchiolitic wheezing. Cochrane Database Syst Rev 2007;(1):CD004881.
79. Jat KR, Chawla D. Surfactant therapy for bronchiolitis in critically ill infants. Cochrane Database Syst Rev 2012;(9):CD009194.
80. LeVine AM, Elliott J, Whitsett JA, et al. Surfactant protein-d enhances phagocytosis and pulmonary clearance of respiratory syncytial virus. Am J Respir Cell Mol Biol 2004;31(2):193–9.
81. Tibby SM, Hatherill M, Wright SM, et al. Exogenous surfactant supplementation in infants with respiratory syncytial virus bronchiolitis. Am J Respir Crit Care Med 2000;162(4 Pt 1):1251–6.
82. Prendiville A, Green S, Silverman M. Ipratropium bromide and airways function in wheezy infants. Arch Dis Child 1987;62(4):397–400.
83. Panickar J, Lakhanpaul M, Lambert PC, et al. Oral prednisolone for preschool children with acute virus-induced wheezing. N Engl J Med 2009;360(4): 329–38.
84. Kim IK, Phrampus E, Sikes K, et al. Helium-oxygen therapy for infants with bronchiolitis: a randomized controlled trial. Arch Pediatr Adolesc Med 2011;165(12): 1115–22.

85. Plint AC, Johnson DW, Patel H, et al. Pediatric Emergency Research Canada (PERC). Epinephrine and dexamethasone in children with bronchiolitis. N Engl J Med 2009;360(20):2079–89.
86. Perrotta C, Ortiz Z, Roque M. Chest physiotherapy for acute bronchiolitis in paediatric patients between 0 and 24 months old. Cochrane Database Syst Rev 2007;(1):CD004873.
87. Al-Ansari K, Sakran M, Davidson B, et al. Nebulized 5% or 3% hypertonic or 0.9% saline for treating acute bronchiolitis in infants. J Pediatr 2010;157(4): 630–4.
88. McKiernan C, Chua LC, Visintainer PF, et al. High flow nasal cannulae therapy in infants with bronchiolitis. J Pediatr 2010;156(4):634.

Asthma Update

Kyle A. Nelson, MD, MPH[a,b,*], Joseph J. Zorc, MD, MSCE[c,d]

KEYWORDS

- Acute • Asthma • Treatment • Pediatric • Emergency

KEY POINTS

- Acute asthma management involves prompt recognition of severity and treatment using short-acting β-agonists (SABAs), anticholinergics, and systemic corticosteroids (SCSs).
- Children with severe exacerbations should receive high-dose SABAs mixed with ipratropium bromide as well as SCSs.
- Children with less-severe exacerbations may benefit from SCSs based on chronic asthma severity reflecting significant airway inflammation.
- Patients not improving after multiple high-dose SABA treatments should receive adjunctive therapy, such as intravenous (IV) magnesium.
- Many children treated for asthma in the emergency department (ED) have significant morbidity and infrequent primary asthma care; prescription of inhaled corticosteroids (ICSs) is appropriate.

INTRODUCTION

Management of acute asthma exacerbations has evolved over recent decades, with an expanding body of research driving advances in therapeutics. Asthma is a heterogeneous chronic inflammatory condition with variable phenotype, influenced by genetic and environmental determinants. Although differences in response to therapy may occur, standard treatment has been defined in the National Asthma Education and Prevention Program (NAEPP) guidelines and involves inhaled bronchodilators and SCSs.[1] Prompt recognition of severity and initiation of therapy are important goals.

Funding Source: None.
Conflicts of Interest: K.A.N., Spouse employed at Vertex Pharmaceuticals, Inc; J.J.Z., None.
[a] Emergency Medicine, Boston Children's Hospital, 300 Longwood Avenue, Boston, MA 02115, USA; [b] Pediatrics, Harvard Medical School, 25 Shattuck Street, Boston, MA 02115, USA; [c] Emergency Medicine, Emergency Information System, The Children's Hospital of Philadelphia, 3401 Civic Center Boulevard, Philadelphia, PA 19146, USA; [d] Pediatrics, Perelman School of Medicine, University of Pennsylvania, 3620 Hamilton Walk, Philadelphia, PA 19104, USA
* Corresponding author. Emergency Medicine, Boston Children's Hospital, 300 Longwood Avenue, Boston, MA 02115.
E-mail address: Kyle.nelson@childrens.harvard.edu

Despite advances in chronic and acute care, asthma remains a major public health issue. It is important to appreciate its epidemiology, including the significant disease burden and health disparities according to race and socioeconomic status. There are aspects of chronic care beyond the ED visit, including prescription of controller therapy and access to primary asthma care, that are also important considerations.[1]

This article discusses current recommendations and evidence for acute asthma management.

EPIDEMIOLOGY

According to recent United States statistics, lifetime prevalence of asthma is estimated at 13% of all children, with 6.7 million experiencing active disease.[2] More than 3.5 million children have greater than or equal to 1 exacerbation per year, resulting in approximately 600,000 ED visits.[2] Children younger than 4 years have the highest rates of ED visits, ambulatory visits, and hospitalizations.[2]

Asthma is uncommonly diagnosed before 12 months of age, and some clinicians hesitate to diagnose asthma in children younger than 24 months, when the diagnosis relies on history and symptoms and overlaps with transient viral bronchiolitis. A diagnosis of asthma is appropriate, however, if a child has compatible history of recurrent episodes of cough, respiratory distress, and wheezing, suggesting the characteristic features of airway obstruction, bronchial hyper-responsiveness, and airway inflammation.[1]

Asthma disproportionately affects minority children, those in urban areas, and those of lower socioeconomic status.[2–7] Puerto Rican children in the United States have the highest prevalence, at 19.2%.[2] Black children have the highest rates of both ED visits and death, however.[2] Moreover, with regard to preventative care, minority children have fewer ambulatory visits compared with white children and lower rates of controller medication use.[2,6,7]

DIFFERENTIAL DIAGNOSIS

Asthma is characterized clinically by a pattern of periodic episodes of cough, wheeze, respiratory distress, and reversible bronchospasm. Although wheezing is the most obvious symptom, asthma may also present as cough without significant wheeze. Asking a family about typical symptoms for a child can provide clarification. Pulmonary function testing can identify airway obstruction in children able to complete it (usually children older than 5 years), although often a clinical diagnosis is made.

Considering the symptoms common for asthma are nonspecific, an appropriate differential diagnoses list should be considered (**Box 1**). A diagnosis of asthma during the first episode of wheezing can be challenging, and clinical presentation overlaps with bronchiolitis in young children.

SEVERITY ASSESSMENT

Rapid determination of severity is important to direct appropriate therapy. Severity is a spectrum—mild, moderate, severe, and impending respiratory failure **Table 1**.

Clinical scores using predominantly subjective measures, such as the pediatric asthma severity score (see **Table 1**), modified pulmonary index, and pulmonary score, have been shown valid and reliable.[8–10] The NAEPP guidelines recommend objectively measuring airway obstruction using spirometry or peak expiratory flow rate (PEFR),[1] although this may be impossible in young or severely ill children. In assessing severity

---

Box 1
Differential diagnosis

Upper respiratory tract infection with wheezing

Bronchiolitis

Pneumonia

Pneumothorax

Congenital cardiac abnormality with heart failure

Congenital pulmonary abnormality

Foreign body

Cystic fibrosis

α_1-Antitrypsin deficiency

Gastroesophageal reflux disease

Tracheoesophageal fistula

Allergic reaction/anaphylaxis

Vocal cord dysfunction

Toxic exposure

---

and formulating treatment plans, patient history and response to medications already used for that exacerbation should be considered.

INITIAL STANDARD THERAPY

The main goals of acute asthma treatment are 2-fold—to rapidly reverse bronchospasm and to treat underlying airway inflammation. Severity-based treatment should be initiated as soon as possible.

Short-acting β-Agonist

Albuterol or levalbuterol

Inhaled SABAs cause bronchodilation of airway smooth muscle through activation of β_2-adrenergic receptors (**Table 2**). Albuterol is the most commonly used SABA, a racemic mixture of 2 enantiomers—(R)-albuterol (binds β_2-receptor and causes bronchodilation plus adverse effects of tachycardia and tremor) and (S)-albuterol (thought to have detrimental effect on airway function). Levalbuterol is a purified form of the (R)-enantiomer, marketed as an alternative with fewer adverse effects than racemic albuterol. Studies comparing racemic albuterol and levalbuterol have not consistently reported superiority over racemic albuterol, however, in improved pulmonary function or clinical outcomes,[11–14] raising questions about cost effectiveness. The updated NAEPP guidelines list levalbuterol as an option for SABA treatment at half the dose of (racemic) albuterol.[1]

Delivery device

Albuterol can be administered using metered dose inhalers (MDIs) that have either valved holding chambers (spacer) or nebulizers; use of each requires proper technique. Although there are potential differences in lung deposition between devices, in general, studies of clinical outcomes have found equivalency or favor MDI with spacer due to shorter ED length of stay (LOS) and less tachycardia.[15–21] Although

Table 1
Acute asthma severity assessment

	Mild	Moderate	Severe	Respiratory Arrest Imminent
Key examination elements (pediatric asthma severity score)				
Wheezing	*None or mild (0)* None or end of expiration only	*Moderate (1)* Throughout expiration	*Severe (2)* Inspiratory/ expiratory or absent due to poor air exchange	Diminished due to poor air exchange
Work of breathing	*None or mild (0)* Normal or minimal retractions	*Moderate (1)* Intercostal retractions	*Severe (2)* Suprasternal retractions, abdominal breathing	Tiring, inability to maintain work of breathing
Prolonged expiration	*None or mild (0)* Normal or minimally prolonged	*Moderate (1)*	*Severe (2)*	Severely prolonged
Other examination elements				
Breath Sounds/ aeration	Normal	Decreased at bases	Widespread decrease	Absent/minimal
Symptoms				
Breathlessness	With activity or agitation	While at rest For infants: soft or shorter cry, difficulty feeding, prefers sitting	While at rest For infants: stops feeding, sits upright	
Talks in	Sentences	Phrases	Words	
Alertness	Alert	May be agitated	Agitated	Drowsy, confused
Measurements				
Pulse oximetry	>94%	Variable	Variable	Variable
PEF (% of predicted by height)	≥70%	40%–69%	<40%	

Data from The Children's Hospital of Philadelphia—ED Pathway for Evaluation/Treatment of Children with Asthma. Based on "Guidelines for the Diagnosis and Management of Asthma." National Asthma Education and Prevention Program, United States National Heart Lung Blood Institute; 2007.

nebulizers have traditionally been the preferred devices, MDI with spacer may be considered an option for children with mild and moderate exacerbations (see **Table 2**).

Data on MDI with spacer use for severe asthma are limited. Patients with severe exacerbations have significant lower airway obstruction, which limits drug deposition in the lung, and higher overall doses using nebulizer are often necessary.

Continuous nebulized SABA treatment
Continuous nebulized albuterol treatment is recommended for patients with severe exacerbations or poor response to intermittent or back-to-back dosing (see

Table 2
First-line medications for acute asthma by acute severity level

		Mild	Moderate	Severe
Albuterol				
Delivery device		MDI with valved holding chamber	MDI with valved holding chamber or nebulizer	Nebulizer
Frequency		Intermittent treatment every 20 min up to 3 doses in 60 min		Intermittent or continuous treatment
Dosing	Weight (kg)	MDI	Nebulizer (intermittent)	Nebulizer (continuous)
	<5	2 Puffs	1.25 mg	5 mg/h
	5–10	4 Puffs	2.5 mg	10 mg/h
	10–20	6 Puffs	3.75 mg	15 mg/h
	>20	8 Puffs	5 mg	20 mg/h
Ipratropium bromide		(Mix with albuterol)		
Comment		Not proved effective	Likely effective when added to β-agonist	Effective, particularly multiple doses
Delivery device	Weight (kg)	Nebulizer		
Dosing	<10	250 µg × 3 doses		
	>10	500 µg × 2 doses		
Systemic corticosteroids				
Comment		Consider if incomplete response to initial therapy	Administer as early as possible for maximal benefit	
Route		Oral	Oral route as effective as parenteral	
Dose		Prednisone or prednisolone 2 mg/kg (max 60 mg)	Prednisone or prednisolone or methylprednisolone 2 mg/kg (max 60 mg)	

Data from The Children's Hospital of Philadelphia—ED Pathway for Evaluation/Treatment of Children with Asthma. Based on "Guidelines for the Diagnosis and Management of Asthma." National Asthma Education and Prevention Program, United States National Heart Lung Blood Institute; 2007.

Table 2). A systematic review found that continuous albuterol was associated with greater PEFR improvement and lower hospitalization rate, most pronounced for those with moderate or severe exacerbations.[22] In that review, continuous albuterol was not associated with more adverse effects (palpitations, tremors, nausea and vomiting, and potassium level when tested).[22] Continuous nebulized levalbuterol has not been found superior to continuous albuterol.[14,23]

Ipratropium Bromide

Ipratropium bromide causes bronchodilation by blocking muscarinic cholinergic receptors (see **Table 2**). It is associated with lower admission rate for children with severe exacerbations and may reduce ED LOS.[24–26] Multidose protocols are associated with greater forced expiratory volume in the first second of expiration improvement and lower hospitalization rates compared with single-dose protocols.[24,25]

Corticosteroids

Corticosteroids block formation of potent inflammatory mediators and reduce airway inflammation. SCSs are proved effective for moderate and severe exacerbations and should be administered as early as possible for maximum benefit (see **Table 2**).[27,28] One systematic review found the reduction in hospitalization rate was most significant after 2 hours, which may be an important consideration when assessing response to therapy.[27] Another review found that SCSs reduced relapse visits, a major ED quality outcome.[28] Adverse events were similar between study groups in these reviews.[27,28] Patients with mild exacerbations should receive SCSs if they have incomplete response to inhaled SABA.

For many ED patients, the potential benefits of SCSs outweigh the potential harms, including patients who have recently completed an SCS course but have recurrence of symptoms. Although SCS courses have been reported to be associated with alteration in bone metabolism and bone mineral density, they were not associated with increased fracture rates.[29–31] Patients requiring more than 1 course of SCS in 6 months should be prescribed ICSs.

Route, dosing, duration

Oral administration of SCSs is the preferred route because of similar bioavailability compared with the parenteral route and less pain (see **Table 2**). Patients with severe exacerbations or significant vomiting may require parenteral administration. Intramuscular (IM) dexamethasone is an option. Studies report similar outcomes with IM dexamethasone compared with oral prednisone.[32,33] The current recommended dose of oral prednisone or prednisolone is 1 mg to 2 mg per kg (maximum 60 mg) per day for 3 to 10 days (NAEPP). In a recent study, a 3-day course of prednisone had similar outcomes compared with a 5-day course.[34]

One or 2 days of oral dexamethasone is reported to have similar ED relapse rates and less vomiting compared with multiple days of prednisolone and may be considered an option, although current studies are limited due to differences in protocols and variable dexamethasone and prednisolone dosing.[35–37]

Inhaled corticosteroid

ICSs are beneficial for long-term asthma control, and administration during acute exacerbations may also be effective but research has some limitations. Systematic reviews have found single-dose ICS protocols similar to SCSs for some outcomes, whereas multidose protocols were associated with greater early (within 60 minutes) PEFR improvement and reduction in hospitalization rate, although these studies had significant heterogeneity.[38,39] At this point, results of studies do not support replacing SCSs with ICSs in ED management of acute exacerbations.

Studies have also not found ICSs superior to SCSs for immediate post-ED outcomes.[40,41] Considering the beneficial effects in chronic asthma, however, initiation or continuation of ICSs along with a short course of OCS at time of discharge should be considered.

REASSESSMENT

Careful reassessment should be conducted after initial treatment, taking into consideration the timing of SCS dosing (**Table 3**). If response to treatment is incomplete or poor, further treatment with SABAs is indicated. Patients with severe exacerbations

Table 3
Reassessment and further management

Response to initial treatment		
Good	**Incomplete**	**Poor**
Mild features	Moderate features	Severe features
PEFR ≥70%	PEFR 40%–69%	PEFR <40%
Further management		
Observe for 30 min after single albuterol treatment	Albuterol every 2 h or continuous	Continuous albuterol
Observe 1–2 h after 3 albuterol treatments	Consider adjunctive therapy	Adjunctive therapy
Discharge *if mild features*	Hospitalization *if not mild features*	Consider ICU admission

require close monitoring and reassessment to determine response and need for adjunctive therapies.

ADJUNCTIVE THERAPIES

Adjunctive therapies are usually administered in addition to (but not instead of) inhaled bronchodilators, and timing may vary according to severity. Anticipating their need is essential to avoid delays in care. Most patients requiring adjunctive therapy will require hospitalization, and many of these therapies should be administered in an ICU setting.

Magnesium Sulfate

Magnesium sulfate is associated with improved pulmonary function and reduced hospitalization rate.[42,43] Its mechanism of action is unclear but it is thought to cause bronchodilation by decreasing intracellular calcium concentration resulting in respiratory smooth muscle relaxation.[42] It is most commonly administered as a single IV bolus, and a dose-response effect has been reported.[44] The recommended dose is 50 mg/kg to 75 mg/kg (maximum 2 g). There is limited pediatric data on inhaled magnesium sulfate and systematic reviews report no clear benefit.[43,45] In practice, most clinicians hospitalize patients who require magnesium.[46]

Helium-oxygen–Delivered SABA

Heliox is a mixture of helium and oxygen, thought to improve drug delivery in obstructed airways due to its lower density and airflow resistance. A recent systematic review found that delivery of aerosolized medication with heliox may improve outcomes in severe exacerbations.[47] The commonly used mixtures (helium:oxygen) are 70:30 or 80:20, and use in patients with significant hypoxemia is, therefore, limited.

Systemic (Injected) β-Agonists

Epinephrine, given subcutaneously or IM, should be considered an option for severe exacerbations, particularly as initial treatment of patients with significant airway obstruction when delivery of inhaled medications to the lower airways may be limited. Terbutaline may be administered subcutaneously and is also commonly administered as a continuous IV infusion, although pediatric studies evaluating such protocols are limited.[48,49]

Noninvasive Ventilatory Support

Noninvasive ventilatory support bilevel positive airway pressure may benefit patients tiring from increased work of breathing and with impending respiratory failure. Pediatric studies are limited but suggest it is generally well tolerated and may reduce need for ICU admission.[50–52] In practice, most patients who require biphasic positive airway pressure are treated in ICU settings.

Other Medications

Aminophylline and theophylline are not recommended for routine exacerbations. They are usually reserved for ICU settings and patients not responsive to other adjunctive therapies. Although studies suggest possible benefit in pulmonary function, LOS did not differ and there were more adverse events, such as vomiting, compared with β-agonists.[53]

Montelukast, a leukotriene receptor antagonist, is an effective controller medication for chronic asthma, but pediatric studies have not consistently shown effectiveness for oral or IV montelukast in the ED.[54–56]

Ketamine is a dissociative anesthetic that is an option during rapid sequence induction for intubation of children with asthma in respiratory failure. It has not, however, been found associated with added benefit during standard acute therapy.[57]

CHEST RADIOGRAPHS

Use of chest radiographs (CXRs) during ED visits with wheezing diagnoses varies in the United States, estimated between 14% and 56% of such visits.[58] Studies seeking to identify predictors of pathologic CXRs (most frequently pneumonia) among children with wheezing have shown that fever, hypoxia, and focal rales or wheezing may be indicators.[59–61] In a study of children of all ages with wheezing who had CXR for possible pneumonia, 4.9% of CXRs showed pneumonia.[61]

In children with first-time wheezing episodes, rates of pathologic CXRs ranged from 6% to 24% with similar predictors as described previously.[62–64] In a prospective study of young children with bronchiolitis, the rate of CXRs inconsistent from bronchiolitis was less than 1%.[65]

The potential risks of CXR include radiation exposure and false-positive results, leading to unnecessary antibiotic therapy. In general, a high threshold for imaging is appropriate for patients with typical asthma exacerbation given the low rate of abnormality.

CLINICAL PRACTICE GUIDELINES

Implementation of clinical practice guidelines for acute asthma is associated with improved efficiency and quality of care, including shorter time to SABAs and SCSs, increased rates of SCSs, decreased LOS, lower hospitalization rate, and fewer prescription errors.[66–70]

POST–EMERGENCY DEPARTMENT CARE
Improving Preventive Therapy

Poor adherence to prescribed ICSs is well documented in patients seeking asthma care in EDs, and studies have reported up to two-thirds of children presenting to EDs have persistent chronic asthma severity, indicating poor long-term control.[68,69] A majority of children treated in EDs, however, are not prescribed ICSs.[71–74]

The NAEPP guidelines recommend ED providers consider initiating controller medications to appropriate patients.[1] A brief assessment of asthma control can assist clinicians in identifying such patients—assess impairment (>2 d/wk of asthma symptoms or SABA use or 1 to 2 nighttime awakenings due to asthma per month) and risk (>1 SCS course in last 6 mo or >3 acute wheezing episodes lasting >1 d each in last 12 mo).[1]

Written Asthma Care Plans

Written asthma care plans are associated with improved outcomes, including increased adherence to ICSs.[75,76] Although discharge instructions should include information regarding care after the acute visit, this is an opportunity for clinicians to provide appropriate care plans to assist patients with future exacerbations and to encourage partnership with primary care physicians and ongoing discussions of home asthma care.

Follow-up After an Acute Visit

Primary care physician visits, both follow-up after the ED and periodically to monitor asthma control, are important for optimal care, because studies have shown that NAEPP guideline-based asthma care reduces morbidity.[77,78] Patients discharged from EDs should have primary care physician follow-up visits within 2 to 4 weeks. Unfortunately, studies have shown unacceptably poor follow-up rates in urban populations.[79,80] Interventions, such as scheduling follow-up at the time of an ED visit, can improve adherence.[79]

SUMMARY

- Acute asthma management involves prompt recognition of severity and treatment using SABAs, anticholinergics and SCSs.
- Children with severe exacerbations should receive high-dose SABAs mixed with ipratropium bromide as well as SCSs.
- Children with less-severe exacerbations may benefit from SCSs based on chronic asthma severity reflecting significant airway inflammation.
- Patients not improving after multiple high-dose SABA treatments should receive adjunctive therapy, such as IV magnesium.
- Many children treated for asthma in EDs have significant morbidity and infrequent primary asthma care; prescription of ICSs is appropriate.

REFERENCES

1. National Asthma Education and Prevention Program. Expert panel report 3: guidelines for the diagnosis and management of asthma—summary report 2007. J Allergy Clin Immunol 2007;120:S94–138.
2. Akinbami LJ, Moorman JE, Garbe PL, et al. Status of childhood asthma in the United States, 1980-2007. Pediatrics 2009;123:S131–45.
3. Centers for Disease Control and Prevention (CDC). Asthma prevalence and control characteristics by race/ethnicity—United States, 2002. MMWR Morb Mortal Wkly Rep 2004;53:145–8.
4. Gold DR, Wright R. Population disparities in asthma. Annu Rev Public Health 2005;26:89–113.
5. Gupta RS, Carrion-Carire V, Weiss KB. The widening black/white gap in asthma hospitalizations and mortality. J Allergy Clin Immunol 2006;117:351–8.

6. Lieu TA, Lozano P, Finkelstein JA, et al. Racial/ethnic variation in asthma status and management practices among children with managed Medicaid. Pediatrics 2002;109(5):857–65.
7. Finkelstein JA, Lozano P, Farber HJ, et al. Underuse of controller medications among Medicaid-insured children with asthma. Arch Pediatr Adolesc Med 2002;156(6):562–7.
8. Gorelick MH, Stevens MW, Schultz TR, et al. Performance of a novel clinical score, the Pediatric Asthma Severity Score (PASS), in the evaluation of acute asthma. Acad Emerg Med 2004;11:8–10.
9. Carroll CL, Sekaran AK, Lerer TJ, et al. A modified pulmonary index score with predictive value for pediatric asthma exacerbations. Ann Allergy Asthma Immunol 2005;94:355–9.
10. Smith SR, Baty JD, Hodge D 3rd. Validation of the pulmonary score: an asthma severity score for children. Acad Emerg Med 2002;9:99–104.
11. Carl JC, Myers TR, Kirchner HL, et al. Comparison of racemic albuterol and levalbuterol for treatment of acute asthma. J Pediatr 2003;143:731–6.
12. Qureshi F, Zaritsky A, Welch C, et al. Clinical efficacy of racemic albuterol versus levalbuterol for the treatment of acute pediatric asthma. Ann Emerg Med 2005; 46:29–36.
13. Hardasmalani MD, DeBari V, Bithoney WG, et al. Levalbuterol versus racemic albuterol in the treatment of acute exacerbation of asthma in children. Pediatr Emerg Care 2005;21:415–9.
14. Andrews T, McGintee E, Mittal MK, et al. High-dose continuous nebulized levalbuterol for pediatric status asthmaticus: a randomized trial. J Pediatr 2009;155:205–10.
15. Mazhar SH, Ismail NE, Newton DA, et al. Relative lung deposition of salbutamol following inhalation from a spacer and a sidestream jet nebulizer following an acute exacerbation. Br J Clin Pharmacol 2008;65(3):334–7.
16. Silkstone VL, Corlett SA, Chrystyn H. Relative lung and total systemic bioavailability following inhalation from a metered dose inhaler compared with a metered dose inhaler attached to a large volume plastic spacer and a jet nebuliser. Eur J Clin Pharmacol 2002;57(11):781–6.
17. Cates CJ, Crilly JA, Rowe BH. Holding chambers (spacers) versus nebulisers for beta-agonist treatment of acute asthma. Cochrane Database Syst Rev 2006;(2):CD000052.
18. Castro-Rodriguez JA, Rodrigo GJ. Beta-agonists through metered-dose inhaler with valved holding chamber versus nebulizer for acute exacerbation of wheezing or asthma in children under 5 years of age: a systematic review with meta-analysis. J Pediatr 2004;145:172–7.
19. Dolovich MB, Ahrens RC, Hess DR, et al. Device selection and outcomes of aerosol therapy: evidence-based guidelines. Chest 2005;127:335–71.
20. Laube BL, Swift DL, Wagner HN Jr, et al. The effect of bronchial obstruction on central airway deposition of a saline aerosol in patients with asthma. Am Rev Respir Dis 1986;133:740–3.
21. Isawa T, Teshima T, Hirano T, et al. Effect of bronchodilation on the deposition and clearance of radioaerosol in bronchial asthma in remission. J Nucl Med 1987;28:1901–6.
22. Camargo CA Jr, Spooner CH, Rowe BH. Continuous versus intermittent beta-agonists in the treatment of acute asthma. Cochrane Database Syst Rev 2003;(4):CD0011115.
23. Wilkinson M, Bulloch B, Garcia-Filion P, et al. Efficacy of racemic albuterol versus levalbuterol used as a continuous nebulization for the treatment of acute

asthma exacerbations: a randomized, double-blind, clinical trial. J Asthma 2011;48(2):188–93.

24. Plotnick LH, Ducharme FM. Acute asthma in children and adolescents: should inhaled anticholinergics be added to beta(2)-agonists? Am J Respir Med 2003;2:109–15.

25. Rodrigo GJ, Castro-Rodriguez JA. Anticholinergics in the treatment of children and adults with acute asthma: a systematic review with meta-analysis. Thorax 2005;60:740–6.

26. Zorc JJ, Pusic MV, Ogborn CJ, et al. Ipratropium bromide added to asthma treatment in the pediatric emergency department. Pediatrics 1999;103(4 Pt 1): 748–52.

27. Rowe BH, Spooner CH, Ducharme FM, et al. Early emergency department treatment of acute asthma with systemic corticosteroids. Cochrane Database Syst Rev 2001;(1):CD002178.

28. Rowe BH, Spooner CH, Ducharme FM, et al. Corticosteroids for preventing relapse following acute exacerbations of asthma. Cochrane Database Syst Rev 2007;(3):CD000195.

29. Mori H, Tanaka H, Ohno Y, et al. Effect of intermittent systemic corticosteroid on bone metabolism in bronchial asthma patients. J Asthma 2009;46:142–6.

30. Kelly HW, Van Natta ML, Covar RA, et al. Effect of long-term corticosteroid use on bone mineral density in children: a prospective longitudinal assessment in the childhood Asthma Management Program (CAMP) study. Pediatrics 2008; 122:e53–61.

31. Holm IA. Do short courses of oral corticosteroids and use of inhaled corticosteroids affect bone health in children? Nat Clin Pract Endocrinol Metab 2009;5: 132–3.

32. Gries DM, Moffitt DR, Pulos E, et al. A single dose of intramuscularly administered dexamethasone acetate is as effective as oral prednisone to treat asthma exacerbations in young children. J Pediatr 2000;136:298–303.

33. Gordon S, Tompkins T, Dayan PS. Randomized trial of single-dose intramuscular dexamethasone compared with prednisolone for children with acute asthma. Pediatr Emerg Care 2007;23:521–7.

34. Chang AB, Clark R, Sloots TP, et al. A 5- versus 3-day course of oral corticosteroids for children with asthma exacerbations who are not hospitalised: a randomised controlled trial. Med J Aust 2008;189:306–10.

35. Qureshi F, Zaritsky A, Poirer MP. Comparative efficacy of oral dexamethasone versus oral prednisone in acute pediatric asthma. J Pediatr 2001;139(1):20–6.

36. Altamimi S, Robertson G, Jastaniah W, et al. Single-dose oral dexamethasone in the emergency management of children with exacerbations of mild to moderate asthma. Pediatr Emerg Care 2006;22(12):786–93.

37. Greenberg RA, Kerby G, Roosevelt GE. A comparison of oral dexamethasone with oral prednisone in pediatric asthma exacerbations treated in the emergency department. Clin Pediatr (Phila) 2008;47(8):817–23.

38. Edmonds ML, Milan SJ, Camargo CA Jr, et al. Early use of inhaled corticosteroids in the emergency department treatment of acute asthma. Cochrane Database Syst Rev 2012;(12):CD002308.

39. Rodrigo GJ. Rapid effects of inhaled corticosteroids in acute asthma: an evidence-based evaluation. Chest 2006;130:1301–11.

40. Edmonds ML, Milan SJ, Brenner BE, et al. Inhaled steroids for acute asthma following emergency department discharge. Cochrane Database Syst Rev 2012;(12):CD002316.

41. Schuh S, Dick PT, Stephens D, et al. High-dose inhaled fluticasone does not replace oral prednisolone in children with mild to moderate acute asthma. Pediatrics 2006;118:644–50.
42. Rowe BH, Bretzlaff JA, Bourdon C, et al. Magnesium sulfate for treating exacerbations of acute asthma in the emergency department. Cochrane Database Syst Rev 2000;(1):CD001490.
43. Mohammed S, Goodacre S. Intravenous and nebulised magnesium sulphate for acute asthma: systematic review and meta-analysis. Emerg Med J 2007;24: 823–30.
44. Ciarallo L, Brousseau D, Reinert S. Higher-dose intravenous magnesium therapy for children with moderate to severe acute asthma. Arch Pediatr Adolesc Med 2000;154:979–83.
45. Rowe BH, Camargo CA Jr. The role of magnesium sulfate in the acute and chronic management of asthma. Curr Opin Pulm Med 2008;14:70–6.
46. Schuh S, Macias C, Freedman SB, et al. North American practice patterns of intravenous magnesium therapy in severe acute asthma in children. Acad Emerg Med 2010;17(11):1189–96.
47. Rodrigo G, Pollack C, Rodrigo C, et al. Heliox for nonintubated acute asthma patients. Cochrane Database Syst Rev 2006;(4):CD002884.
48. Travers AH, Rowe BH, Barker S, et al. The effectiveness of IV beta-agonists in treating patients with acute asthma in the emergency department: a meta-analysis. Chest 2002;122:1200–7.
49. Bogie AL, Towne D, Luckett PM, et al. Comparison of intravenous terbutaline versus normal saline in pediatric patients on continuous high-dose nebulized albuterol for status asthmaticus. Pediatr Emerg Care 2007;23:355–61.
50. Akingbola OA, Simakajornboon N, Hadley EF Jr, et al. Noninvasive positive-pressure ventilation in pediatric status asthmaticus. Pediatr Crit Care Med 2002;3:181–4.
51. Carroll CL, Schramm CM. Noninvasive positive pressure ventilation for the treatment of status asthmaticus in children. Ann Allergy Asthma Immunol 2006;96: 454–9.
52. Beers SL, Abramo TJ, Bracken A, et al. Bilevel positive airway pressure in the treatment of status asthmaticus in pediatrics. Am J Emerg Med 2007;25: 6–9.
53. Mitra A, Bassler D, Goodman K, et al. Intravenous aminophylline for acute severe asthma in children over two years receiving inhaled bronchodilators. Cochrane Database Syst Rev 2005;(2):CD001276.
54. Harmanci K, Bakirtas A, Turktas I, et al. Oral montelukast treatment of preschool-age children with acute asthma. Ann Allergy Asthma Immunol 2006;96:731–5.
55. Nelson KA, Smith SR, Trinkaus K, et al. Pilot study of oral montelukast added to standard therapy for acute asthma exacerbations in children aged 6 to 14 years. Pediatr Emerg Care 2008;24:21–7.
56. Morris CR, Becker AB, Piñieiro A, et al. A randomized, placebo-controlled study of intravenous montelukast in children with acute asthma. Ann Allergy Asthma Immunol 2010;104(2):161–71.
57. Allen JY, Macias CG. The efficacy of ketamine in pediatric emergency department patients who present with acute severe asthma. Ann Emerg Med 2005; 46:43–50.
58. Neuman MI, Graham D, Bachur R. Variation in the use of chest radiography for pneumonia in pediatric emergency departments. Pediatr Emerg Care 2011; 27(7):606–10.

59. Mahabee-Gittens EM, Dowd MD, Beck JA, et al. Clinical factors associated with focal infiltrates in wheezing infants and toddlers. Clin Pediatr (Phila) 2000;39(7): 387–93.
60. Mahabee-Gittens EM, Bachman DT, Shapiro ED, et al. Chest radiographs in the pediatric emergency department for children <or = 18 months of age with wheezing. Clin Pediatr (Phila) 1999;38(7):395–9.
61. Mathews B, Shah S, Cleveland RH, et al. Clinical predictors of pneumonia among children with wheezing. Pediatrics 2009;124(1):e29–36.
62. Walsh-Kelly CM, Hennes HM. Do clinical variables predict pathologic radiographs in the first episode of wheezing? Pediatr Emerg Care 2002;18(1): 8–11.
63. Walsh-Kelly CM, Kim MK, Hennes HM. Chest radiography in the initial episode of bronchospasm in children: can clinical variables predict pathologic findings? Ann Emerg Med 1996;28(4):391–5.
64. Roback MG, Dreitlein DA. Chest radiograph in the evaluation of first time wheezing episodes: review of current clinical practice and efficacy. Pediatr Emerg Care 1998;14(3):181–4.
65. Schuh S, Lalani A, Allen U, et al. Evaluation of the utility of radiography in acute bronchiolitis. J Pediatr 2007;150(4):429–33.
66. Emond SD, Woodruff PG, Lee EY, et al. Effect of an emergency department asthma program on acute asthma care. Ann Emerg Med 1999;34(3):321–5.
67. Dalcin Pde T, da Rocha PM, Franciscatto E, et al. Effect of clinical pathways on the management of acute asthma in the emergency department: five years of evaluation. J Asthma 2007;44(4):273–9.
68. Norton SP, Pusic MV, Taha F, et al. Effect of a clinical pathway on the hospital-isation rates of children with asthma: a prospective study. Arch Dis Child 2007;92(1):60–6.
69. Self TH, Usery JB, Howard-Thompson AM, et al. Asthma treatment protocols in the emergency department: are they effective? J Asthma 2007;44(4):243–8.
70. Cunningham S, Logan C, Lockerbie L, et al. Effect of an integrated care pathway on acute asthma/wheeze in children attending hospital: cluster randomized trial. J Pediatr 2008;152(3):315–20.
71. Scarfone RJ, Zorc JJ, Capraro GA. Patient self-management of acute asthma: adherence to national guidelines a decade later. Pediatrics 2001;108:1332–8.
72. Sills M, Ginde AA, Clark S, et al. Multicenter study of chronic asthma severity among emergency department patients with acute asthma. J Asthma 2010; 47(8):920–8.
73. Scarfone RJ, Zorc JJ, Angsuco CJ. Emergency physicians' prescribing of asthma controller medications. Pediatrics 2006;117:821–7.
74. Garro AC, Asnis L, Merchant RC, et al. Frequency of prescription of inhaled corticosteroids to children with asthma in U.S. emergency departments. Acad Emerg Med 2011;18(7):767–70.
75. Zemek RL, Bhogal SK, Ducharme FM. Systematic review of randomized controlled trials examining written action plans in children: what is the plan? Arch Pediatr Adolesc Med 2008;162:157–63.
76. Ducharme FM, Zemek RL, Chalut D, et al. Written action plan in pediatric emergency room improves asthma prescribing, adherence, and control. Am J Respir Crit Care Med 2011;183(2):195–203.
77. Cloutier MM, Hall CB, Wakefield DB, et al. Use of asthma guidelines by primary care providers to reduce hospitalizations and emergency department visits in poor, minority, urban children. J Pediatr 2005;146:591–7.

78. Cloutier MM, Wakefield DB, Sangeloty-Higgins P, et al. Asthma guideline use by pediatricians in private practices and asthma morbidity. Pediatrics 2006;118: 1880–7.

79. Zorc JJ, Scarfone RJ, Li Y, et al. Scheduled follow-up after a pediatric emergency department visit for asthma: a randomized trial. Pediatrics 2003;111: 495–502.

80. Smith SR, Jaffe DM, Fisher EB, et al. Improving follow-up for children with asthma after an acute Emergency Department visit. J Pediatr 2004;145:772–7.

Evaluation of Child with Fever Without Source
Review of Literature and Update

Rajan Arora, MD[a], Prashant Mahajan, MD, MPH, MBA[b],*

KEYWORDS

- Fever • Serious bacterial infection • Fever without source • Tissue culture

KEY POINTS

- Fever is a common reason for visits to the emergency department for children 36 months of age and younger.
- Although laboratory testing is routinely used and hospitalization is frequent, especially for the young febrile infant, there is substantial variation in their evaluation and management.
- This variation in practice has significant implications in terms of cost and, potentially, safety, owing to possible iatrogenic overuse of invasive procedures (lumbar punctures), empiric antibiotics, and unnecessary hospitalizations.
- Routinely used screening tests in the evaluation of serious bacterial infection (SBI) in young febrile infants are inaccurate, and cannot be relied upon to distinguish between those with bacterial and those with nonbacterial infections.
- Newer pathogen-detection techniques are likely to evolve rapidly and to affect the way SBI as an entity is evaluated.

INTRODUCTION

Fever is a common complaint in infants and children, and represents 10.5% to 25% of pediatric emergency department (ED) visits.[1–3] Although most febrile children have self-limited viral infections, a small but not insignificant proportion (especially infants 3 months of age and younger) will have serious bacterial infection (SBI), including bacteremia, bacterial meningitis, urinary tract infection (UTI), pneumonia, septic arthritis, osteomyelitis, and enteritis.[4,5] Incidence of SBI has been estimated at 6%

Funding Sources: Nil.
Conflict of Interest: Nil.
[a] Division of Emergency Medicine, Carman and Ann Adam Department of Pediatrics, Children's Hospital of Michigan, Wayne State University School of Medicine, 3901 Beaubien Boulevard, Detroit, MI 48201, USA; [b] Division of Emergency Medicine, Carman and Ann Adam Department of Pediatrics, Center for Quality and Innovation, Children's Hospital of Michigan, Wayne State University School of Medicine, 3901 Beaubien Boulevard, Detroit, MI 48201, USA
* Corresponding author.
E-mail address: pmahajan@dmc.org

to 10% in infants younger than 3 months and 5% to 7% of children between 3 and 36 months of age.[6,7] However, during the past 2 decades, routine vaccinations against *Haemophilus influenzae* type b and *Streptococcus pneumoniae* have significantly changed the epidemiology of SBI. The evaluation of the young febrile infant is more challenging because the infant's immune system is relatively immature during the first 2 to 3 months of life; chemotactic responses such as opsonin activity, macrophage function, and neutrophil activity are decreased, making the infant more susceptible to bacterial infection.[8] The risk of SBI decreases with age, and increases with height and duration of fever. The evaluation and management of febrile infants and children who are ill-appearing or have an evident focus of infection is straightforward. It is the otherwise well-appearing subset of febrile infants and children without a localizing focus that poses a diagnostic dilemma. Febrile illness in children results in significant parental anxiety. Management decisions about febrile children are further complicated by the fact that parents and physicians weigh the risks and costs differently.[9] Despite many studies aimed at identifying individual biomarkers or a combination of clinical and laboratory tests, to date there is no single test or combinations of tests and clinical findings that have characteristics adequate to reliably identify SBI in the febrile child. It is, therefore, not surprising that the clinical priority, recently identified by emergency physicians, is the need for development of clinical decision rules for the evaluation and management of the febrile child younger than 36 months.[10]

This article reviews the literature on the evaluation and management of the febrile child, and comments on recent advances that may have potential to change the paradigm for detection of pathogens. The authors discuss evaluation of the febrile child in 2 age groups, febrile infants 3 months or younger and those between 3 and 36 months of age.

OCCULT BACTEREMIA

Occult bacteremia (OB) is defined as the presence of bacteria in the blood of an otherwise well-appearing febrile child in the absence of an identifiable focal bacterial source of infection. This term was introduced in the 1970s when bacteremia was identified in febrile children (3–36 months) who were at risk for developing systemic or focal infections such as sepsis, meningitis, and osteomyelitis, despite a relatively benign clinical appearance, but.[11] In the prevaccine era, the prevalence of OB was 2.4% to 11.6% in all children with fever without source (FWS), with *Streptococcus pneumoniae* accounting for most cases (50%–90%); 3% to 25% were due to *Haemophilus influenzae* type b, with the remainder due to *Salmonella* species and *Neisseria meningitidis*.[12,13]

The impact of conjugate vaccines has been highest in the 3- to 36-month group of well-appearing febrile children. Not only has the overall incidence of bacteremia dropped to 0.17% to 0.36%, the nonvaccinated population has also benefited through the phenomenon known as "herd protection." Indeed, in well-appearing children 3 to 36 months of age with FWS, overall OB rates of less than 0.5% have been reported in studies with pneumococcal conjugate vaccine (PCV7) coverage in the general population of approximately 80%.[14,15] Although there are surveillance data suggesting a relative increase in infections caused by a limited number of nonvaccine serotypes, particularly serotype 19A, which is often multidrug resistant, the majority of cases of bacteremia are due to *Streptococcus pyogenes*, *Enterococcus* spp, *N meningitidis*, non–type b *H influenzae*, *Escherichia coli*, *Moraxella. catarrhalis*, *Salmonella* spp, and *Staphylococcus aureus*.[14–17]

A shift in epidemiology of OB has also been identified in febrile infants younger than 3 months, largely attributable to advances in medical practices, prenatal screening, and intrapartum chemoprophylaxis against Group B *Streptococcus* (GBS). A large epidemiologic study on 4122 infants 1 week to 3 months of age revealed that *E coli* accounted for 56% of all cases of bacteremia, followed by GBS (21%), *S aureus* (8%), *Streptococcus viridans* (3%), *S pneumoniae* (3%), *Klebsiella* (2%), and *Salmonella* (2%). There were no cases of *Listeria monocytogenes* bacteremia, or meningococcemia, with only 1 case of enterococcal bacteremia.[18]

URINARY TRACT INFECTION

Pediatric UTIs account for 0.7% of physician office visits and 5% to 14% of ED visits by children annually.[19] The overall prevalence of UTI in febrile infants younger than 24 months has been estimated as from 5% to 7%, however, certain subgroups of children are at higher risk for UTIs.[20,21] In 2008, Shaikh and colleagues[21] pooled estimates for 18 studies that examined the rate of culture-positive bacteriuria in febrile infants, breaking down the results by age group and sex. There was a prevalence of 7.5% and 8.7%, respectively, among febrile girls and boys younger than 3 months, whereas corresponding numbers for febrile children aged 3 to 12 months were 8.3% and 1.7%, respectively. Among febrile children aged 12 to 24 months, only data for girls were available, suggesting a rate of 2.1%. UTI rates in uncircumcised febrile male infants younger than 3 months was the highest for any group, at 20.1% (95% confidence interval [CI] 16.8–23.4), and was 10 times higher than their circumcised counterparts who had the lowest rates. UTI rates were significantly higher among white infants than among black infants (8.0% vs 4.7%).

The updated 2011 American Academy of Pediatrics guidelines recommend aggressive diagnosis, treatment, and investigation of possible UTI, with the goal of reducing renal scarring and, thus, kidney damage.[20] It provides an initial algorithm to estimate the risk of UTI in febrile children aged 2 to 24 months that is based on clinical and demographic characteristics. The major risk factor for febrile infant boys is whether they are circumcised. The probability of UTI ($\leq$1% or $\leq$2%) can be estimated according to the number of risk factors present, namely, non–black race, temperature of at least 39°C, fever for more than 24 hours, and absence of another source of infection. In girls, risk factors such as white race, age under 12 months, temperature greater than 39°C, fever longer than 2 days, and absence of another source of infection will determine the probability or likelihood of UTI, with each additional risk factor increasing the probability.[22] Diagnosis of UTI requires the presence of both pyuria and bacteriuria and at least 50,000 colonies per mL of a single uropathogenic organism in an appropriately collected (straight catheterization) specimen of urine.[20] It should be noted that the guidelines exclude infants 2 months of age and younger.

MENINGITIS

Incidence of pneumococcal meningitis in children younger than 2 years has decreased by 64% following widespread use of PCV7 vaccine as reported from an extensive review of the Nationwide Inpatient Sample (1994–2004).[23,24] The investigators also report a 17.5%, 54%, and 50% decrease in meningitis due to GBS, meningococcus, and *H influenzae*. Most experts do not recommend obtaining cerebrospinal fluid (CSF) studies in the evaluation of an alert, febrile child 3 to 36 months of age with a normal neurologic examination. Performance of lumbar puncture continues to vary in the younger febrile infant, and no firm recommendations can be made because of paucity of large and geographically diverse studies in this age group.[25]

PNEUMONIA

The diagnosis of pneumonia in the pediatric population remains challenging. Despite its common occurrence, accurate diagnosis of bacterial pneumonia is difficult because most lower respiratory tract infections are viral in etiology, and findings on routine chest radiographs are nondiagnostic (ie, it is often difficult to ascribe cause, bacterial or nonbacterial, on "positive" chest radiograph findings in the absence of positive cultures). Indeed, blood cultures are rarely positive, and obtaining sputum/pleural fluid aspirates for etiologic diagnosis is impractical. Moreover, there is substantial variation in interpretation of chest radiographs among ED physicians and even among trained radiologists.[25]

Similarly to bacteremia and meningitis, the incidence of pneumococcal pneumonia has reduced substantially (a 65% decline in hospital admissions for pneumococcal pneumonia and a 39% decline in admissions for pneumonia in all pediatric age groups). In an extensive analysis, Murphy and colleagues[26] reveal the following factors that increase the likelihood of a radiographic pneumonia: increasing duration of fever (likelihood ratio [LR+] 1.62 for fever longer than 3 days and LR+ 2.24 for fever longer than 5 days), presence of cough (LR+ 1.24), prolonged cough (>10 days, LR+ 2.25), and a white blood cell (WBC) count greater than 20,000/mm^3 (LR+ 2.17). A different study revealed that the incidence of pneumonia increased with age (odds ratio [OR] 2.62 for infants >12 months; 95% CI 1.04–6.60), C-reactive protein (CRP) level greater than 100 mg/L (OR 3.18; 95% CI 1.19–8.51), and absolute neutrophil count greater than 20×10^9/L (OR 3.52; 95% CI 1.37–9.06).[27]

In summary, pneumonia as an SBI in the absence of signs and symptoms of lower respiratory tract involvement is highly unlikely, and routine chest radiographs should not be performed.

FEBRILE CHILDREN WITH CONFIRMED VIRAL ILLNESS

Because fever in most febrile children will have a viral source, identification of the presence of virus by rapid bedside tests have been incorporated for both epidemiologic and management purposes.[28] The advent of rapid testing for viral pathogens has resulted in changes in the management of febrile infants younger than 90 days, as well as older febrile infants and children, including decreased ancillary testing, decreased use of antibiotics, and shorter hospital stays.[29,30] Febrile children with documented viral infections had a lower prevalence of SBI, with the investigators recommending that blood cultures may not be necessary in their evaluation.[31] In a recent study on children aged 2 to 36 months, 1 or more viruses were detected in 76% (n = 75) of children with FWS. Adenovirus, human herpesvirus 6, enterovirus, and parechoviruses accounted for 57% of all viruses.[28] It was concluded that future studies should explore the utility of testing for the implicated viruses, as better recognition of viruses that cause undifferentiated fever in young children may help limit unnecessary antibiotic use.

However, detection of specific viral infections (especially respiratory syncytial virus [RSV]) has been shown to decrease, but not completely eliminate the risk of SBIs in very young febrile infants, especially those 60 days of age and younger. One multicenter prospective study of 1248 febrile infants 60 days and younger revealed that there was no significant difference in the prevalence of bacteremia and meningitis in febrile infants with documented RSV infection than in those without RSV (1.1% vs 2.3%, risk difference: 1.2%; 95% CI: 0.4%–2.7%).[32] Similar results were demonstrated by the same investigators when rates of SBI were compared among febrile infants with and without influenza infection.[33] An evidence-based review conducted by the Agency for Healthcare Research and Quality (AHRQ) demonstrated a significantly reduced risk of SBI among infants who tested positive for the presence of viral infection or clinical bronchiolitis when compared with infants who tested negative for the presence of viral infection or bronchiolitis, but cautioned that this finding may not be applicable to neonates.[34]

In summary, identification of a virus in a febrile child may help clinicians to reduce the need for further testing to identify a bacterial cause in the older febrile child. Clinicians should consider obtaining urine studies to rule out UTIs, especially in young children (females <2 years old, uncircumcised males <1 year old, and circumcised males <6 months old), and as part of a comprehensive evaluation for SBI including blood and CSF samples in febrile infants 60 days of age and younger.

ROLE OF SCREENING TESTS

To date there is no ideal test for identifying young, febrile children with occult SBIs, although much research has been performed on complete WBC count, and differential counts including absolute neutrophil count (ANC), band counts, CRP, interleukins (IL) (IL-6, IL-1, and IL-8), and serum procalcitonin (PCT).[35]

Complete WBC count continues to remain the most commonly used screening test for SBI and various algorithms suggest a cutoff value between 15,000 and 20,0000/mm^3 to stratify febrile infants as low or high risk.[36] However, the test characteristics remain suboptimal, with sensitivities ranging from 50% to 69% and specificity from 53% to 80%.[37] Studies in the post-PCV7 era have shown that a WBC count of greater than 15,000/mm^3 yields a positive predictive value of only 1.5% to 3.2%.[34] It is important to recognize that traditionally accepted WBC cutoffs may no longer be relevant as the epidemiology of OB shifts away from *S pneumoniae*.[38,39] Zaidi and colleagues[39] retrospectively reviewed nontyphi *Salmonella* bacteremia and showed that 54% had a median WBC count of 10,000/mm^3. Furthermore, WBC counts by themselves are of limited value for "ruling in" SBI (positive likelihood ratio 0.87–2.43) and for ruling out SBI (negative likelihood ratio 0.61–1.14).[40]

Both CRP and serum PCT have been studied in the evaluation of the febrile child. Several studies have demonstrated that serum PCT levels increase more rapidly in bacterial infections when compared with CRP and other biomarkers such as the interleukins. Furthermore, serum PCT levels correlate with severity of disease and mortality.[35,41] Studies on the accuracy of PCT in screening febrile children for SBI in the ED setting have revealed inconsistent results. Two separate studies demonstrated that PCT was the single best laboratory screening test when compared with IL-6, IL-8, and IL-1 receptor antagonists, CRP, and other routinely used laboratory screening tests for distinguishing those with viral and bacterial infections.[42,43] By contrast, the findings of another study of 72 febrile children 1 to 36 months of age suggest that the diagnostic accuracy of PCT, CRP, and WBC are comparable with that of clinical scoring (Yale Observational Scale [YOS]) and do not change posttest probabilities to a clinically useful extent.[44] Evidence-based reviews of published studies on the use of PCT as a screening test for SBI in febrile children younger than 3 years concluded that PCT is still not sufficiently sensitive to be used as a single screening tool to exclude the possibility of SBI.[45–47] PCT seems promising and may have some utility in identifying SBI, but it is not clear if the marginal benefit over routinely obtained screening tests is sufficient to be included in the evaluation of the febrile child.

ROLE OF PREDICTION RULES

Clinical-decision rules or prediction rules use clinical findings (history, physical examination, and test results) to make a diagnosis or predict outcomes, and when appropriately applied can "change clinical behavior and reduce unnecessary costs while maintaining quality of care and patient satisfaction."[48] Reliance on clinical examination alone is insufficient, as demonstrated by the suboptimal performance of the YOS in very young febrile infants. Craig and colleagues[49] evaluated 40 clinical features to construct a multivariate model to identify SBI in 15,781 febrile children younger than 5 years, and demonstrated that clinical signs and symptoms contribute differently to predicting the risk of SBI. Overall ill/unwell appearance was found to be the strongest diagnostic marker for all SBI. Other clinical parameters such as raised temperature, no fluid intake in the previous 24 hours, increased capillary refill time, and chronic disease were also predictive of SBI. Bachur and Harper[6] developed a model that sequentially used 4 clinical parameters to define high-risk patients: positive urinalysis, WBC count greater than 20,000/mm^3 or less than 4100/mm^3, temperature greater than 39.6°C, and age younger than 13 days. The sensitivity of the model for SBI is 82% (95% CI 78%–86%) and the negative predictive value is 98.3% (95% CI 97.8%–98.7%). The negative predictive value for bacteremia or meningitis is 99.6% (95% CI 99.4%–99.8%).

Some of the more well-known algorithms/rules in the evaluation of the febrile infant are described in **Table 1**. A comprehensive review was recently conducted by the AHRQ, which concludes that the 3 more well-known rules (ie, Boston, Philadelphia, and Rochester) were fairly accurate in identifying a low-risk group for SBI in infants younger than 3 months.[34] Recently, biological markers such as PCT and CRP have been incorporated along with other routine screening tests in patient-evaluation algorithms. For instance, the "lab-score" combines PCT, CRP, and urine dipstick. It has been derived and validated for predicting SBIs in children 7 days to 36 months of age with FWS.[50,51] **Table 2** details the elements and test characteristics of a lab-score cutoff of 3 or greater in predicting the risk of SBI by age. In their validation article, the Bressan and colleagues[51] compared the characteristics of the lab-score with individual biomarkers, and demonstrated superior performance of combined lab-score over individual biomarkers. Another study investigated the accuracy and usefulness of the lab-score in predicting SBI in well-appearing infants younger than 3 months with FWS, and found it more useful for ruling in, rather than ruling out SBI.[52]

This approach, however, has significant implications in terms of cost and, potentially, safety, because of the possible iatrogenic overuse of invasive procedures (lumbar punctures), empiric antibiotics, and unnecessary hospitalizations.[53,54] Considerable debate exists, and much has been written, about these guidelines because: (1) most research studies pertaining to febrile infants have been conducted in a single or small groups of academic centers; (2) many studies have used retrospective study designs and different inclusion criteria (eg, with respect to age and temperature cutoffs to define fever), and different laboratory criteria for distinguishing high-risk from low-risk infants; and (3) increasing evidence questions the discriminatory ability of commonly used screening tests in young febrile infants. Consequently, variation continues to exist, and multiple laboratory testing is common, in the evaluation of febrile infants. Variation in approach is determined by several factors, including the clinical setting (academic vs community EDs vs general pediatric practices) and clinician training (emergency medicine vs general pediatrics vs pediatric emergency medicine).[6,7,53]

CULTURES AS REFERENCE STANDARDS: TIME TO REEVALUATE OUR APPROACH?

Cultures of relevant tissue fluids are a part of the evaluation for SBI and constitute the current reference standard. However, reliance on blood cultures is problematic for

Table 1
Commonly used algorithms and pathways for risk stratification in management of febrile infants 3 months of age and younger

Low-Risk Criteria	Boston[a]	Philadelphia[a]	Rochester[a]	Pittsburgh Criteria	Boston Predictive Model	Milwaukee[a] Criteria
Age (d)	28–89	29–56	0–60	<60	<90	28–56
Temperature (°C)	≥38.0	≥38.2	≥38.0	>38.0	>39.6	≥38.0
Clinical appearance or YOS	Well	Well	Well	No	No	Well
CBC	>5000 or <20,000	<15,000	>5000 or <15,000	>5000 or <15,000	>20,000 or <40,100	<15,000
Band counts	NA	<0.2 B:N ratio	<1500	<1500	NA	NA
UA	<10 WBC/hpf	<10 WBC/hpf	<10 WBC/hpf	Enhanced WBC <9	>5/Dip(+)	UA <5–10 WBC/hpf (no bacteria, negative LE/nitrite)
Urine Gram stain	NA	Yes	NA	Yes	NA	NA
CSF	<10 WBC/mm^3	<8 WBC/mm^3	Not required	<5, (−) GM	NA	<10 WBC/mm^3
Stools	If diarrhea	If diarrhea	If diarrhea	<5	NA	NA
Chest radiograph	If done	All	If done	Yes	NA	If done

Abbreviations: B:N, Bands: Neutrophil; CBC, complete blood count; CSF, cerebrospinal fluid; GM, gram stain; hpf, high-power field; LE, Leukocyte Esterase; NA, no data available; UA, urinalysis; WBC, white blood cells; YOS, Yale Observational Scale.
[a] Reliable caretaker and follow-up required within 24 hours if patient is discharged home from the ED.

Table 2
Lab-score and its test characteristics

Predictors	Sensitivity (95% CI)	Specificity (95% CI)	Cutoff Values	PPV (95% CI)	NPV (95% CI)	LR + (95% CI)	LR − (95% CI)	Points
Procalcitonin (ng/mL)			<0.5					0
			>0.5					2
			>2					4
C-reactive protein (mg/L)			<40					0
			40–99					2
			≥100					4
Urine dipstick (leukocyte esterase and/or nitrite)			Negative					0
			Positive					1
	Sensitivity (95% CI)	Specificity (95% CI)		PPV (95% CI)	NPV (95% CI)	LR + (95% CI)	LR − (95% CI)	
Lab-score ≥3 (N = 406)	86 (77–92)	83 (79–87)		60 (51–68)	95 (92–97)	5.1 (3.9–6.6)	0.17 (0.1–0.28)	
Age <3 mo (n = 106)	78 (59–89)	90 (81–95)		72 (54–85)	92 (84–96)	7.7 (3.9–15.3)	0.25 (0.12–0.50)	
Age 3–12 mo (n = 138)	79 (62–90)	85 (78–91)		59 (43–73)	94 (87–97)	5.4 (3.3–8.8)	0.24 (0.12–0.50)	
Age >12 mo (n = 162)	97 (86–100)	77 (69–84)		55 (43–67)	99 (94–100)	4.2 (3.1–5.8)	0.04 (0.01–0.25)	

Abbreviations: CI, confidence interval; LR, likelihood ratio; NPV, negative predictive value; PPV, positive predictive value.
Data from Lacour AG, Zamora SA, Gervaix A. A score identifying serious bacterial infections in children with fever without source. Pediatr Infect Dis J 2008;27:654–6; and Galetto-Lacour A, Zamora SA, Andreola B, et al. Validation of a laboratory risk index score for the identification of severe bacterial infection in children with fever without source. Arch Dis Child 2010;95:968–73.

several reasons. In the postconjugate vaccine era, a majority of blood cultures are false positive and reflect the growth of "contaminants." The likelihood of obtaining false-positive cultures increased after the introduction of PCV7 from 62.5% to 87.8% (OR 4.3; 95% CI 1.44–13.38).[55] Other studies have revealed that contaminants are 10 times more likely than pathogens to be isolated in the evaluation of a febrile child.[14,15] False-positive cultures are also a common occurrence in young febrile infants, as demonstrated by a study of 4255 blood cultures in infants younger than 3 months, which revealed that 73% of positive culture results were contaminants, potentially leading to increased treatments, iatrogenic complications, and costs.[18] The ability of culture techniques to identify true pathogens depends on various factors including time between sample collection and incubation, volume of blood collected, the duration inoculated blood-culture bottles are left at room temperature, the presence of fastidious pathogens that grow slowly or require complex culture media, and prior antimicrobial therapy. Also, a significant number of clinically important microbial pathogens remain unrecognized because they are resistant to cultivation in the laboratory.[56] Thus the false-negative rate of cultures is largely unknown, further limiting their usefulness in the clinical realm. Another consideration in the clinical use of blood-culture testing is the time to growth of pathogens, which frequently leads to hospitalization or use of long-acting antibiotics until lack of growth can be confirmed. In addition, blood cultures may also be false negative if bacteremia is transient or intermittent. Indeed, the false-positive and false-negative rates of cultures will affect the duration and cost of care.

Experts suggest that it may no longer be cost-effective to obtain routine blood cultures in the evaluation of SBI in febrile children between 3 and 36 months of age. Furthermore, newer pathogen-detection techniques or quantification of the host response as an alternative approach for disease identification has been investigated to overcome the limitations of cultures. Although exhaustive review of recent advances in microbiological detection is beyond the scope of this article, 2 technologies need to be highlighted. First, application of molecular assays for pathogen identification, the promising universal polymerase chain reaction (PCR) assay based on the detection of the bacterial 16S ribosomal RNA gene, has shown some promise but does have its limitations. An integrated diagnostic platform, the "Film array," a multiplex PCR system that fully automates detection of multiple organisms from a single sample with a turnaround time of approximately 1 hour, is being investigated.[57,58] Second, it is now possible to detect the presence of infection by assessing the specific host responses, as different pathogens induce distinct transcriptional "biosignatures" in the RNA of blood leukocytes that can be reliably measured by microarray analysis using small blood samples. Recent data reveal that pathogens can be detected with approximately 95% accuracy, and this technique is currently being investigated in the context of the febrile infant.[59]

MANAGEMENT OF THE FEBRILE CHILD WITH FWS
Management of Febrile Child 3 to 36 Months Old

No single algorithm, guideline, or combination of laboratory screening tests can be recommended in the evaluation of SBI in this age group because of the impact of conjugate vaccines on the epidemiology of SBI and the suboptimal test characteristics of the screening biomarkers. Clinicians should perform urine analysis and cultures on appropriately collected samples, especially in febrile female children younger than 24 months, uncircumcised males younger than 12 months, and circumcised males younger than 6 months. Chest radiographs should not be obtained in the absence of signs and symptoms suggestive of a lower respiratory tract involvement. Blood and CSF studies should be obtained on individual cases based on history, physical examination, and social situation.

Management of Febrile Infant 3 Months and Younger

Clinicians have typically subdivided febrile infants into 2 categories: febrile neonates (28 days or 4 weeks and younger) and febrile infants 28 to 90 days old.

Febrile neonate (28 days or 4 weeks and younger)
The management of febrile neonates is less controversial because of the relative immaturity of their immune system; these infants have a higher incidence of SBI compared with other age categories and their examination is unreliable. Thus, even for a well-appearing febrile neonate, most experts would advocate a complete sepsis evaluation including a lumbar puncture and hospitalization for parenteral antimicrobial therapy pending the results of the assessment. If herpes simplex virus is suspected on clinical or epidemiologic grounds, acyclovir therapy should be strongly considered. Results of rapid viral testing do not alter the management in this age group.

Febrile infant between 4 weeks and 12 weeks old
The authors anticipate that the evaluation for SBI in this age group will continue to vary in its comprehensiveness and application based on practice setting, training of providers, and the availability of ancillary tests including comprehensive rapid viral panels and screening tests such as PCT and CRP. At present, no single algorithm or treatment pathway can be recommended, but readers are directed to a comprehensive evidence-based analysis conducted by the AHRQ that details the shortcomings of various evaluation approaches. It is likely that the younger febrile infant (ie, those between 4 weeks and 8 weeks of age) will obtain analysis of blood and urine with or without CSF, empiric parenteral third-generation cephalosporins, and may or may not be hospitalized until culture negative. Given the higher prevalence of UTI, urine analysis and culture should be performed via either bladder catheterization or suprapubic aspiration. Clinicians could choose to include a complete blood count, CRP, and PCT along with results of viral studies when available to make treatment and disposition decisions for infants between 4 weeks and 12 weeks of age. It is imperative that a reliable follow-up within 24 hours is assured among those febrile infants who are managed on an outpatient basis, especially those who do not get a CSF analysis. It is likely that individual institutions will modify currently available guidelines/algorithms to reduce variation in care. A variety of these guidelines are available in the peer-reviewed literature.

SUMMARY

Fever is a common reason for ED visits by children 36 months and younger. Although laboratory testing is routinely used and hospitalization is frequent, especially in the young febrile infant, there is substantial variation in their evaluation and management. In practice, however, this variation has significant implications in terms of cost and, potentially, safety because of possible iatrogenic overuse of invasive procedures (lumbar punctures), empiric antibiotics, and unnecessary hospitalizations. Considerable debate exists, and much has been written about, clinical-evaluation guidelines because: (1) most research studies pertaining to febrile infants have been conducted in a single center or small groups of academic centers; (2) many studies have used retrospective study designs, different inclusion criteria (eg, with respect to age and temperature cutoffs to define fever), and different laboratory criteria for distinguishing high-risk from low-risk infants; and (3) increasing evidence questions the discriminatory ability of commonly used screening tests in young febrile infants. Routinely used screening tests in the evaluation of young febrile infants for SBIs are inaccurate, and cannot be relied on to distinguish between those with bacterial and those with nonbacterial infections. The value of newer screening tests, such as PCT levels, in this population is not clear, and needs to be evaluated in a large, multicenter study including sufficient numbers of patients to obtain precise estimates of test accuracy. Finally, newer pathogen-detection techniques are likely to evolve rapidly and to affect the way SBI as an entity is evaluated. Given the current state of research and epidemiology of SBI in well-appearing febrile children, a complete evaluation for SBI including blood, urine, and CSF studies along with hospitalization and use of broad-spectrum antibiotics should be pursued in the febrile infant up to 6 weeks of age. Routine blood tests and blood cultures should not be performed in the 3-month-old to 36-month-old febrile infant unless there are specific indications including, but not limited to, inadequate immunization, constrained family support, or resources. Algorithms that are modified for local application may be pursued in the well-appearing febrile infant aged 6 to 12 weeks.

REFERENCES

1. Chamberlain JM, Patel KM, Pollack MM. Association of emergency department care factors with admission and discharge decisions for pediatric patients. J Pediatr 2006;149(5):644–9.
2. Mahajan P, Knazik S, Chen X. Evaluation of febrile infants <60 days of age: review of NHAMCS data. PAS: Pediatric Academic Societies Annual Meeting, May 6, 2008. Toronto.
3. McCaig LF, Nawar EW. National Hospital Ambulatory Medical Care Survey: 2004 emergency department summary. Adv Data 2006;(372):1–29.
4. Baraff LJ, Bass JW, Fleisher GR, et al. Practice guideline for the management of infants and children 0 to 36 months of age with fever without source. Agency for Health Care Policy and Research. Ann Emerg Med 1993;22(7):1198–210.
5. Lee GM, Fleisher GR, Harper MB. Management of febrile children in the age of the conjugate pneumococcal vaccine: a cost-effectiveness analysis. Pediatrics 2001;108:835–44.
6. Bachur RG, Harper MB. Predictive model for serious bacterial infections among infants younger than 3 months of age. Pediatrics 2001;108(2):311–6.
7. Harper M. Update on the management of the febrile infant. Clin Pediatr Emerg Med 2004;5(1):5–12.
8. Baker MD, Avner JR. The febrile infant: what's new? Clin Pediatr Emerg Med 2008;9(4):213–20.
9. Kramer MS, Etezadi-Amoli J, Ciampi A, et al. Parents' versus physicians' values for clinical outcomes in young febrile children. Pediatrics 1994;93:697–702.
10. Eagles D, Stiell IG, Clement CM, et al. International survey of emergency physicians' priorities for clinical decision rules. Acad Emerg Med 2008;15(2):177–82.
11. Burke JP, Klein JO, Gezon HM, et al. Pneumococcal bacteremia. Review of 111 cases, 1957-1969, with special reference to cases with undetermined focus. Am J Dis Child 1971;121(4):353–9.
12. Jaffe DM, Tanz RR, Davis AT, et al. Antibiotic administration to treat possible occult bacteremia in febrile children. N Engl J Med 1987;317(19):1175–80.
13. Bass JW, Steele RW, Wittler RR, et al. Antimicrobial treatment of occult bacteremia: a multicenter cooperative study. Pediatr Infect Dis J 1993;12(6):466–73.

14. Waddle E, Jhaveri R. Outcomes of febrile children without localizing signs after pneumococcal conjugate vaccine. Arch Dis Child 2009;94(2):144–7.
15. Wilkinson M, Bulloch B, Smith M. Prevalence of occult bacteremia in children aged 3 to 36 months presenting to the emergency department with fever in the postpneumococcal conjugate vaccine era. Acad Emerg Med 2009;16(3):220–5.
16. Mintegi S, Benito J, Sanchez J, et al. Predictors of occult bacteremia in young febrile children in the era of heptavalent pneumococcal conjugated vaccine. Eur J Emerg Med 2009;16(4):199–205.
17. Herz AM, Greenhow TL, Alcantara J, et al. Changing epidemiology of outpatient bacteremia in 3- to 36-month-old children after the introduction of the heptavalent-conjugated pneumococcal vaccine. Pediatr Infect Dis J 2006; 25(4):293–300.
18. Greenhow TL, Hung YY, Herz AM. Changing epidemiology of bacteremia in infants aged 1 week to 3 months. Pediatrics 2012;129(3):e590–6.
19. Freedman AL. Urologic diseases in North America project: trends in resource utilization for urinary tract infections in children. J Urol 2005;173:949–54.
20. American Academy of Pediatrics, Subcommittee on Urinary Tract Infection, Steering Committee on Quality Improvement and Management. Urinary tract infection: clinical practice guideline for the diagnosis and management of the initial UTI in febrile infants and children 2 to 24 months. Pediatrics 2011;128(3):595–610.
21. Shaikh N, Morone NE, Bost JE, et al. Prevalence of urinary tract infection in childhood: a meta-analysis. Pediatr Infect Dis J 2008;27(4):302–8.
22. Gorelick MH, Shaw KN. Clinical decision rule to identify febrile young girls at risk for urinary tract infection. Arch Pediatr Adolesc Med 2000;154(4):386–90.
23. Kaplan SL, Mason EO Jr, Wald ER, et al. Decrease of invasive pneumococcal infections in children among 8 children's hospitals in the United States after the introduction of the 7-valent pneumococcal conjugate vaccine. Pediatrics 2004;113(3):443–9.
24. Tsai CJ, Griffin MR, Nuorti JP, et al. Changing epidemiology of pneumococcal meningitis after the introduction of pneumococcal conjugate vaccine in the United States. Clin Infect Dis 2008;46(11):1664–72.
25. American College of Emergency Physicians Clinical Policies Committee, American College of Emergency Physicians Clinical Policies Subcommittee on Pediatric Fever. Clinical policy for children younger than three years presenting to the emergency department with fever. Ann Emerg Med 2003;42:530–45.
26. Murphy CG, van de Pol AC, Harper MB, et al. Clinical predictors of occult pneumonia in the febrile child. Acad Emerg Med 2007;14(3):243–9.
27. Mintegi S, Benito J, Pijoan JI, et al. Occult pneumonia in infants with high fever without source a prospective multicenter study. Pediatr Emerg Care 2010;26(7): 470–4.
28. Colvin JM, Muenzer JT, Jaffe DM, et al. Detection of viruses in young children with fever without an apparent source. Pediatrics 2012;130(6):e1455–62.
29. Ramers C, Billman G, Hartin M, et al. Impact of a diagnostic cerebrospinal fluid enterovirus polymerase chain reaction test on patient management. JAMA 2000; 283(20):2680–5.
30. Benito-Fernandez J, Vazquez-Ronco MA, Morteruel-Aizkuren E, et al. Impact of rapid viral testing for influenza A and B viruses on management of febrile infants without signs of focal infection. Pediatr Infect Dis J 2006;25(12):1153–7.
31. Smitherman HF, Caviness AC, Macias CG. Retrospective review of serious bacterial infections in infants who are 0 to 36 months and have influenza A infection. Pediatrics 2005;115(3):710–8.

32. Levine DA, Platt SL, Dayan PS, et al. Risk of serious bacterial infection in young febrile infants with respiratory syncytial virus infections. Pediatrics 2004;113(6): 1728–34.
33. Krief W, Levine D, Platt S, et al. Influenza virus infection and the risk of serious bacterial infections in young febrile infants. Pediatrics 2009;124(1):30–9.
34. Hui C, Neto G, Tsertsvadze A, et al. Diagnosis and management of febrile infants (0-3 months). Rockville (MD): Agency for Healthcare Research and Quality (US); 2012 (Evidence Report/Technology Assessments, No. 205). Available at: http://www.ncbi.nlm.nih.gov/books/NBK92690/. Accessed March 4, 2013.
35. Hsiao AL, Baker MD. Fever in the new millennium: a review of recent studies of markers of serious bacterial infection in febrile children. Curr Opin Pediatr 2005; 17(1):56–61.
36. Kuppermann N. Occult bacteremia in young febrile children. Pediatr Clin North Am 1999;46(6):1073–109.
37. Galetto-Lacour A, Gervaix A. Identifying severe bacterial infection in children with fever without source. Expert Rev Anti Infect Ther 2010;8(11):1231–7.
38. Kuppermann N, Malley R, Inkelis SH, et al. Clinical and hematologic features do not reliably identify children with unsuspected meningococcal disease. Pediatrics 1999;103(2):E20.
39. Zaidi E, Bachur R, Harper M. Non-typhi *Salmonella* bacteremia in children. Pediatr Infect Dis J 1999;18(12):1073–7.
40. Van den Bruel A, Thompson MJ, Haj-Hassan T, et al. Diagnostic value of laboratory tests in identifying serious infections in febrile children: systematic review. BMJ 2011;342:d3082.
41. Carrol ED, Newland P, Riordan FA, et al. Procalcitonin as a diagnostic marker of meningococcal disease in children presenting with fever and a rash. Arch Dis Child 2002;86(4):282–5.
42. Fernández Lopez A, Luaces Cubells C, García García JJ, et al. Procalcitonin in pediatric emergency departments for early diagnosis of invasive bacterial infections in febrile infants: results of a multicenter study and the utility of a rapid qualitative test for this marker. Pediatr Infect Dis J 2003;22(10):895–903.
43. Lacour AG, Gervaix A, Zamora SA, et al. Procalcitonin, IL-6, IL-8, IL-1 receptor antagonist and C-reactive protein as identificators of serious bacterial infections in children with fever without localizing signs. Eur J Pediatr 2001;160(2):95–100.
44. Thayyil S, Shenoy M, Hamaluba M, et al. Is procalcitonin useful in early diagnosis of serious bacterial infections in children? Acta Paediatr 2005;94(2):155–8.
45. Sanders S, Barnett A, Correa-Velez I, et al. Systematic review of the diagnostic accuracy of C-reactive protein to detect bacterial infection in non-hospitalized infants and children with fever. J Pediatr 2008;153(4):570–4.
46. Herd D. In children under age three does procalcitonin help exclude serious bacterial infection in fever without focus? Arch Dis Child 2007;92(4):362–4.
47. Jones AE, Fiechtl JF, Brown MD, et al. Procalcitonin test in the diagnosis of bacteremia: a meta-analysis. Ann Emerg Med 2007;50(1):34–41.
48. McGinn TG, Guyatt GH, Wyer PC, et al. Users' guides to the medical literature: XXII: how to use articles about clinical decision rules. Evidence-Based Medicine Working Group. JAMA 2000;284:79–84.
49. Craig JC, Williams GJ, Jones M, et al. The accuracy of clinical symptoms and signs for the diagnosis of serious bacterial infection in young febrile children: prospective cohort study of 15781 febrile illnesses. BMJ 2010;340:c1594.
50. Lacour AG, Zamora SA, Gervaix A. A score identifying serious bacterial infections in children with fever without source. Pediatr Infect Dis J 2008;27:654–6.

51. Galetto-Lacour A, Zamora SA, Andreola B, et al. Validation of a laboratory risk index score for the identification of severe bacterial infection in children with fever without source. Arch Dis Child 2010;95:968–73.
52. Bressan S, Gomez B, Mintegi S, et al. Diagnostic performance of the lab-score in predicting severe and invasive bacterial infections in well-appearing young febrile infant. Pediatr Infect Dis J 2012;31(12):1239–44.
53. Pantell RH, Newman TB, Bernzweig J, et al. Management and outcomes of care in fever in early infancy. JAMA 2004;291(10):1203–12.
54. DeAngelis C, Joffe A, Wilson M, et al. Iatrogenic risks and financial costs of hospitalizing febrile infants. Am J Dis Child 1983;137(12):1146–9.
55. Sard B, Bailey MC, Vinci R. An analysis of pediatric blood cultures in the post-pneumococcal conjugate vaccine era in a community hospital emergency department. Pediatr Emerg Care 2006;22:295–300.
56. Relman DA. The human body as microbial observatory. Nat Genet 2002;30(2):131–3.
57. Azzari C, Moriondo M, Indolfi G, et al. Molecular detection methods and serotyping performed directly on clinical samples improve diagnostic sensitivity and reveal increased incidence of invasive disease by *Streptococcus pneumoniae* in Italian children. J Med Microbiol 2008;57:1205–12.
58. Poritz MA, Blaschke AJ, Byington CL, et al. Film array, an automated nested multiplex PCR system for multi-pathogen detection: development and application to respiratory tract infection. PLoS One 2011;6(10):e2604.
59. Ramilo O, Allman W, Chung W, et al. Gene expression patterns in blood leukocytes discriminate patients with acute infections. Blood 2007;109(5):2066–77.

Skin and Soft Tissue Infections

Rakesh D. Mistry, MD, MS

KEYWORDS

- Skin infection • Cutaneous abscess • Cellulitis • *Staphylococcus aureus*

KEY POINTS

- The incidence of skin and soft tissue infections has rapidly increased in the previous decade, concomitant with the emergence of community-acquired methicillin-resistant *Staphylococcus aureus* (CA-MRSA) as a pathogen.
- The mainstay of therapy for skin abscesses remains incision and drainage; the role of wound packing and adjuvant antibiotics appears to be diminishing.
- Systemic antibiotics are indicated for treatment of cellulitis, and group A streptococcus remains a primary pathogen in this infection; the role of CA-MRSA is unknown.
- Bedside ultrasonography is superior to clinical examination in diagnosis of skin infections, and use of this modality improves emergency department management.
- The link between *Staphylococcus aureus* colonization and infection is unclear, although decolonization using a multifaceted approach may be used in cases of recurrent household infection.

INTRODUCTION

Infections of the skin and soft tissues are frequently encountered in ambulatory settings such as the emergency department (ED) and primary care offices.[1-3] Skin and soft tissue infections (SSTIs) encompass a wide range of severity, from impetigo to fulminant "flesh-eating" invasive infection, better known as necrotizing fasciitis.[4] However, the predominant skin infections encountered by pediatric practitioners include cutaneous abscesses and cellulitis. This article focuses on the current status of the ambulatory management of these 2 infections, as more benign infections such as impetigo, pustulosis, and folliculitis are less challenging for the clinician, and discussion of invasive infections are beyond the scope of this article.

A cutaneous, or skin abscess, is defined as a focal, contained, purulent infection with a clear "cavity" and surrounding inflammation involving the deep subcutaneous tissues. On physical examination, abscesses are typically tender, indurated, erythematous, and fluctuant. Fluctuance is a sign of purulence within the abscess cavity,

Disclosures: None.
Section of Pediatric Emergency Medicine, Department of Pediatrics, Children's Hospital Colorado, University of Colorado School of Medicine, 13123 East 16th Avenue, Box B251, Aurora, CO 80045, USA
E-mail address: rakesh.mistry@childrenscolorado.org

Pediatr Clin N Am 60 (2013) 1063–1082
http://dx.doi.org/10.1016/j.pcl.2013.06.011
0031-3955/13/$ – see front matter © 2013 Elsevier Inc. All rights reserved.

although in some cases this finding may be difficult to detect, owing to induration and depth of the lesion. Occasionally, a pustule may be visible at the "point" of the abscess when the cavity is close to the skin surface; this pustule may erupt and produce spontaneous drainage of pus from the lesion (**Fig. 1**). Mild systemic symptoms may be present in the setting of cutaneous abscess, including fever and malaise; toxicity is rare.

Cellulitis is pyogenic infection of the skin without an organized cavity and is typically limited to the epidermis, dermis, and superficial subcutaneous tissues (**Fig. 2**).[5] The hallmark physical findings of cellulitis include erythema, warmth, induration, and tenderness, although all criteria need not be present to make the diagnosis. In most cases, the margins of the infection are ill defined, although well-demarcated margins occur in group A streptococcal erysipelas.[5–7] Cellulitis may present with fever and malaise, and severe toxicity is exceedingly uncommon. Clinical parameters of cellulitis overlap with skin abscess, because these infections lie within a spectrum; cases of cellulitis may evolve into abscess, and nearly all skin abscesses have some component of cellulitis immediately surrounding the abscess cavity. As a result of this overlap, SSTI diagnosis and treatment is challenging.

Microbiology

Most SSTIs result from infection with gram-positive cocci, specifically *Staphylococcus aureus* and group A streptococci.[5,8,9] Although typical commensal organisms of the skin, bacteria infect the skin and soft tissues via direct inoculation, typical through disruption of the skin barrier. Proliferation of bacteria and development of cellulitis or abscess do not occur in a predictable fashion, and the clinical differentiation of superficial and dermal involvement versus presence of an abscess cavity may be difficult. Gram-negative organisms may also infect the skin and soft tissues, particularly in the buttock and axillary regions.[10,11] Anaerobic bacteria are not typically present in cellulitis but are commonly implicated in necrotizing fasciitis as coinfecting organisms with *S. aureus* or group A streptococci.[4,12]

Epidemiology and Emergence of CA-MRSA

In the United Sates, the incidence of SSTIs among the pediatric population has increased substantially in the previous 15 years.[1,3,9,13–15] This upsurge is concomitant with emergence of community-associated strains of methicillin-resistant *Staphylococcus aureus* (CA-MRSA). Different from previous "hospital-acquired" or nosocomial

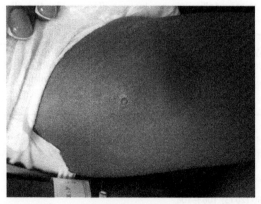

Fig. 1. Clinical appearance of a typical cutaneous abscess of the thigh. Note the presence of a central pustule that is nearing spontaneous drainage.

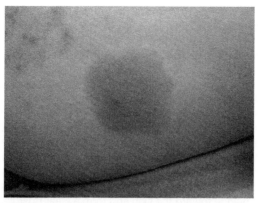

Fig. 2. A patient with a simple cellulitis of the upper extremity. The lesion is erythematous, warm, tender, and indurated.

strains (HA), CA-MRSA is a genetically distinct organism.[16–18] The genes coding for methicillin resistance lie within the staphylococcal chromosomal cassette, or SCC*mec* gene, of which there are 4 predominant types. SCC*mec* type IV codes for CA-MRSA, and is a small, mobile genetic element, which facilitates transfer of methicillin resistance more readily than the larger elements coding for hospital-acquired methicillin-resistant *Staphylococcus aureus* (HA-MRSA). Clinical manifestations also differ, as CA-MRSA most commonly presents as skin infections, whereas HA-MRSA produces invasive infections, such as pneumonia and sepsis.[15,19] It should be noted that the terms of "community" and "hospital" strains have become blurred, because CA-MRSA has been increasingly implicated in hospitalized and chronically ill populations.[20–24]

Among SSTIs, cutaneous abscesses have had the most demonstrable increase in the era of CA-MRSA.[1,3,25] Previously, skin abscesses were a result of methicillin-sensitive strains of *S. aureus* (MSSA); isolation of CA-MRSA from abscesses has since far surpassed that of MSSA. Because wound cultures are readily available after drainage, the microbiology of skin abscesses is well established, allowing for accurate epidemiologic surveillance. In the United States, the prevalence of CA-MRSA from cultured lesions is nearly universally greater than 50% and is as high as 70% to 80% in municipalities such as Chicago, Houston, and San Francisco.[8–10,26–28]

Although great attention has been paid to CA-MRSA and SSTI in the United States, descriptions of CA-MRSA are occurring worldwide.[29] The CA-MRSA strain ubiquitous across the United States were derived from the precursor strain USA300, although others are present around the world.[8,9,29,30] Recent surveillance data have revealed that CA-MRSA is present on 6 continents and that prevalence in areas of Europe and South America rival that of the United States.[29,31–34] In fact, analysis of CA-MRSA isolates across the Atlantic Ocean and Pacific Ocean have shown conservation of highly expressed virulence factors, such as Panton-Valentine leukocidin.[29] Although CA-MRSA is present across the globe, similar dramatic increases in the incidence of SSTI as in the United States have yet to be documented.

CLINICAL AND DIAGNOSTIC APPROACH
Clinical Evaluation

The usual approach to SSTI involves assessment of clinical findings, and at extremes of cellulitis and abscess, clinical assessment alone is useful in evaluation. Cellulitis involves the dermal and subcutaneous layers of skin, with erythema and signs of inflammation present: warmth, tenderness, and induration (hardness or firmness of the soft tissues).[5] Most often, cellulitis develops after traumatic introduction of bacteria into the skin, from minor trauma (eg, scratching from fingernails, insect bites) or more significant penetrating injury. Rarely, cellulitis develops from direct extension local foci (eg, osteomyelitis) or from hematogenous seeding, with the latter more frequent in neonates. It is often helpful to demarcate the margins of the lesion using a pen or skin marker, as extent of the lesion is useful in determining progression of infection, response to therapy, and clinical resolution. Skin abscesses are clinically defined by findings similar to cellulitis, accompanied by fluctuance. Fluctuance often corresponds with the presence of a fluid-filled cavity. Skin abscesses frequently exist under pressure with surrounding inflammation, can cause pain, and may impair common activities in children depending on location; for example, buttock abscesses often preclude young children from sitting down. As pressure builds within the cavity, the infection may advance toward the skin and form a clear pustule, which may eventually "erupt" and produce spontaneous drainage of purulent material.

As previously mentioned, cellulitis and abscess exist as a spectrum of infections; therefore, there are many children present with SSTIs that are difficult to differentiate from a diagnostic perspective. In recent years, the advent of bedside ultrasound (US) has permitted enhanced diagnosis of SSTIs in the ED setting. Early studies in adults determined that US, in the hands of trained emergency medicine clinicians, was superior to physical examination in determining the presence of abscess.[35–37] Furthermore, clinical management is positively affected, with improved accuracy of US documented in 48% of cases of suspected nondrainable lesions and 73% of suspected abscess.[36,38,39] Increasingly, bedside US has been adopted by pediatric emergency physicians and exhibited similar promise in management in children with SSTI.[36,39,40] Considering benefits, including low expense, rapidity of assessment, and diagnostic accuracy, bedside US will have an increasing role in ED management of pediatric SSTI.

Microbiologic Diagnosis

In the case of cutaneous abscess, pus is readily accessible for culture either spontaneously or following drainage, easily permitting isolation of the offending bacterium for clinical and surveillance purposes. Accordingly, the current bacteriology of skin abscess is well established, with the overwhelming majority cases resulting from S. aureus, either CA-MRSA or methicillin-sensitive Staphylococcus aureus (MSSA). Notably, there is little distinction between abscesses resulting from CA-MRSA or MSSA in terms of clinical presentation, risk factors, or abscess size; therefore, determination of the infecting organism is not possible without isolation in culture.[41–44]

On the other hand, the bacteriology of cellulitis is not as well understood, in the absence of readily obtainable purulent material. The lack of microbiologic data for cellulitis has posed a dilemma for clinicians. Before the emergence of CA-MRSA, attempts to identify bacterial organisms have been made using needle aspiration, via insertion and aspiration of infected skin tissue either at the leading edge or point of maximal inflammation of the lesion.[45–53] In addition, injection of a small amount of bacteriostatic saline (0.5 cc), followed by aspiration, has been postulated as a potential method.[47] Unfortunately, yield of pathogens from these needle aspiration methods are highly variable, with infecting organisms identified anywhere from 10% to 60% of attempts.[45,46,48–52]

Recently the approach to cellulitis has become even more confusing, as the prevalence of CA-MRSA among cellulitis is unknown. Nonetheless, emergency physicians are increasingly instituting CA-MRSA active therapy in cases of simple cellulitis.[25,54]

However, many experts maintain that group A streptococcus remains a primary cause of cellulitis and erysipelas; therefore emergency clinicians should maintain suspicion for these organisms. Recent data have supported this claim, at least in adults, with more than 70% of patients with cellulitis having serology consistent with group A streptococcal infection.[55]

SURGICAL THERAPY

Once the presence of a skin abscess has been determined, the mainstay of therapy remains incision and drainage of the lesion.[18,56–58] Removal of purulent material provides immediate relief from pain and improves healing. Incision and drainage procedures are frequently performed in the ED setting, in the hands of general and pediatric emergency physicians. Consultation with general surgery may be obtained in situations where the abscess is close to sensitive structures (eg, face, perineum, and genitalia) or in cases where an extremely deep, complex lesion is suspected. Performance of an incision and drainage procedure is discussed later in this article.

Sedation and Analgesia

Before drainage of cutaneous abscess, consideration should always be given regarding analgesia, because these infections produce substantial pain for children. Removal of purulent material reduces pain in children, although drainage procedures are often painful as well. Therefore, adjunctive sedation and analgesia is necessary when the procedure is completed in the ED. Literature specific to sedation and analgesia for abscess management is very limited, although the approach used for procedures such as laceration repair is often used. Topical anesthetic, specifically eutectic mixture of local anesthetics, has been used for superficial anesthesia and to promote drainage through maceration of thin skin or pustules at a site of eruption.[59] Topical anesthesia is only adjunctive, however, as the maximal depth of action in healthy tissue is just 3 mm after 60 minutes of application.[60]

Local anesthesia, with infiltrated lidocaine, is often used. Smaller lesions, which do not require extensive debridement, are often excellent candidates for local anesthesia alone. Larger lesions may be more challenging because injection directly into the abscess may not result in adequate anesthesia owing to the inflamed and necrotic tissue.[61] Infiltration around the lesion into healthy tissue is an option; so-called "field block" can provide sufficient analgesia in older children and adolescents who can tolerate injection, allowing for incision, drainage, and debridement of the wound. Local anesthesia is often difficult to use for lesions in sensitive areas (eg, genitourinary) or in young children.

Procedural sedation is often instituted for ED abscess drainage in the pediatric population. The primary goal of procedural sedation in the context of skin abscesses is to permit adequate drainage; therefore, the level of sedation achieved should only be that necessary for completion of the procedure. Procedural sedation is often of greater utility for young children or for larger-sized lesions.[62] Comprehensive review of the approach to sedation, including method of administration and choice of pharmacologic agents is beyond the scope of this article, although commonly selected approaches include oral, intranasal, or intravenous benzodiazepines, intravenous, ketamine, or propofol, or a combination approach.

Method of Incision and Drainage

Removal of purulent material from skin abscesses is best accomplished in an organized and stepwise fashion (**Table 1**).[61,63] Sterile preparation of the area, including

Table 1
Recommended steps for incision and drainage procedure

Recommended Steps	Materials	Comment
Analgesia and sedation		Dependent on many variables, including lesion size, patient age, and clinician preference
Sterile preparation	Povidone-iodine	
Incision	11-blade scalpel	Incise ½–2/3 or fluctuance
Manual expression		
Wound culture	Bacterial culturette	Recommended by CDC and IDSA
Lysis of intracavitary septae	Blunt or curved hemostat	Define margin of lesion to assure septations are disrupted
Manual expression		
Saline irrigation (optional)	20 cc syringe, 18–20 g angiocath, normal saline	No literature to support, although may be used to clear debris
Wound stent (optional)	Strip of iodoform gauze, vessel loop, section of penrose drain	Suggested for large lesions-packing not recommended

Abbreviations: CDC, Centers for Disease Control and Prevention; IDSA, Infectious Diseases Society of America.

antiseptic solution, sterile draping, and sterile gloves, is typically been recommended. Incision of the lesion at the area of maximal fluctuance is performed using a scalpel (usually a 11-blade), creating a linear opening across the length of the fluctuance (**Fig. 3**). Larger incisions (>1–2 cm) with sufficient depth may be required to permit sufficient access to the abscess cavity. Expressed pus should be sent for wound culture, both for surveillance and treatment purposes.[18,56,57] After manual expression of purulent material, probing and debridement of the abscess using a blunt instrument, ideally a hemostat, should be performed (**Fig. 4**). Many abscesses are complex, with septations and loculations, and lysis of this tissue may release other collections of

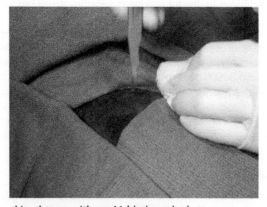

Fig. 3. Incision of a skin abscess with an 11-blade scalpel.

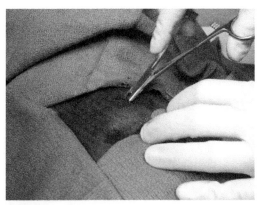

Fig. 4. Lysis of loculations and septations within an abscess cavity, using a blunt hemostat.

purulence. Therefore, aggressive debridement to the margins of the abscess cavity is indicated. Following debridement and repeat expression, forceful irrigation of the cavity with sterile saline may be performed. Management of the open abscess cavity remains controversial and is discussed later.

Wound Management

Among the most controversial debates with respect to abscess management is the utility of wound packing. Complete packing of the abscess cavity with gauze strip (eg, iodoform) has customarily been used to aid in debridement, avoid reaccumulation, and permit healthy tissue growth with closure of the wound. After placement, packing is usually removed within 24 to 48 hours and then replaced if continued purulent or necrotic material is present. Difficulties in the use of wound packing in children, specifically pain incurred with placement, removal, and replacement (if necessary), has led to increasing literature discouraging this practice. Recent randomized clinical trials have found that healing rates are equivalent whether drained abscesses are packed or not packed, although packing was associated with increased pain and analgesic use.[64,65] As a result, this practice is less frequently used in children, with nearly 50% or practitioners avoiding wound packing after drainage.[54]

Alternatives to packing are occasionally used for large lesions. Wound "stents" are an option, involving insertion of a strip of iodoform or section of penrose drain secured into the open incision.[61] The stent is maintained for several days to promote continued drainage of the abscess cavity by preventing premature closure of the incision. Although more commonly used, formal assessments of this method are lacking.

Recently, loop drains have been proposed as an alternative to wound packing.[66-68] Loop drains involve drainage via the recommended method, including debridement and irrigation, followed by tunneling of the tract and passage of a rubber vessel loop between the incision and distal healthy tissue (**Fig. 5**). The ends of the vessel loop are then tied together securely to form an annular wound stent. After approximately 3 days, the loop drain is cut and easily removed. Acceptable outcomes of abscesses treated in this manner have been described, and the literature appears promising.[66-68] However, utility of loop drains have not undergone systematic evaluation.

Although less commonly debated, primary closure of the wound after drainage is not routinely performed, and outcomes have not been shown to be superior to the

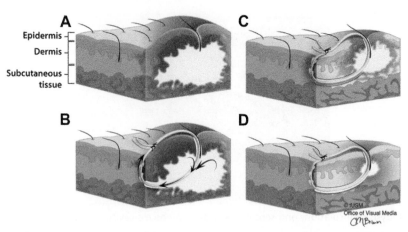

Fig. 5. Placement of "loop drain" for skin abscess. (*A*) Presenting abscess with extensive subdermal necrosis. (*B*) Operative process with drainage through peripheral incisions, followed by drain placement, often in radial pattern. (*C, D*) Abscess decompression following drainage with wound contraction around subdermal drain. (*Courtesy of* Indiana University School of Medicine, with permission.)

usual healing by secondary intention.[69] Healing via secondary intention is presently favored in most settings.

Alternatives to Incision and Drainage

Recognizing the labor and time intensive nature of complete incision and drainage, alternative methods have been evaluated. Needle aspiration, accomplished by introduction of a large bore needle into cavity and removal of purulent material with a syringe, is a commonly selected option. Although less time consuming, complete removal of pus cannot be assured and wound debridement is not possible. In a randomized trial by Gaspari and colleagues,[70] needle aspiration alone was associated with a greater than 50% higher rate of treatment failure than incision and drainage. A noninvasive approach, using mechanical unroofing (eg, lifting using a needle) of the pustule or "point" of the abscess to promote purulent drainage, without incision or debridement, has also been attempted without success.[71] Retrospective studies have also evaluated the utility of topical anesthetic alone to macerate the pustule or scab of an abscess, without instrument manipulation, and produce spontaneous drainage.[59] This method, followed by manual expression of the abscesses, was attempted with the goal of obviate complete incision and drainage. Although fewer patients required formal drainage procedures, there is insufficient outcome data to support this approach.[59] As a result, complete incision and drainage is recommended; methods such as needle aspiration, unroofing, topical anesthetic alone cream should not be used in lieu of formal drainage.

ANTIMICROBIAL THERAPY AND NONSURGICAL MANAGEMENT

The choice of antibiotic therapy is highly dependent on the nature of the infection, the bacteria present, and the local prevalence of these organisms. Although gram-positive cocci produce the overwhelming majority of SSTIs, the role of antimicrobials varies by infection. The approach to abscesses and cellulitis has changed recently subsequent to the increased prevalence of CA-MRSA.

Antibiotics and Skin Abscesses

The role of antimicrobials in skin abscesses that have been drained, also known as adjuvant antibiotic therapy, has been highly debated. Before the ubiquitous prevalence of CA-MRSA, MSSA abscesses were most prevalent, and randomized clinical trials demonstrated that incision and drainage alone was optimal therapy.[72–74] Although drainage alone remained the mainstay of therapy for years, the rising prevalence of CA-MRSA has been accompanied by a rapid increase in the use of adjuvant antibiotics.[8,54,75] Recent national evaluations have found that greater than 90% of emergency physicians are using adjuvant antibiotics, likely a result of concerns for deep-seated infection, recurrence, and invasiveness.[54] In particular, younger patient age and the presence of fever are factors that are associated with increased likelihood to use adjuvant antibiotics, although better outcomes have not been proved.[54]

Evidence in the current CA-MRSA era supports incision and drainage alone as adequate therapy (**Table 2**). Initial evaluations of patients prescribed adjuvant CA-MRSA "active" antibiotics and those prescribed MRSA "ineffective" antibiotics (eg, β-lactams) described similar outcomes, although these data originated from retrospective and uncontrolled trials.[8,76,77] Recent randomized trials offer support for these findings, demonstrating equivalent patient outcomes with and without use of adjuvant antibiotic therapy.[27,78–80] A noninferiority placebo controlled randomized trial by Duong and colleagues[80] demonstrated no difference in failure rates between abscess drainage and placebo (5.3%) compared with drainage and TMP-SMX (4.1%) as adjuvant therapy for pediatric ED abscesses. Without clear risk factors associated with treatment failure, prescription of adjuvant antibiotic therapy remains at the discretion of the clinician. Considerations for adjuvant therapy should be given for children with fever, younger age, large lesions in sensitive areas of the body, and inability to perform an adequate incision and drainage procedure. However, based on current literature, it appears that the "pendulum is swinging" away from use of adjuvant therapy after successful abscess drainage procedures. Presently, current data on withholding adjuvant antibiotics are based on measures of *efficacy*, or performance in ideal randomized trial settings, rather than measures of *effectiveness*: how a therapy performs in the "real-world" setting. Therefore, large-scale clinical effectiveness studies are ongoing to demonstrate that incision and drainage alone is not only equivalent or better than adjuvant antibiotics, but also more effective in preventing clinical failure and recurrence.

When adjuvant antibiotic therapy is to be prescribed for cutaneous abscesses, treatment is focused toward empiric coverage for CA-MRSA, because this organism is most prevalent (>50%) among abscess isolates in the United States. Because prevalence studies have confirmed that greater than 15% of abscesses result from CA-MRSA infection, the Centers for Disease Control recommends empiric treatment should be used for these common infections.[9,57] Therefore, use of common CA-MRSA active antibiotics, including trimethoprim-sulfamethoxazole (TMP-SMX) or clindamycin, for a duration for 7 to 10 days is recommended (**Table 3**).[18] It must be emphasized that rates of clindamycin resistance and inducible resistance remain variable by region; therefore, clinicians should be aware of local microbiology and resistance patterns.[81,82]

Antibiotics and Cellulitis

The role of antibiotics in nonpurulent SSTI and cellulitis is more definitive. In the absence of a collection, treatment includes systemic antimicrobials that effectively reach the skin at the site of infection, for a duration of 7 to 10 days. Traditionally,

Table 2
Recent clinical trials evaluating adjunctive antibiotics for drained skin abscesses

Study	Study Design	Population	N	Time at Assessment for Failure	Comment
Paydar et al,[77] 2006	Retrospective	Adults	376	2 mo	No difference in outcome between sensitivity-concordant and discordant antibiotic therapy
Lee et al,[76] 2004	Prospective cohort	Children	69	1–6 d 6–10 d	No difference in effective vs ineffective therapy for CA-MRSA abscesses
Moran et al,[8] 2006	Prospective cohort	Adults	422	2–3 wk	No difference in outcome between sensitivity-concordant and discordant antibiotic therapy
Rajendran et al,[27] 2007	RCT	Adults	167	7 d	No difference in failure rate with cephalexin vs placebo in high MRSA prevalent population (88%)
Chen et al,[78] 2010	Randomized Contraolled Trial (RCT)	Children	200	48–72 h 7 d	Clinical failure rates not different between clindamycin (3%) vs cephalexin (6%); $P = .33$
Schmitz et al,[79] 2010	RCT	Adults	212	7 d	Clinical failure rates not different between TMP-SMX (17%) vs Placebo (26%); mean difference 9% (95% confidence interval: −2%–21%)
Duong et al,[80] 2010	RCT (noninferiority)	Children	161	10–14 d	Clinical failure rates not different between TMP-SMX (4.1%) vs Placebo (5.3%); mean difference 1.2 (95% confidence interval: $-\infty$ to 6.8%)

use of antibiotics effective against MSSA and group A streptococci (eg, cephalexin) had been recommended for cellulitis.[5] However, surveillance of the microbiology of cellulitis is limited; therefore, the prevalence of CA-MRSA in this infection remains unknown.[5,18,83] As mentioned, the questionable performance of needle aspiration for microbiologic diagnosis has led this practice to fall out of favor. Therefore, clinicians often institute empiric treatment of cellulitis.

Table 3
Common antibiotics prescribed for skin and soft tissue infections

Antibiotic	Method of Administration	Organisms Covered	Pediatric Dosing	Comment
Trimethoprim-Sulfamethoxazole	Oral or IV	CA-MRSA	8–12 mg/kg/d divided q12 h	Not recommended as monotherapy for cellulitis
Clindamycin	Oral or IV	CA-MRSA MSSA GAS	30–40 mg/kg/d divided q8 h	Oral preparation not always tolerated due to palatability; emerging CA-MRSA resistance
Cephalexin	Oral	MSSA GAS	25–50 mg/kg/d divided q6–12 h	Ineffective against CA-MRSA infections
Doxycycline	Oral or IV	CA-MRSA MSSA	2.2 mg/kg/d divided q12 h	Variable resistance and only indicated above >12 y
Rifampin	Oral or IV	MRSA MSSA GAS	15–20 mg/kg/d divided q12 h	Cannot be used as monotherapy; often used in conjunction with other antibiotics for severe infections
Linezolid	Oral or IV	CA-MRSA MSSA GAS	30 mg/kg/d divided q8 h	Expensive and not routinely available
Vancomycin	IV	CA-MRSA MSSA GAS	60 mg/kg/d divided q6 h	Indicated for invasive disease or severe toxicity
Daptomycin	IV	CA-MRSA MSSA GAS	4–10 mg/kg/d q24 h	Cannot be used for pneumonia

Abbreviations: GAS, group A Streptococcus; IV, intravenous.

In recent years, CA-MRSA coverage has been included in treatment regimens for cellulitis, using TMP-SMX or clindamycin,[25,54] which often has occurred at the expense of group A streptococcal coverage, as TMP-SMX is poorly effective against group A streptococci. Recent evaluations have suggested that group A streptococci remains a common cause of cellulitis in the CA-MRSA era.[25,55] Jeng and colleagues[55] used highly specific serum tests for group A streptococcal infection (anti-DNAse B and anti-streptolysin O) to suggest that as many as 73% of cellulitis may still result from this bacterium, even in the current CA-MRSA climate. This postulate is supported by studies demonstrating prescription of TMP-SMX alone as an independent risk factor for treatment failure of nondrained SSTI in children, even in areas of high CA-MRSA prevalence.[25,84] Therefore, current recommendations suggest treatment with antibiotic regimens that include coverage for *S. aureus* and group A streptococcus, such as cephalexin or clindamycin (see **Table 3**).[18,56] In the case of patients with previous CA-MRSA infection, or family history of CA-MRSA infection, inclusion of coverage for this organism is also warranted, and regimens may include clindamycin or dual therapy with cephalexin and TMP-SMX or clindamycin.[85]

Topical Therapy

The most common topical antibiotic recommended for SSTIs is mupirocin, which has excellent activity against *S. aureus*. Although effective for minor skin infections such as pustulosis and folliculitis, mupirocin alone is not recommended for treatment of nondrained SSTI, as systemic therapy is necessary.[56] In cases of nondrained SSTI, combination of mupirocin and warm compresses or soaks several times is often prescribed to promote coalescence and spontaneous drainage. For small nonorganized SSTI, this approach may be initially used successfully for treatment or in some cases lead to abscess formation and facilitate incision and drainage at follow-up.

Hospitalization for SSTI

Inpatient admissions for SSTI have also increased in the previous decade, mirroring the rapid rise in ED visits.[86,87] However, the decision to manage SSTIs as inpatients remains at the discretion of the clinician, owing the lack of evidence defining risk factors for outpatient failure. Admission of patients with SSTI is recommended in children who are acutely toxic, diabetic, or immunocompromised. Consideration for hospitalization should be given for SSTI in the setting of fever, younger age, and large size of lesion. Additional considerations are given for increasing size, associated lymphangitis, and rapidity of spread of the lesion, particularly with cellulitis.[5,54]

COMPLICATIONS
Treatment Failure and Recurrence

The prognosis of skin abscesses and cellulitis evaluated in the ED is universally good. Fortunately, systemic illness resulting from SSTI is rare, and therapy directed at the local infection is often sufficient.[52,88,89] With adequate ED treatment, including drainage procedures, the treatment failure for outpatient management of skin abscesses is estimated at approximately 3% to 8% after 7 to 10 days.[10,78,80,84] Postulated risk factors for treatment failure include the presence of fever, age less than 1 year, and size of lesion greater than 5 cm; presence of these factors occasionally are associated with ED clinicians' decision to hospitalize children with cutaneous abscesses.[54,76,78] Outcome data on simple cellulitis are not as plentiful, although treatment failure does occur. Large lesion, rapid extension, involvement of sensitive structures, and signs of systemic illness are factors considered in evaluating inpatient versus outpatient management. If electing for outpatient therapy, any case of cellulitis and nondrained SSTI should be reevaluated within 48 to 72 hours to determine response to therapy, progression of the infection, and even potential evolution to abscess. Unfortunately, even with adequate therapy, recurrent infections are not uncommon, occurring in 18% to 28% of children after initial ED treatment. Treatment failure and recurrence rates do not differ between CA-MRSA and MSSA, with or without adjuvant antibiotic therapy.[10,78,80,90]

CA-MRSA Colonization

With the increase in primary and recurrent SSTIs among children and families, much attention has been placed on S. aureus colonization. Like MSSA, CA-MRSA has the potential to exist as a commensal skin organism in healthy children in the absence of infection. Colonization occurs in the nares, axilla, skin folds, and fingernails, and organisms may even persist on fomites. Among the US population, rates of S. aureus colonization is common, and similar to the rising incidence of SSTI, CA-MRSA colonization has increased from 0.8% in 2002 to 9% in 2005, to as high as 60%.[91–93] The actual link between colonization and new-onset SSTIs remains debatable. In the setting of acute SSTI, attempts to identify simultaneous colonization have showed high rates of discordance, with more than 40% of S. aureus strains differing between the infection and anterior nares.[94] Additionally, colonization with S. aureus has not been identified as risk factor for SSTI treatment failure.[95]

A principal interest in colonization exists to identify candidates for decolonization, to reduce the burden of recurrent SSTI, and to decrease transmission within households. Interestingly, there is suggestion that colonization may actually have a protective effect on recurrence, although this has yet to be proved. Several varied decolonization protocols have been created and implemented within institutions. Typical decolonization protocols combine methods to eliminate S. aureus from the integument and to prevent transmission (**Box 1**). Serial administration of intranasal mupirocin is typically recommended for the anterior nares, and either chlorhexidine or bleach baths is used for skin antisepsis. The efficacy of chlorhexidine as compared with bleach baths is not well established, although a single study has shown better effectiveness of bleach baths, which are inexpensive and commonly available.[96] When decolonization is instituted, methods should be applied to all members of the household, as this is more effective than isolated treatment of the index case of SSTI.[97]

Box 1
Components of decolonization protocols

Personal Hygiene

Refrain from sharing personal hygiene items (eg, hairbrushes, razors, or towels)

Discard lotions in jars and replace them with pump or pour bottles

Wash towels in hot water after each use

Wash bed linens in hot water once weekly

Topical and Systemic Therapy

Intranasal mupirocin twice daily for 5 days

4% chlorhexadine baths for 5 days

6% sodium hypocholorite (bleach) baths for 5 days

Course of oral clindamycin or TMP-SMX

SUMMARY

SSTIs represent a challenge for emergency physicians owing to the increasing clinical burden, emergence of CA-MRSA, and evolving diagnostic and management strategies. CA-MRSA has contributed greatly to the shifting epidemiology of skin abscesses and to the dilemma posed for nondrained soft tissue infections and cellulitis. Moreover, clinical diagnosis of cellulitis from early abscess may be difficult; bedside US may be effective for these cases. Incision and drainage procedure remains the mainstay of therapy for cutaneous abscesses, and the role of adjuvant antibiotics for abscesses is diminishing. Although all forms of *S. aureus* can produce cellulitis, the continued prevalence of group A streptococcus appears to be substantial, affecting antimicrobial choices. Finally, the impact of *S. aureus* colonization, and accompanying decolonization procedures, on development of recurrent skin infections is actively being investigated.

REFERENCES

1. Hersh AL, Chambers HF, Maselli JH, et al. National trends in ambulatory visits and antibiotic prescribing for skin and soft-tissue infections. Arch Intern Med 2008;168(14):1585–91.
2. Frazee BW, Lynn J, Charlebois ED, et al. High prevalence of methicillin-resistant Staphylococcus aureus in emergency department skin and soft tissue infections. Ann Emerg Med 2005;45(3):311–20.
3. Pallin DJ, Egan DJ, Pelletier AJ, et al. Increased US emergency department visits for skin and soft tissue infections, and changes in antibiotic choices, during the emergence of community-associated methicillin-resistant Staphylococcus aureus. Ann Emerg Med 2008;51(3):291–8.
4. Miller LG, Perdreau-Remington F, Rieg G, et al. Necrotizing fasciitis caused by community-associated methicillin-resistant Staphylococcus aureus in Los Angeles. N Engl J Med 2005;352(14):1445–53.
5. Swartz MN. Clinical practice. Cellulitis. N Engl J Med 2004;350(9):904–12.
6. Bonnetblanc JM, Bédane C. Erysipelas: recognition and management. Am J Clin Dermatol 2003;4(3):157–63.
7. Leppard BJ, Seal DV, Colman G, et al. The value of bacteriology and serology in the diagnosis of cellulitis and erysipelas. Br J Dermatol 1985;112(5):559–67.
8. Moran GJ, Krishnadasan A, Gorwitz RJ, et al. Methicillin-resistant S. aureus infections among patients in the emergency department. N Engl J Med 2006; 355(7):666–74. http://dx.doi.org/10.1056/NEJMoa055356.
9. Kaplan SL, Hulten KG, Gonzalez BE, et al. Three-year surveillance of community-acquired Staphylococcus aureus infections in children. Clin Infect Dis 2005;40(12):1785–91.
10. Mistry RD, Scott HF, Zaoutis TE, et al. Emergency department treatment failures for skin infections in the era of community-acquired methicillin-resistant Staphylococcus aureus. Pediatr Emerg Care 2011;27(1):21–6. http://dx.doi.org/10.1097/PEC.0b013e318203ca1c.
11. Mistry RD, Scott HF, Alpern ER, et al. Prevalence of proteus mirabilis in skin abscesses of the axilla. J Pediatr 2010;156(5):850–1. http://dx.doi.org/10.1016/j.jpeds.2010.01.014.
12. Elliott D, Kufera JA, Myers RA. The microbiology of necrotizing soft tissue infections. Am J Surg 2000;179(5):361–6.
13. Fridkin SK, Hageman JC, Morrison M, et al. Methicillin-resistant Staphylococcus aureus disease in three communities. N Engl J Med 2005;352(14):1436–44.

14. Purcell K, Fergie J. Epidemic of community-acquired methicillin-resistant Staphylococcus aureus infections: a 14-year study at Driscoll Children's Hospital. Arch Pediatr Adolesc Med 2005;159(10):980–5.

15. Zaoutis TE, Toltzis P, Chu J, et al. Clinical and molecular epidemiology of community-acquired methicillin-resistant Staphylococcus aureus infections among children with risk factors for health care-associated infection: 2001-2003. Pediatr Infect Dis J 2006;25(4):343–8.

16. Naimi TS, LeDell KH, Como-Sabetti K, et al. Comparison of community- and health care-associated methicillin-resistant Staphylococcus aureus infection. JAMA 2003;290(22):2976–84.

17. Fritz SA, Garbutt J, Elward A, et al. Prevalence of and risk factors for community-acquired methicillin-resistant and methicillin-sensitive staphylococcus aureus colonization in children seen in a practice-based research network. Pediatrics 2008;121(6):1090–8. http://dx.doi.org/10.1542/peds.2007-2104.

18. Liu C, Bayer A, Cosgrove SE, et al. Clinical practice guidelines by the Infectious Diseases Society of America for the treatment of methicillin-resistant Staphylococcus aureus infections in adults and children: executive summary. Clin Infect Dis 2011;52(3):285–92. http://dx.doi.org/10.1093/cid/cir034.

19. Herold BC, Immergluck LC, Maranan MC, et al. Community-acquired methicillin-resistant Staphylococcus aureus in children with no identified predisposing risk. JAMA 1998;279(8):593–8.

20. Hultén KG, Kaplan SL, Lamberth LB, et al. Hospital-acquired Staphylococcus aureus infections at Texas Children's Hospital, 2001-2007. Infect Control Hosp Epidemiol 2010;31(2):183–90. http://dx.doi.org/10.1086/649793.

21. Matlow A, Forgie S, Pelude L, et al. National surveillance of methicillin-resistant Staphylococcus aureus among hospitalized pediatric patients in Canadian acute care facilities, 1995-2007. Pediatr Infect Dis J 2012;31(8):814–20. http://dx.doi.org/10.1097/INF.0b013e31825c48a0.

22. Simor AE, Ofner-Agostini M, Bryce E, et al. The evolution of methicillin-resistant Staphylococcus aureus in Canadian hospitals: 5 years of national surveillance. CMAJ 2001;165(1):21–6.

23. David MZ, Medvedev S, Hohmann SF, et al. Increasing burden of methicillin-resistant Staphylococcus aureus hospitalizations at US academic medical centers, 2003-2008. Infect Control Hosp Epidemiol 2012;33(8):782–9. http://dx.doi.org/10.1086/666640.

24. Maree CL, Daum RS, Boyle-Vavra S, et al. Community-associated methicillin-resistant Staphylococcus aureus isolates causing healthcare-associated infections. Emerg Infect Dis 2007;13(2):236–42. http://dx.doi.org/10.3201/eid1302.060781.

25. Elliott DJ, Zaoutis TE, Troxel AB, et al. Empiric antimicrobial therapy for pediatric skin and soft-tissue infections in the era of methicillin-resistant Staphylococcus aureus. Pediatrics 2009;123(6):e959–66. http://dx.doi.org/10.1542/peds.2008-2428 pii:peds.2008-2428.

26. Buckingham SC, McDougal LK, Cathey LD, et al. Emergence of community-associated methicillin-resistant Staphylococcus aureus at a Memphis, Tennessee Children's Hospital. Pediatr Infect Dis J 2004;23(7):619–24.

27. Rajendran PM, Young D, Maurer T, et al. Randomized, double-blind, placebo-controlled trial of cephalexin for treatment of uncomplicated skin abscesses in a population at risk for community-acquired methicillin-resistant Staphylococcus aureus infection. Antimicrob Agents Chemother 2007;51(11):4044–8.

28. Talan DA, Krishnadasan A, Gorwitz RJ, et al. Comparison of Staphylococcus aureus from skin and soft-tissue infections in US emergency department

patients, 2004 and 2008. Clin Infect Dis 2011;53(2):144–9. http://dx.doi.org/10.1093/cid/cir308.

29. Vandenesch F, Naimi T, Enright MC, et al. Community-acquired methicillin-resistant Staphylococcus aureus carrying Panton-Valentine leukocidin genes: worldwide emergence. Emerg Infect Dis 2003;9(8):978–84.

30. Orscheln RC, Hunstad DA, Fritz SA, et al. Contribution of genetically restricted, methicillin-susceptible strains to the ongoing epidemic of community-acquired Staphylococcus aureus infections. Clin Infect Dis 2009;49(4):536–42. http://dx.doi.org/10.1086/600881.

31. Nimmo GR. USA300 abroad: global spread of a virulent strain of community-associated methicillin-resistant Staphylococcus aureus. Clin Microbiol Infect 2012;18(8):725–34. http://dx.doi.org/10.1111/j.1469-0691.2012.03822.x.

32. Rossney AS, Shore AC, Morgan PM, et al. The emergence and importation of diverse genotypes of methicillin-resistant Staphylococcus aureus (MRSA) harboring the Panton-Valentine leukocidin gene (pvl) reveal that pvl is a poor marker for community-acquired MRSA strains in Ireland. J Clin Microbiol 2007;45(8):2554–63. http://dx.doi.org/10.1128/JCM.00245-07.

33. Wu D, Wang Q, Yang Y, et al. Epidemiology and molecular characteristics of community-associated methicillin-resistant and methicillin-susceptible Staphy-lococcus aureus from skin/soft tissue infections in a children's hospital in Beijing, China. Diagn Microbiol Infect Dis 2010;67(1):1–8. http://dx.doi.org/10.1016/j.diagmicrobio.2009.12.006.

34. Grundmann H, Aires-de-Sousa M, Boyce J, et al. Emergence and resurgence of meticillin-resistant Staphylococcus aureus as a public-health threat. Lancet 2006;368(9538):874–85. http://dx.doi.org/10.1016/S0140-6736(06)68853-3.

35. Squire BT, Fox JC, Anderson C. ABSCESS: applied bedside sonography for convenient evaluation of superficial soft tissue infections. Acad Emerg Med 2005;12(7):601–6.

36. Ramirez-Schrempp D, Dorfman DH, Baker WE, et al. Ultrasound soft-tissue applications in the pediatric emergency department: to drain or not to drain? Pediatr Emerg Care 2009;25(1):44–8. http://dx.doi.org/10.1097/PEC.0b013e318191d963.

37. Gaspari R, Blehar D, Mendoza M, et al. Use of ultrasound elastography for skin and subcutaneous abscesses. J Ultrasound Med 2009;28(7):855–60 pii: 28/7/855.

38. Tayal VS, Hasan N, Norton HJ, et al. The effect of soft-tissue ultrasound on the management of cellulitis in the emergency department. Acad Emerg Med 2006; 13(4):384–8.

39. Iverson K, Haritos D, Thomas R, et al. The effect of bedside ultrasound on diagnosis and management of soft tissue infections in a pediatric ED. Am J Emerg Med 2011;30(8):1347–51. http://dx.doi.org/10.1016/j.ajem.2011.09.020.

40. Marin JR, Alpern ER, Panebianco NL, et al. Assessment of a training curriculum for emergency ultrasound for pediatric soft tissue infections. Acad Emerg Med 2011;18(2):174–82. http://dx.doi.org/10.1111/j.1553-2712.2010.00990.x.

41. Kuo DC, Chasm RM, Witting MD. Emergency physician ability to predict methicillin-resistant Staphylococcus aureus skin and soft tissue infections. J Emerg Med 2010;39(1):17–20. http://dx.doi.org/10.1016/j.jemermed.2007.09.046 pii:S0736-4679(08)00102-9.

42. Miller LG, Perdreau-Remington F, Bayer AS, et al. Clinical and epidemiologic characteristics cannot distinguish community-associated methicillin-resistant Staphylococcus aureus infection from methicillin-susceptible S. aureus infection: a prospective investigation. Clin Infect Dis 2007;44(4):471–82.

43. Sattler CA, Mason EO, Kaplan SL. Prospective comparison of risk factors and demographic and clinical characteristics of community-acquired, methicillin-resistant versus methicillin-susceptible Staphylococcus aureus infection in children. Pediatr Infect Dis J 2002;21(10):910–7.
44. Mistry RD, Marin JR, Alpern ER. Abscess volume and ultrasound characteristics of community-associated methicillin-resistant Staphylococcus aureus infection. Pediatr Emerg Care 2013;29(2):140–4. http://dx.doi.org/10.1097/PEC.0b013e3182808a41.
45. Epperly TD. The value of needle aspiration in the management of cellulitis. J Fam Pract 1986;23(4):337–40.
46. Liles DK, Dall LH. Needle aspiration for diagnosis of cellulitis. Cutis 1985;36(1):63–4.
47. Traylor KK, Todd JK. Needle aspirate culture method in soft tissue infections: injection of saline vs. direct aspiration. Pediatr Infect Dis J 1998;17(9):840–1.
48. Todd JK. Office laboratory diagnosis of skin and soft tissue infections. Pediatr Infect Dis 1985;4(1):84–7.
49. Fleisher G, Ludwig S. Cellulitis: a prospective study. Ann Emerg Med 1980;9(5):246–9.
50. Goetz JP, Tafari N, Boxerbaum B. Needle aspiration in Hemophilus influenzae type b cellulitis. Pediatrics 1974;54(4):504–6.
51. Howe PM, Eduardo Fajardo J, Orcutt MA. Etiologic diagnosis of cellulitis: comparison of aspirates obtained from the leading edge and the point of maximal inflammation. Pediatr Infect Dis J 1987;6(7):685–6.
52. Hook EW 3rd, Hooton TM, Horton CA, et al. Microbiologic evaluation of cutaneous cellulitis in adults. Arch Intern Med 1986;146(2):295–7.
53. Patel Wylie F, Kaplan SL, Mason EO, et al. Needle aspiration for the etiologic diagnosis of children with cellulitis in the era of community-acquired methicillin-resistant Staphylococcus aureus. Clin Pediatr (Phila) 2011;50(6):503–7. http://dx.doi.org/10.1177/0009922810394652.
54. Mistry RD, Weisz K, Scott HF, et al. Emergency management of pediatric skin and soft tissue infections in the community-associated methicillin-resistant Staphylococcus aureus era. Acad Emerg Med 2010;17(2):187–93. http://dx.doi.org/10.1111/j.1553-2712.2009.00652.x.
55. Jeng A, Beheshti M, Li J, et al. The role of beta-hemolytic streptococci in causing diffuse, nonculturable cellulitis: a prospective investigation. Medicine (Baltimore) 2010;89(4):217–26. http://dx.doi.org/10.1097/MD.0b013e3181e8d635.
56. Stevens DL, Bisno AL, Chambers HF, et al. Practice guidelines for the diagnosis and management of skin and soft-tissue infections. Clin Infect Dis 2005;41(10):1373–406. http://dx.doi.org/10.1086/497143.
57. Gorwitz RJ, Jernigan DB, Powers JH, et al. Strategies for clinical management of MRSA in the community: summary of an experts' meeting convened by the Centers for Disease Control and Prevention. 2006. Available at: http://www.cdc.gov/ncidod/dhqp/ar_mrsa_ca.html. Accessed April 24, 2013.
58. Chambers HF, Moellering RC, Kamitsuka P. Clinical decisions. Management of skin and soft-tissue infection. N Engl J Med 2008;359(10):1063–7.
59. Cassidy-Smith T, Mistry RD, Russo CJ, et al. Topical anesthetic cream is associated with spontaneous cutaneous abscess drainage in children. Am J Emerg Med 2012;30(1):104–9. http://dx.doi.org/10.1016/j.ajem.2010.10.020.
60. Bjerring P, Arendt-Nielsen L. Depth and duration of skin analgesia to needle insertion after topical application of EMLA cream. Br J Anaesth 1990;64(2):173–7.

61. Daly L. Incision and drainge of a cutaneous abscess. In: Henretig F, King C, editors. Textbook of Pediatric Emergency Procedures. 2nd edition. Lippincott, Williams, Wilkins; 2008. p. 1079–84.
62. Uspal NG, Marin JR, Alpern ER, et al. Factors associated with the use of procedural sedation during incision and drainage procedures at a children's hospital. Am J Emerg Med 2013;31(2):302–8. http://dx.doi.org/10.1016/j.ajem.2012.07.028.
63. Halvorson GD, Halvorson JE, Iserson KV. Abscess incision and drainage in the emergency department–Part I. J Emerg Med 1985;3(3):227–32.
64. O'Malley GF, Williams E, Dominici P, et al. Packing simple cutaneous abscess after incision and drainage is painful and probably unecessary. Ann Emerg Med 2007;50(Suppl 3):S58.
65. Kessler DO, Krantz A, Mojica M. Randomized trial comparing wound packing to no wound packing following incision and drainage of superficial skin abscesses in the pediatric emergency department. Pediatr Emerg Care 2012;28(6):514–7. http://dx.doi.org/10.1097/PEC.0b013e3182587b20.
66. Tsoraides SS, Pearl RH, Stanfill AB, et al. Incision and loop drainage: a minimally invasive technique for subcutaneous abscess management in children. J Pediatr Surg 2010;45(3):606–9. http://dx.doi.org/10.1016/j.jpedsurg.2009.06.013 pii:S0022-3468(09)00471-0.
67. Ladd AP, Levy MS, Quilty J. Minimally invasive technique in treatment of complex, subcutaneous abscesses in children. J Pediatr Surg 2010;45(7):1562–6. http://dx.doi.org/10.1016/j.jpedsurg.2010.03.025 pii:S0022-3468(10)00299-X.
68. McNamara WF, Hartin CW Jr, Escobar MA, et al. An alternative to open incision and drainage for community-acquired soft tissue abscesses in children. J Pediatr Surg 2011;46(3):502–6. http://dx.doi.org/10.1016/j.jpedsurg.2010.08.019.
69. Singer AJ, Taira BR, Chale S, et al. Primary versus secondary closure of cutaneous abscesses in the emergency department: a randomized controlled trial. Acad Emerg Med 2013;20(1):27–32. http://dx.doi.org/10.1111/acem.12053.
70. Gaspari RJ, Resop D, Mendoza M, et al. A randomized controlled trial of incision and drainage versus ultrasonographically guided needle aspiration for skin abscesses and the effect of methicillin-resistant Staphylococcus aureus. Ann Emerg Med 2011;57(5):483–491.e1. http://dx.doi.org/10.1016/j.annemergmed.2010.11.021 pii:S0196-0644(10)01763-4.
71. Sørensen C, Hjortrup A, Moesgaard F, et al. Linear incision and curettage vs. deroofing and drainage in subcutaneous abscess. A randomized clinical trial. Acta Chir Scand 1987;153(11–12):659–60.
72. Llera JL, Levy RC. Treatment of cutaneous abscess: a double-blind clinical study. Ann Emerg Med 1985;14(1):15–9.
73. Macfie J, Harvey J. The treatment of acute superficial abscesses: a prospective clinical trial. Br J Surg 1977;64(4):264–6.
74. Stewart MP, Laing MR, Krukowski ZH. Treatment of acute abscesses by incision, curettage and primary suture without antibiotics: a controlled clinical trial. Br J Surg 1985;72(1):66–7.
75. Rajendran PM, Young DM, Maurer T, et al. Antibiotic use in the treatment of soft tissue abscesses: a survey of current practice. Surg Infect (Larchmt) 2007;8(2):237–8.
76. Lee MC, Rios AM, Aten MF, et al. Management and outcome of children with skin and soft tissue abscesses caused by community-acquired methicillin-resistant Staphylococcus aureus. Pediatr Infect Dis J 2004;23(2):123–7.

77. Paydar KZ, Hansen SL, Charlebois ED, et al. Inappropriate antibiotic use in soft tissue infections. Arch Surg 2006;141(9):850–4. http://dx.doi.org/10.1001/archsurg.141.9.850 [discussion: 855–6].
78. Chen AE, Carroll KC, Diener-West M, et al. Randomized controlled trial of cephalexin versus clindamycin for uncomplicated pediatric skin infections. Pediatrics 2011;127(3):e573–80. http://dx.doi.org/10.1542/peds.2010-2053.
79. Schmitz GR, Bruner D, Pitotti R, et al. Randomized controlled trial of trimethoprim-sulfamethoxazole for uncomplicated skin abscesses in patients at risk for community-associated methicillin-resistant Staphylococcus aureus infection. Ann Emerg Med 2010;56(3):283–7. http://dx.doi.org/10.1016/j.annemergmed.2010.03.002 pii:S0196-0644(10)00218-0.
80. Duong M, Markwell S, Peter J, et al. Randomized, controlled trial of antibiotics in the management of community-acquired skin abscesses in the pediatric patient. Ann Emerg Med 2010;55(5):401–7. http://dx.doi.org/10.1016/j.annemergmed.2009.03.014.
81. Frank AL, Marcinak JF, Mangat PD, et al. Clindamycin treatment of methicillin-resistant Staphylococcus aureus infections in children. Pediatr Infect Dis J 2002;21(6):530–4.
82. Frank AL, Marcinak JF, Mangat PD, et al. Community-acquired and clindamycin-susceptible methicillin-resistant Staphylococcus aureus in children. Pediatr Infect Dis J 1999;18(11):993–1000.
83. Eady EA, Cove JH. Staphylococcal resistance revisited: community-acquired methicillin resistant Staphylococcus aureus–an emerging problem for the management of skin and soft tissue infections. Curr Opin Infect Dis 2003;16(2):103–24.
84. Williams DJ, Cooper WO, Kaltenbach LA, et al. Comparative effectiveness of antibiotic treatment strategies for pediatric skin and soft-tissue infections. Pediatrics 2011;128(3):e479–87. http://dx.doi.org/10.1542/peds.2010-3681.
85. Daum RS. Clinical practice. Skin and soft-tissue infections caused by methicillin-resistant Staphylococcus aureus. N Engl J Med 2007;357(4):380–90.
86. Lautz TB, Raval MV, Barsness KA. Increasing national burden of hospitalizations for skin and soft tissue infections in children. J Pediatr Surg 2011;46(10):1935–41. http://dx.doi.org/10.1016/j.jpedsurg.2011.05.008 pii:S0022-3468(11)00435-0.
87. Gerber JS, Coffin SE, Smathers SA, et al. Trends in the incidence of methicillin-resistant Staphylococcus aureus infection in children's hospitals in the United States. Clin Infect Dis 2009;49(1):65–71. http://dx.doi.org/10.1086/599348.
88. Sigurdsson AF, Gudmundsson S. The etiology of bacterial cellulitis as determined by fine-needle aspiration. Scand J Infect Dis 1989;21(5):537–42.
89. Sadow KB, Chamberlain JM. Blood cultures in the evaluation of children with cellulitis. Pediatrics 1998;101(3):e4. http://dx.doi.org/10.1542/peds.101.3.e4.
90. Fritz SA, Epplin EK, Garbutt J, et al. Skin infection in children colonized with community-associated methicillin-resistant Staphylococcus aureus. J Infect 2009;59(6):394–401. http://dx.doi.org/10.1016/j.jinf.2009.09.001.
91. Kuehnert MJ, Kruszon-Moran D, Hill HA, et al. Prevalence of Staphylococcus aureus nasal colonization in the United States, 2001-2002. J Infect Dis 2006;193(2):172–9.
92. Creech CB 2nd, Kernodle DS, Alsentzer A, et al. Increasing rates of nasal carriage of methicillin-resistant Staphylococcus aureus in healthy children. Pediatr Infect Dis J 2005;24(7):617–21.
93. Fritz SA, Hogan PG, Hayek G, et al. Staphylococcus aureus colonization in children with community-associated Staphylococcus aureus skin infections

and their household contacts. Arch Pediatr Adolesc Med 2012;166(6):551–7. http://dx.doi.org/10.1001/archpediatrics.2011.900.

94. Chen AE, Cantey JB, Carroll KC, et al. Discordance between Staphylococcus aureus nasal colonization and skin infections in children. Pediatr Infect Dis J 2009;28(3):244–6. http://dx.doi.org/10.1097/INF.0b013e31818cb0c4.

95. Reber A, Moldovan A, Dunkel N, et al. Should the methicillin-resistant Staphylococcus aureus carriage status be used as a guide to treatment for skin and soft tissue infections? J Infect 2012;64(5):513–9. http://dx.doi.org/10.1016/j.jinf.2011.12.023.

96. Fritz SA, Camins BC, Eisenstein KA, et al. Effectiveness of measures to eradicate Staphylococcus aureus carriage in patients with community-associated skin and soft-tissue infections: a randomized trial. Infect Control Hosp Epidemiol 2011;32(9):872–80. http://dx.doi.org/10.1086/661285.

97. Fritz SA, Hogan PG, Hayek G, et al. Household versus individual approaches to eradication of community-associated Staphylococcus aureus in children: a randomized trial. Clin Infect Dis 2012;54(6):743–51. http://dx.doi.org/10.1093/cid/cir919.

Approach to Syncope and Altered Mental Status

Emily C. MacNeill, MD[a],*, Sudhir Vashist, MBBS, MD[b]

KEYWORDS

- Pediatric • Syncope • Transient altered mental status
- Persistent altered mental status • Seizure

KEY POINTS

- Although altered mental status (AMS), transient or persistent, can cause a great deal of anxiety for patients and providers, a rational approach to these patients is essential to avoid underuse or excessive use of testing.
- An age-based approach is important, because the various diseases are common in different age groups.
- In patients with transient AMS, differentiating true syncope from other causes is the first step; a stepwise approach, guided by the history and physical examination, can then proceed.
- Persistent AMS, on the other hand, is a life-threatening presentation and time is of the essence.
- The differential diagnosis is broad and, rather than trying to recall long lists of highly specific causes, it is more helpful to consider broad categories of disease: structural lesions, insufficient delivery of appropriate substrate to the brain, metabolic imbalance, inflammation, infection, and abnormal electrical activity.
- Maintaining a broad differential and evaluating for multiple diseases simultaneously is critical in the care of these patients.

INTRODUCTION: NATURE OF THE PROBLEM

Altered mental status (AMS), whether transient (t-AMS) or persistent (p-AMS), presents a diagnostic challenge. With a broad differential diagnosis, a wide range of severity, and potential involvement of any organ system, this presentation is complicated by

Funding Sources: None.
Conflict of Interest: None.
[a] Department of Emergency Medicine, Carolinas Medical Center, Carolinas Healthcare System, 1000 Blythe Boulevard, 3rd Floor Medical Education Building, Charlotte, NC 28203, USA;
[b] Department of Pediatrics, Children's Heart Program, University of Maryland School of Medicine, 110 South Paca Street, 7th Floor, Baltimore, MD 21201, USA
* Corresponding author.
E-mail address: Emily.macneill@carolinas.org

an inability of the patient to give an accurate history. For the purposes of this article, the term AMS is used to describe any change in the way a patient interacts with their environment. What is distinguished is the concept of t-AMS and p-AMS, because the differential is different for these presentations.

For teaching purposes, mnemonics have been developed to help clinicians consider all possible causes of AMS. This long list of possible diagnoses is cumbersome and difficult to remember. Instead, it may be simpler to consider broader categories of disease. For the brain to function normally, it requires adequate perfusion with appropriate delivery of oxygen, nutrients, and balanced electrolytes. In addition, there cannot be structural disease; masses, blood, and excessive cerebrospinal fluid (CSF), which can all impede normal function. It cannot be plagued by infection or inflammation, and electrical activity has to be organized. Some causes more commonly cause t-AMS (moments of inadequate perfusion, abnormal electrical activity), whereas others cause persistent symptoms (structural, metabolic, or infectious).

A detailed description of all causes of AMS is beyond the scope of this article; trauma and toxicology are not discussed. Instead, a description of some of the more common causes is delineated. As these potential causes are reviewed, there are some key themes that must be considered. First, the differential diagnosis for AMS changes with age (**Table 1**). Second, t-AMS is common and usually benign, whereas p-AMS is less common, carries a higher morbidity and mortality, and requires rapid diagnosis and treatment. There is no substitute for a thorough history and physical examination with these patients; it is essential for guiding diagnostic workup.

Table 1
Breakdown of common causes of t-AMS and p-AMS by age

Infants/Toddlers	School Age	Adolescents
t-AMS		
Seizure	Seizure	Seizure
Trauma	Trauma	Trauma
Sepsis	Migraine	Psychiatric causes
ALTE	Syncope	Syncope
BHSs	—	—
p-AMS		
Seizure	Seizure	Seizure
Trauma	Trauma	Trauma
Shock	Shock	Shock
Toxicologic	Toxicologic	Toxicologic
Electrolyte abnormality	Electrolyte abnormality	Electrolyte abnormality
Sepsis/encephalitis	Encephalitis	Encephalitis
Inborn errors of metabolism	Hyperglycemia or hypoglycemia	Hyperglycemia or hypoglycemia
Hypoglycemia	Brain mass	Brain mass
BHSs	Postictal state	Postictal state
Intussusception	Shigellosis	Posterior reversible encephalopathy syndrome

CAUSES FOR T-AMS
Apparent Life-Threatening Event

Defined in 1986 by the National Institutes of Health as an episode that is "frightening to the observer" and has some combination of apnea, color change, change in motor tone, and choking or gagging, Apparent life-threatening events (ALTEs) are the most common presentation of t-AMS in young infants. As is evident by the definition itself, it is impossible to distinguish whether these ALTEs were caused by a cerebral perfusion problem or abnormal electrical activity, and they are difficult to assign to a particular disease.[1] In the neonate, it is prudent to consider sepsis as a possible cause; however, recent literature[1] has shown that bacterial infections, cardiac abnormalities, and structural neurologic diseases are rare. Child abuse and neglect should be considered in these patients, because they have a higher incidence than the general population. The workup for these children is controversial; most of the literature points to a varied, expensive, and low-yield evaluation when these cases are looked at retrospectively. A prudent workup for the child in whom neither sepsis nor nonaccidental trauma is a concern, is a hemoglobin test, electrocardiography (ECG), and a brief period of observation.[2]

Breath Holding

Breath-holding spells (BHSs) present in young children from 6 months to 6 years of age; 80% to 90% present by the time the child is 18 months of age. The classic presentation of BHS is a toddler who throws a tantrum, suddenly holds their breath, turns blue, and then passes out. When consciousness is regained, the child seems fine. The term BHS is inaccurate because it implies that it is an act of volition when it is involuntary.[3] There are 2 varieties of BHS: pallid (after minor trauma and related to bradycardia) and cyanotic (failure to inhale after forced expiration); both start with an inciting event such as emotional upset or minor trauma. In both cases, the child can have loss of consciousness, seizurelike activity, including tonic-clonic movements, and urinary incontinence. Children can have both types of spells and can have numerous episodes per day. Diagnosis is made by historical features. Various treatments have been found to be effective, including supplemental iron for those children who have iron deficiency anemia, serotonin reuptake inhibitors, and pacemaker placement for those with frequent and severe spells.[4,5]

Seizure

Seizures are a common phenomenon, with an estimated lifetime prevalence of 5 to 10/1000.[6] In 1 multicenter study of adults and children,[7] seizure was the presenting diagnosis for 1.2% of visits to the emergency department (ED). Distinguishing seizure from syncope and BHSs can be difficult. The patient can be found in a postictal state, or the seizure type itself can be subtle. There are some pediatric partial seizure types, such as Panayiotopoulos syndrome, which cause episodes that seem to be syncopal. Patients with this benign form of epilepsy can present with sudden loss of muscle tone and unresponsiveness as their only symptom.[8] Although it is tempting to order a computed tomography (CT) scan for patients who present with first-time seizure, if the infant is asymptomatic at the time of presentation, this is unlikely to show any disease and exposes children to unnecessary radiation. A more prudent evaluation would be referral to a pediatric neurologist for magnetic resonance imaging (MRI) and electroencephalography (EEG) as an outpatient.

Syncope

Syncope is the most common cause of t-AMS. It is characterized by rapid onset, short duration, and spontaneous complete recovery.[9] The mechanism for syncope is global decrease in cerebral perfusion, resulting from a decrease in systemic blood pressure (BP). This mechanism differentiates syncope from other causes of transient loss of consciousness (T- LOC) (**Fig. 1**). Because BP is determined by cardiac output and total peripheral vascular resistance, any decrease in either the cardiac output (cardiac syncope) or total peripheral vascular resistance (syncope secondary to orthostatic hypotension) can result in cerebral hypoperfusion. However, the most common type of syncope, reflex syncope, is a combination of both these pathophysiologic mechanisms (**Fig. 2**).

Syncope is usually benign. **Box 1** summarizes various causes of syncope based on mechanism. Reflex syncope, the most common form, is rare in children younger than 10 years but then increases in incidence dramatically, with a peak around 15 years of age.[10] As many as 15% to 20% of all children may experience a syncopal episode before the end of their second decade of life, and lifetime cumulative incidence of reflex syncope in young subjects is 18% to 47%. This finding is in contrast to that of epilepsy (0.5%) or cardiac syncope.[11] Cardiac syncope or syncope secondary to cardiovascular disease (whether structural or arrhythmogenic) is less common, making up 2% to 6% of all cases of pediatric syncope (**Box 2**).[10]

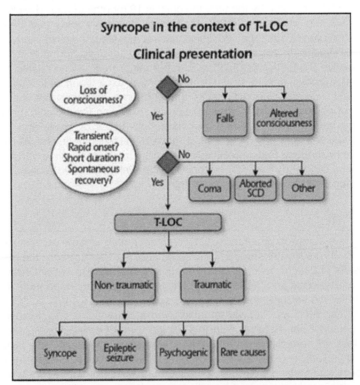

Fig. 1. Syncope in the context of transient AMS. SCD, sudden cardiac death. (*From* Moya A, Sutton R, Ammirati F, et al, The Task Force for the Diagnosis and Management of Syncope, European Society of Cardiology (ESC). Guidelines for the diagnosis and management of syncope (version 2009). Eur Heart J 2009;30(21):2635; with permission.)

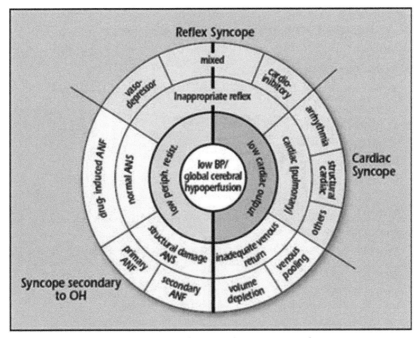

Fig. 2. Pathophysiologic basis of the classification of various types of syncope. ANF, autonomic nervous failure; ANS, autonomic nervous system. (*From* Moya A, Sutton R, Ammirati F, et al, The Task Force for the Diagnosis and Management of Syncope, European Society of Cardiology (ESC). Guidelines for the diagnosis and management of syncope (version 2009). Eur Heart J 2009;30(21):2637; with permission.)

Box 1
Pathophysiologic classification of syncope

1. Neurally mediated/reflex syncope (most common cause in children)

    A. Vasovagal

        a. Orthostatic stress (common trigger)

        b. Other triggers (fear, pain, sight of blood)

    B. Situational (cough, sneeze, defecation, micturition, postprandial, postexercise)

    C. Atypical forms (without apparent trigger or atypical presentation)

2. Cardiac syncope (risk of SCD) (see **Box 2** for complete list of causes)

    A. Arrhythmia as the primary cause

    B. Structural/functional heart disease

3. Syncope caused by orthostatic hypotension (uncommon cause in children)

    A. Autonomic failure (primary or secondary)

    B. Drug induced (vasodilators, diuretics, phenothiazines, antidepressants)

    C. Volume depletion (hemorrhage, diarrhea, vomiting)

Box 2
Causes of cardiovascular syncope: potentially fatal if unrecognized

1. Arrhythmias
   A. Bradyarrhythmias
      a. Sinus node dysfunction (especially in patients with congenital heart defects)
      b. AV block
      c. Kearnes-Sayre syndrome
      d. Pacemaker malfunction
   B. Tachyarrhythmias
      a. Supraventricular
         1. WPW
         2. Supraventricular tachycardia/atrial arrhythmias (especially in patients with congenital heart defects)
      b. Ventricular: ventricular tachycardia/torsades/ventricular fibrillation
         1. Channelopathies
            a. Long QT syndrome
            b. Catecholaminergic polymorphic ventricular tachycardia
            c. Brugada syndrome
            d. Short QT syndrome
         2. Drug induced
         3. Idiopathic
            a. Ventricular fibrillation
            b. Outflow tract
2. Structural/functional heart disease
   A. Cardiomyopathy
      a. Hypertrophic cardiomyopathy
      b. Dilated cardiomyopathy
   B. Coronary anomalies
      a. Anomalous origin
      b. Kawasaki disease
   C. Valvar aortic stenosis
   D. Arrhythmogenic right ventricular dysplasia
   E. Acute myocarditis
   F. Congenital heart disease (repaired and unrepaired)
   G. Pulmonary hypertension, pulmonary embolus
   H. Aortic dissection (Marfan syndrome)
   I. Cardiac masses

Reflex Syncope

Reflex syncope is also known as neurally mediated, neurocardiogenic, or vasovagal syncope. Cardiovascular reflexes that control the circulation become intermittently inappropriate, in response to a trigger, resulting in vasodilatation from a decrease in efferent sympathetic activity or bradycardia or asystole from an increase in the vagal discharge and thereby in a decrease in arterial BP and global cerebral perfusion (see **Fig. 2**).

Cardiac Syncope

Many of the children with cardiovascular disorders who go on to experience sudden cardiac arrest (SCA) have syncope or presyncope as the warning symptom. Identifying this subset amongst all patients who present with syncope is challenging. In a study evaluating warning signs in children and young adults with SCA, 72% had at least 1 cardiovascular symptom before their cardiac arrest (recent fatigue, near-syncope, lightheadedness, chest pain, palpitations, and shortness of breath); nearly a quarter of the SCA victims had at least 1 objective warning event (syncope or unexplained seizure activity), which remained undiagnosed as a cardiac disorder before the cardiac arrest.[12] Previous literature has reported 17% to 25% of young athletes with sudden nontraumatic death have a previous history of syncope.[13,14]

Syncope and Sudden Cardiac Death in Athletes

Because incidence of syncope peaks in adolescence, syncope is not uncommon is athletes. However, exertional syncope is a major red flag and warrants high index of suspicion for underlying cardiac disease. It is critical to differentiate if the syncopal event was unrelated to physical activity (most likely benign reflex syncope), was post-exertional (most likely postexertional postural hypotension and again benign) or truly exertional (high chance of an underlying cardiac disease). In 1 study,[15] nearly 6% of all athletes had syncope, of which 13% had exercise-related syncope. However, exertional syncope was only in 1.3% of all athletes who fainted, and 2 of 6 (ie, one-third of the athletes with true exertional syncope) had a cardiac diagnosis. One study summarizing the cause of death in young competitive athletes in the United States over a 27-year period[16] found a cardiovascular cause in 1049 (56%) of all 1866 deaths. Hypertrophic cardiomyopathy (HCM) (36%), coronary anomalies (17%), myocarditis, arrhythmogenic right ventricular cardiomyopathy, and channelopathies were the most common cause identified (see **Box 2**).

HCM

HCM is an autosomal-dominant condition that affects 0.1% to 0.2% of the general population and is the most common cause of sudden cardiac death (SCD) in the young. HCM has a wide clinical spectrum, ranging from asymptomatic patients to patients with heart failure, left ventricular outflow tract obstruction, atrial arrhythmias, or syncope/sudden death as the initial presentation. Nearly 21% of athletes who died of HCM had some signs or symptoms of cardiovascular disease before death.[14] Arrhythmias are responsible for syncope and sudden death in these patients. There may be a history of exertional symptoms or a family history of HCM or sudden death. Physical examination is mostly normal. An ejection systolic murmur pronounced on standing can be heard in the obstructive form. ECG is helpful in the diagnosis and is abnormal in nearly 95% of patients with HCM, with findings of left ventricle hypertrophy, left axis deviation, T wave abnormalities, or abnormal Q waves. However, echocardiography is diagnostic. All patients should avoid competitive sports. Treatments modalities include β-blockers, calcium channel blockers, heart failure management, myectomy, antiarrhythmics, and implantable cardioverter defibrillator (ICD) placement depending on the clinical status.

Coronary Artery Anomalies

Reported incidence of anomalous origin of coronary artery from opposing sinus is 0.17% and it is the second most common cause of SCD in athletes.[17] As with HCM, SCD can be the initial presenting event. However, nearly half of the patients may have signs of cardiovascular disease before their death.[18] Syncope with exercise is the hallmark clinical feature, because hemodynamic changes during exercise may exacerbate compromised myocardial perfusion. Ventricular arrhythmia (**Fig. 3**) is the cause of syncope or death. Echocardiography can miss these anomalies if not evaluated carefully and patients may have a negative ECG stress test. Thus, in a patient with exertional syncope, if the echocardiogram cannot convincingly show the origin of the coronary arteries, CT angiography of the coronary arteries should be performed. Patients have excellent outcomes after surgical repair, which can include unroofing the vessel from its intramural course.

Long QT Syndrome

Long QT syndrome (LQTS) is an inherited channelopathy affecting 1:2500 patients. Alterations in the potassium and sodium channels result in ventricular repolarization abnormalities and a predisposition toward the development of ventricular arrhythmias. The incidence of cases of SCD caused by LQTS in young athletes is estimated to be from 0.5% to 8%.[19–21] Diagnosing LQTS can be complex. In general, a QTc of more than 470 milliseconds in males and more than 480 milliseconds in females requires further investigation (**Fig. 4**).[22] Persons with LQTS may present with syncopal events during periods of stress, emotion, exercise, swimming, loud auditory stimuli, or relative bradycardia (ie, during sleep or rest), depending on the subtype of LQTS that the patient has.

There are several challenges with LQTS diagnosis, because one-third of the patients with LQTS may have normal QT interval at baseline and 10% to 15% of healthy individuals may have QTc greater than 440 milliseconds. In a study of pediatric ED patients with presyncope/syncope, one-third had QTc values of 440 milliseconds or greater. Of the patients who followed up with a pediatric cardiologist, no patient received a diagnosis of LQTS with normalization of QTc values.[23] Although isolated finding of borderline QT intervals on an ECG obtained after a syncopal episode must be interpreted with caution, it is prudent to refer these patients to a pediatric cardiologist for further evaluation. Treatment of this disorder includes avoidance of triggers, avoidance of QT-prolonging medications (visit http://www.qtdrug.org for comprehensive lists) β-blockers, and ICD placement.

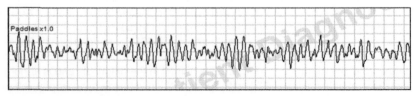

Fig. 3. Ventricular fibrillation in a young athlete with anomalous left coronary artery from the right sinus who collapsed on the field while playing.

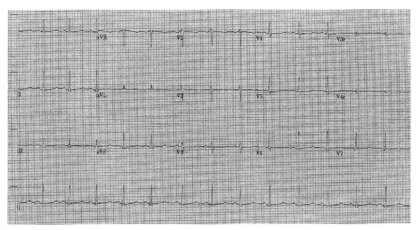

Fig. 4. ECG showing LQTS.

Brugada Syndrome

Manifested by right bundle branch block and ST elevation in V1 to V3 (**Fig. 5**), Brugada syndrome (BS) could be responsible for 4% of all SCD and up to 20% of SCD in structurally normal hearts. Arrhythmias, fast polymorphic ventricular tachycardia (VT) degenerating into ventricular fibrillation (VF), can occur at any age. Patients can present with palpitations, dizziness, syncope, nocturnal agonal respiration, or aborted SCD. Arrhythmias occur at rest and when vagal tone is augmented such as nighttime during sleep. Eighty percent of patients with VT/VF have a history of syncope. Fever is another important trigger for arrhythmias in BS. Although fever itself can be associated with orthostatic hypotension and syncope, ECG should be carefully evaluated to rule out BS.[24] Patients with BS should be admitted for observation during febrile illness and should avoid triggers. Medications such as quinidine and ICD placement are the mainstays of therapy (see http://www.brugada.org for medications to avoid in patients with BS).

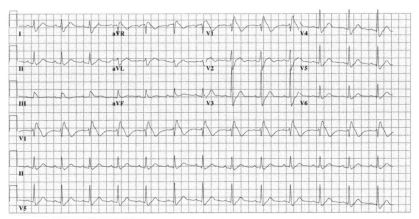

Fig. 5. ECG of Brugada syndrome: type 1, the most common, is characterized by >2 mm J point elevation followed by down-sloping ST segment and negative T waves in the right precordial leads. (*Courtesy of* Dr P.G. Postema, Amsterdam, Netherlands and ECGpedia.org.)

Catecholaminergic Polymorphic VT

Catecholaminergic polymorphic VT (CPVT) is another rare cause of sudden death among persons with structurally normal hearts, with an estimated prevalence of 1:10,000 persons.[25] It is an inherited disorder, with both autosomal-dominant and autosomal-recessive forms. Most events occur in the first and second decade of life. Patients present with syncope/SCD caused by bidirectional VT (**Fig. 6**) or polymorphic VT triggered by exercise or emotional stress. Baseline ECG is usually normal, and a stress test must be obtained. Treatment of this disorder includes β-blockers, trigger avoidance, verapamil, and ICD placement.

Arrhythmogenic Right Ventricular Dysplasia or Cardiomyopathy

Arrhythmogenic right ventricular dysplasia (ARVD) is an autosomal-dominant genetic cardiomyopathy affecting 1:2000 to 1:5000 people, which causes ventricular arrhythmias, resulting in syncope or sudden death.[26] Exercise is a common trigger, and the disease usually presents in the second to fifth decade of life. There is progressive replacement of right ventricular myocardium with fibrofatty tissue, which is diagnosed by MRI. The diagnosis of ARVD can be difficult, and clinical criteria should be used to aid in the diagnosis. Baseline ECG (**Fig. 7**) is abnormal in 90% of the patients. Competitive sports are contraindicated for these patients, and all symptomatic patients should receive an ICD.

Myocarditis

Myocarditis can also result in SCD secondary to fatal arrhythmias, which can occur in both the acute and healing phase of the illness.[27] Any patient presenting with syncope with recent history of febrile illness, rash, fatigue, and chest pain should be evaluated for myocarditis. Clinical examination may be normal, or patients may have a regurgitant murmur, pericardial rub, and muffled heart sounds on auscultation. ECG can show ventricular ectopy or nonspecific ST/T wave abnormalities. Cardiac enzyme levels may be increased, and echocardiogram may show decreased function, atrioventricular (AV) valve regurgitation, or pericardial effusion. Delayed gadolinium-

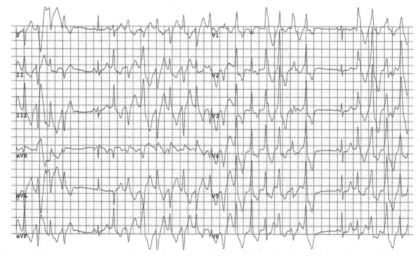

Fig. 6. ECG showing CPVT. (*Courtesy of* Dr van der Werf, Amsterdam, Netherlands and ECGpedia.org.)

A

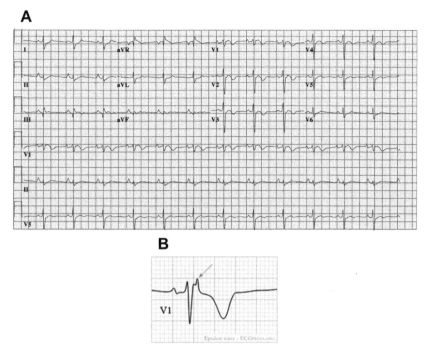

B

Fig. 7. (*A*) ARVD ECG: note the inverted T waves in the right precordial leads, late potentials (ε waves), widened QRS complex in right precordial leads and prolonged S wave upstroke in V1 >55 milliseconds (*B*) V1 shown with ε wave. (*Courtesy of* ECGpedia.org.)

enhanced cardiac MRI has high sensitivity and specificity in diagnosing this condition. Treatment is mostly supportive; however, a subset of patients develop dilated cardiomyopathy, which may require medical management or cardiac transplant. Patients should avoid all competitive sports for 6 months after the onset, and they should be evaluated for arrhythmias and residual cardiac dysfunction before resuming training and competition.

Wolff-Parkinson-White Syndrome

Wolff-Parkinson-White syndrome (WPW) is a result of an accessory pathway with both antegrade and retrograde conduction properties (**Fig. 8A**). Prevalence of WPW is estimated to be 1 to 3/1000 individuals, with an incidence of SCD of 0.2 to 15 per 1000 patient years.[28] The mechanism of SCD is rapid antegrade conduction over the accessory pathway in the setting of atrial fibrillation, resulting in VF. Any patient presenting with symptoms of palpitations or syncope who has irregular wide complex rhythm should be assumed to have atrial fibrillation with WPW (see **Fig. 8B**). Catheter ablation is a safe and usually effective treatment option. All patients who present with WPW, even if asymptomatic, should be referred to a pediatric cardiologist for risk assessment and further management.

Postoperative Arrhythmias in the Setting of Repaired Congenital Heart Defects

A major success story of pediatric cardiology is that more patients with complex congenital heart defects (CHD) survive into adulthood. Arrhythmogenic substrate created by the defect itself or from the surgery predisposes these patients to cardiac

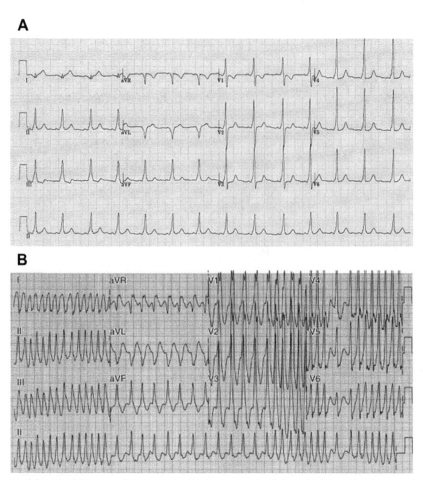

Fig. 8. (*A*) WPW ECG: note the pre-excitation or δ wave and short PR interval. (*B*) Pre-excited atrial fibrillation.

arrhythmias (**Fig. 9**). Patients with Senning/Mustard and Fontan procedures are likely to have atrial arrhythmias and sinus node dysfunction. Patients after tetralogy of Fallot repair are predisposed to both VT and atrial flutter. Heart block can occur after ventricular septal defect or AV canal repair. Any syncopal episode in a patient with previous cardiac history or surgery should be carefully evaluated for these arrhythmias, which can be hemodynamically compromising. Treatment of these dysrhythmias is complex and should be undertaken by a pediatric cardiologist.

Migraine

Migraines affect as much as 8.6% of the pediatric population.[29] Although commonly described as paroxysms of pain associated with nausea, vomiting, or abdominal pain and relieved by sleep, there are variants that can present with t-AMS; 3% of migraines are acute confusional migraines.[30] This diagnosis should be considered in patients with a family history of migraines, a personal history of migraines, or a concurrent headache. Episodes can last from a few minutes to hours. Treatments for this type

A

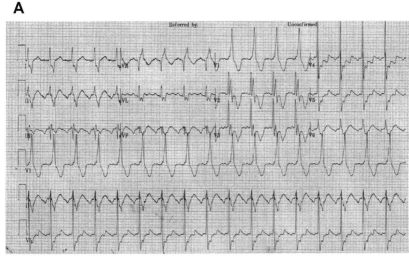

B

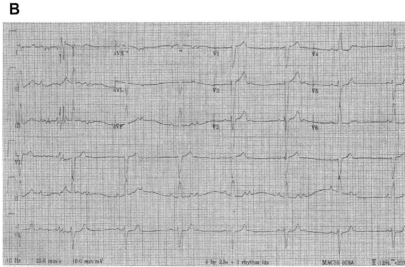

Fig. 9. (*A*) Atrial flutter in a 6-year-old patient after ventricular septal defect and interrupted aortic arch repair in infancy (*B*) Late complete heart block after AV canal repair in infancy.

of migraine are not well studied, given the rarity of the occurrence and because the diagnosis is made after return to baseline; however, 1 small study[31] implied that these episodes may be treatable with common migraine medications such as prochlorperazine.

Conversion

Conversion disorder and malingering are diagnoses of exclusion for patients who present with t-AMS. However, they are on the differential, especially in otherwise healthy adolescents, who present with recurrent syncopal episodes. The true incidences of these causes are unknown; however, in studies of patients referred for further evaluation, between 10% and 20% were believed to have psychogenic causes of t-AMS.[32,33] Historical clues that can help with this diagnosis include occurrence during times of secondary gain and lack of self-injury. Although the role of head-up tilt table testing is controversial in the evaluation of reflex syncope, it can be useful in evaluating for conversion. In reflex syncope, whe n the patient is tilted upright, their BP should decrease and they should experience a syncopal event. Conversely, conversion can be diagnosed if the patient experiences a syncopal event when tilted, without a corresponding change in BP.[34]

CAUSES FOR P-AMS
Infants and Young Children

As noted in the introduction, p-AMS occurs when the brain has a structural issue, an inadequate supply of oxygen, an imbalance in key electrolytes, inflammation from metabolic or infectious causes, or problems with the way electricity is conducted through the tissue. Because of their higher surface area/volume ratio and increased metabolic rate in combination with small glycogen stores and inefficient gluconeogenesis, infants are at higher risk for AMS from inadequate perfusion and hypoglycemia. This situation is true even from mild insults such as gastroenteritis, feeding intolerance, fevers, and so forth. In addition, the risk of direct infection of the central nervous system (CNS) is higher because of an immature immune system. Metabolic abnormalities are usually diagnosed at this time of life as well. Thus, the incidence of AMS is higher in infants.

Sepsis
When any young infant presents to a physician with a deviation from their normal activity, infection is always a concern. Sepsis alone in a neonate can cause AMS for several reasons: poor cerebral perfusion from distributive shock; insufficient glucose delivery to the brain from hypermetabolic state in the setting of low reserves; metabolic derangements such as severe metabolic acidosis, respiratory acidosis, or hyponatremia; and direct infectious involvement of the brain. Fever is not always present, even in the setting of overwhelming infection.

Inborn errors of metabolism
Most children who are born in hospitals in the United States undergo extensive testing for inborn errors of metabolism (IEM). Thus, it is not often that a clinician comes into contact with a previously undiagnosed problem. However, there are situations in which a child may have a metabolic disorder that is unknown, especially in the first few days of life, and it is imperative that clinicians think of IEM in infants who present with p-AMS. IEMs that present with AMS, especially in the first few days of life, are the organic acidemias or urea cycle disorders. These disorders of normal protein catabolism lead to profound acidosis or a buildup of neurotoxic ammonia. These infants present in the first few days/weeks of life with lethargy and vomiting. Rapid realization of the presence of an IEM, and prompt treatment, leads to marked improvement in morbidity and mortality.[35] Before initiation of treatment, evaluation of these patients should include blood and urine for amino acid levels, a comprehensive metabolic panel, blood gas, and ammonia level. Rapid initiation of treatment is paramount for survival and for optimal neurologic outcome. This treatment includes shutting down the catabolic state regardless of blood sugar with the administration of glucose-containing intravenous (IV) fluids. If the ammonia level is increased, the patient requires emergent hemodialysis.

Nonaccidental trauma
In infants and young children, the possibility of nonaccidental trauma (NAT) should always be considered. The incidence of inflicted brain injury in children younger than 2 years is slightly higher and associated with a worse outcome than that of accidental brain injury.[36,37] This situation can be challenging for practitioners, because these children may have few signs of external trauma. There may be associated symptoms and signs, such as irritability, focal neurologic deficits, or a bulging fontanel; however, these findings do not need to be present for clinicians to consider intracranial injury.[36] It is always important to consider NAT in an infant who presents with p-AMS, regardless of signs of trauma. Although judicious use of CT is always recommended, the exception comes in the evaluation for NAT, for which it is the most rapidly available and sensitive examination for acute intracranial hemorrhage. After ensuring that there is no acute neurosurgical emergency, if there is a concern for trauma, these infants should be admitted for skeletal surveys, retinal examinations, and potentially an MRI to evaluate for more subtle or chronic injuries.

Intussusception
The classic presentation of intussusception is an infant with colicky abdominal pain and bloody stool. However, AMS and hypotonia are well-described presenting symptoms; in 1 study,[38] 19% of all patients with intussusception presented with lethargy or somnolence. Although intussusception can occur in older patients, AMS is a presenting symptom more commonly seen in the infant age group. One theory for this finding is endogenous opioid release causing AMS.[39] Infants with intussusception who present with AMS often have symptoms of gastrointestinal illness, such as vomiting, irritability, abdominal pain, melena, or palpable mass. In the evaluations of patients for intussusception, ultrasonography has proved to be a readily available, safe, and sensitive tool. If findings are positive, patients should receive a therapeutic air enema performed by a radiologist.[40]

Infections (shigellosis)
One of the known complications of shigellosis is seizure or encephalopathy not secondary to CNS infection or as a direct effect of the Shiga toxin. In 1 study of 71 pediatric patients with *Shigella* infections, 9% were unconscious and 5% had documented seizure. Children with AMS tended to have shorter durations of illness, higher fevers, more severe dehydration, and lower serum sodium levels.[41,42] Diagnosing *Shigella* involves isolation of the bacteria from the stool or blood. Although shigellosis is usually a mild, self-limited disease, presentation with AMS should be treated with antibiotics. Although resistance is increasing, first-line therapy includes trimethoprim-sulfamethoxazole or ampicillin.[43]

Encephalitis
Encephalitis means inflammation of the brain. Although encephalitis is often thought of as an infectious process, there are also parainfectious and inflammatory causes. Infectious causes cause direct pathogen-mediated cell death and mechanical injury, and both infectious and parainfectious causes can cause immune-mediated effects, including demyelination and neurotransmitter disturbances. Fever is not always present, even with a later confirmed infectious source.[44] Emergent lumbar puncture and initiation of broad-spectrum antibiotics and antivirals are indicated in encephalopathic patients in whom infection is a concern. When the meninges are involved, patients can have associated headache, photophobia, and stiff neck; however, when they are not inflamed, these helpful clues may be absent. Thus, encephalitis must always be considered as a cause of p-AMS. Acute demyelinating

encephalomyelitis is a well-described cause of noninfectious encephalitis. It is most commonly described after an antecedent infection, and it can present with or without fever. It is a diagnosis made by MRI after negative serologic evaluation.

Seizure

Seizures are common, with an annual incidence of 84 per 100,000 persons, half of whom go on to develop epilepsy.[45] Although epilepsy is a complex diagnosis, with many subtypes and presentations, the focus of this section is nonconvulsive status epilepticus (NCSE) and the postictal state. NCSE can be difficult to identify clinically. These patients can present with stable AMS and a waxing and waning mental status or be critically ill. In 1 pediatric retrospective study,[45] the incidence of NCSE in patients with AMS was 14%. Although NCSE is most common in patients with a known seizure disorder, it should be considered in all children with AMS without obvious traumatic, metabolic, structural, or infectious cause. Emergent bedside EEG is the diagnostic study of choice, and treatment should include antiepileptic drugs and potentially barbiturate anesthesia.[46] A prolonged postictal state is also a consideration in patients with p-AMS.[47] Prolonged postictal states can persist for days, especially in patients who have had multiple complex seizures, who have developmental delay or cortical abnormalities, and in those with underlying psychiatric diagnoses.[48]

Metabolic derangement (glucose, sodium)

Abnormal blood glucose levels, high or low, can cause AMS. In the case of hypoglycemia, there are 2 mechanisms for this process: autonomic dysfunction and neuroglycopenia. Although the most common cause of hypoglycemia in older children is a misadventure with insulin, in younger infants, increased metabolic rate and metabolic stresses such as infections or dehydration can lead to profound hypoglycemia. In hyperglycemic patients with diabetic ketoacidosis (DKA), AMS from cerebral edema is an ominous sign. It occurs in only 1% of episodes of DKA but it has a high mortality (20%–50%).[49] The mechanism of this AMS is believed to be secondary to a combination of multiple metabolic abnormalities, including dehydration and decreased cerebral perfusion caused by circulatory collapse; acidosis; hyperosmolality; and decreased glucose use by cerebral tissue.[50,51] Treatment of this disorder involves careful insulin administration and restoration of euvolemia.

Because brain volume is regulated by equal osmolality of intracellular and extracellular sodium, rapid changes in sodium, most commonly hyponatremia, can cause p-AMS. In children, the cause of hyponatremia can come from total fluid losses (gastroenteritis, postoperative), excessive sodium loss from the kidneys (mineralocorticoid deficiency, cerebral salt wasting), excessive water retention by the kidneys (SIADH [syndrome of inappropriate antidiuretic hormone secretion]), or conditions in which there is excessive free water (cirrhosis, nephritic syndrome, or heart failure).[52] Young children are at increased risk of hyponatremic encephalopathy secondary to a larger brain/intracranial volume ratio, with less room for swelling.[52] The correct historical clues, in the presence of p-AMS and marked hyponatremia, are diagnostic for this condition. Normalization of sodium levels is critical but must be performed carefully and slowly to avoid rapid osmotic shifts.

Intracranial tumor/mass

Space-occupying lesions of the brain, whether blood or a mass or a combination, cause depressed level of consciousness by the same mechanism. There can be mass effect, which directly increases intracranial pressure, obstruction of drainage of the cerebral spinal fluid, or acute herniation.[53] It is critical for physicians to consider stroke in children, in whom the incidence equals that of brain tumor (2/100,000).[54] Half of strokes are hemorrhagic, and 50% of those present with AMS.[55] Imaging with CT is the first step in diagnostic testing and should be followed by emergent neurosurgical consultation.

Posterior reversible encephalopathy syndrome

Posterior reversible encephalopathy syndrome (PRES), formally hypertensive encephalopathy, is an increasingly recognized disease thanks to the ready availability of MRI studies. PRES occurs when acute hypertension exceeds the vasoconstrictive and regulatory processes in the brain, causing a vasogenic edema. Patients can present with headache, seizure, and AMS. In children, there is often an underlying cause; nephrotic syndrome, Henoch-Schönlein purpura, and therapies for malignancies are some of the many culprits.[56] The treatment of PRES includes cessation of offending agents and prompt management of BP.

APPROACH TO THE PATIENT WITH TRANSIENT AMS
Patient History

Accurate, detailed, and thorough history is the most important part of the evaluation of a patient presenting to the ED with t-AMS and should establish the diagnosis correctly. Every effort should be made to obtain a direct history from the eyewitnesses, asking questions pertaining to circumstances before the attack, about the actual episode and details of events after the episode. An age-based approach to patients with t-AMS is critical to avoid excessive workups and not miss any life-threatening causes. In neonates, one should consider sepsis and ask about sick contacts, group B β *Streptococcus* status of the mother, and temperature instability. A broad family history is important (**Box 3C**). Indicators of seizure include abnormal movements, eye rolling, and a postictal period. As the patient enters toddlerhood, BHSs enter into the differential. The clinician needs to ask about temporal proximity to an emotionally stressful event or minor trauma. A patient or family history of migraines can point a clinician toward an atypical or acute confusional migraine.

An important distinction to make for the diagnostic workup is whether this event was true syncope and if so, was it a common, benign reflex syncope episode or a more ominous cause. Many of the children with cardiovascular disorder who go on to experience SCA have syncope or presyncope as a warning symptom. Identifying this small subset amongst all patients who present with syncope is difficult. See **Box 3** for historical features that can help differentiate benign neurally mediated syncope from cardiac syncope. In contrast to reflex syncope, which is often triggered by specific events and has premonitory symptoms, individuals with syncope from a cardiac disorder at risk for SCA usually have an abrupt collapse without warning, because of the onset of a potentially lethal ventricular arrhythmia. Syncope occurring during exercise is an ominous sign and warrants a high index of suspicion for underlying cardiac disease. Distinguishing between neurocardiogenic syncope and seizures is a common clinical dilemma faced by care providers. **Table 2** provides diagnostic clues differentiating syncope from seizure. A careful history of the event and details of the past medical and family history should eliminate most of the causes of cardiac syncope.

Physical Examination

After an episode of t-AMS, the patient likely has a normal physical examination. As with all physical examinations, careful attention must be paid to the vital signs. Hypothermia as well as hyperthermia can be indications of sepsis in neonates. Heart rate and BP should be compared with age-appropriate norms. Neurologic examination

> **Box 3**
> **Historical features that may help differentiate reflex syncope versus cardiac syncope.**
> (*A*) Clinical feature of neurally mediated syncope; (*B*) clinical features of cardiac syncope; and
> (*C*) family history features concerning for cardiac syncope
>
> A. Reflex syncope
>   1. Long history of recurrent syncope
>   2. Absence of heart disease
>   3. Typical triggers (**Table 2**) such as prolonged standing in hot, crowded places
>   4. After exertion
>   5. With head rotation or pressure on carotid sinus (tight collars, shaving, backing up a car)
>   6. Associated with nausea or vomiting
>   7. Prodrome of lightheadedness, dizziness, diaphoresis, nausea, and tunnel vision
>
> B. Cardiac syncope: red flags
>   1. Presence of heart disease or previous cardiac surgery
>   2. Family history of hereditary cardiomyopathy or channelopathy (**Box 2**)
>   3. Sudden onset of palpitation, shortness of breath, or chest pain followed by syncope
>   4. Episodes during exertion, swimming, or supine
>   5. ECG abnormality
>   6. Episodes brought on by sudden startle or loud noise such as alarm clock (LQTS)
>   7. Acute or subacute history of febrile illness, exercise intolerance, or fatigue (cardiomyopathy, myocarditis)
>   8. Abrupt syncope with no premonitory symptoms
>   9. Injury with syncope
>   10. Event triggers: extreme emotional stress (LQTS)
>   11. Young age at presentation (<10 years of age, especially <6 years of age)
>   12. Unexplained seizure in the past
>
> C. Cardiac syncope: red flags in the family history
>   1. Sudden unexpected unexplained death at a young age (<30 years)
>   2. Unexplained fainting spells or seizures
>   3. Unexplained driving or drowning accidents
>   4. Sudden infant death syndrome
>   5. Congenital deafness
>   6. Hereditary cardiomyopathies (HCM, dilated cardiomyopathy, ARVD)
>   7. Hereditary channelopathies (LQTS, Brugada, CPVT, short QTS)
>   8. Pacemaker or defibrillator implants at a young age
>   9. Marfan syndrome

can be difficult in young infants; careful attention to development, tone, and pupil examination is a must. Cardiovascular examination should focus on evaluation for dysrhythmia and murmurs. Because infants with ALTEs have a higher frequency of NAT, these patients should be examined from head to toe to evaluate for other signs

Table 2
Clinical clues helpful in differentiating syncope from seizures

	Syncope	Seizure
Triggers	Typical	Rarely (flashing lights)
Prodrome/aura	1. Sweating and pallor 2. Nausea, vomiting, and abdominal discomfort 3. Lightheadedness, blurring	1. Rising sensation in abdomen 2. Smell
Movements	1. Last few seconds, <15 s 2. Asynchronous 3. Nonrhythmical 4. After fall and unconsciousness	1. Last ~1 min 2. Synchronous 3. Rhythmical 4. Before fall
Flaccidity	Often complete	Unlikely
Tongue bite	1. Rare 2. Middle	1. Common 2. On the side
Recovery	1. Immediate clear headedness 2. Nausea, vomiting and pallor	1. Prolonged confusion 2. Muscle aches and headaches

Adapted from Moya A, Sutton R, Ammirati F, et al, The Task Force for the Diagnosis and Management of Syncope, European Society of Cardiology (ESC). Guidelines for the diagnosis and management of syncope (version 2009). Eur Heart J 2009;30(21):2655; with permission.

of trauma. Physical examination is unremarkable in all cases of reflex syncope and most cases of cardiac syncope. However, clinical features (detailed in **Box 4**) can impart important diagnostic clues to a potentially serious cause of syncope.

Imaging and Additional Testing

In neonates, a full septic evaluation should be considered if there are any changes from normal behavior. If there is concern for NAT, if there are any neurologic abnormalities on examination, or if the patient has any complaint of headache, a CT scan of the head should be performed. A finger-stick glucose measurement is obtained for many patients who present after an episode of t-AMS; however, this is unlikely to be helpful, because a patient who has returned to baseline is unlikely to be persistently hypoglycemic. Hemoglobin should be measured to diagnose anemia, and a urine pregnancy test in the adolescent female is mandatory. Although the workup for an ALTE is controversial, and beyond the scope of this article, an ECG should be obtained to evaluate for dysrhythmia potential.

Box 4
Physical examination findings that indicate cardiovascular cause of syncope

Key points to assess and to look for in physical examination

1. Heart rate and orthostatic BP

2. Sternotomy scar points toward past cardiac surgery, device pocket

3. Right ventricular heave with loud second heart sound suggest pulmonary hypertension

4. Gallop heard in dilated cardiomyopathy and congestive heart failure

5. Midsystolic murmur that increases in intensity with standing suggestive of HCM

6. Systolic murmur of aortic stenosis

7. Tumor plop of left atrial myxoma

Careful clinician judgment has to be used when considering imaging, because all modalities carry some inherent risks. CT exposes children to radiation and should be reserved for concerns of trauma or intracranial bleeding. For other possible intracranial causes of t-AMS, MRI might be a better option, because of its increased sensitivity for small and posterior lesions, keeping in mind that in young children, this test requires sedation and cannot be performed quickly.

The single most clinically useful and cost-effective test to evaluate syncope is the 12-lead ECG (**Box 5**). All patients presenting to the ED with syncope should receive ECG with a rhythm strip. In 1 review of 480 pediatric patients who presented with syncope,[57] a cardiac cause for syncope was identified in 22 patients (5%), 21 of whom were identified by an abnormal history (exercise-induced syncope or family history of sudden death), physical examination, or ECG. If the history and physical examination are typical for neurocardiogenic syncope and the ECG is normal, further testing generally is not needed.

Referral to a pediatric cardiologist should be for atypical history, red flags, abnormal ECG, and abnormal murmurs, as detailed in **Boxes 3–5**. Additional testing may include continuous in-hospital ECG monitoring when the patient is at high risk for a life-threatening arrhythmia, Holter monitoring, loop recorders, and echocardiography to assess for cardiac function and structural abnormalities. The role of tilt table testing is debatable, because of issues of low reproducibility and a high false-negative rate. Exercise stress testing is important in evaluating exertional syncope. An electrophysiology study may sometimes be indicated in patients with structural heart disease.

APPROACH TO THE PATIENT WITH P-AMS
Patient History

As with any initial presentation, physicians must assess the patient for respiratory and cardiovascular stability and they must establish a Glasgow Coma Score if trauma is considered. Once the patient has been stabilized, the provider can move on to a more detailed history and physical examination. In infants, key questions focus on signs or symptoms of infection (fever, sick contacts, cough, coryza, vomiting, diarrhea, and rashes), a family history, and a birth history to evaluate for the potential of

---

Box 5
ECG abnormalities to look for in a patient presenting with syncope

1. LVH, ST/T wave abnormality

2. Nonsustained VT

3. Wide QRS (left bundle branch block, right bundle branch block, bifascicular block, intraventricular conduction delay)

4. Bradycardia, AV block, or prolonged pauses

5. Corrected QT interval to assess for LQTS, short QT syndrome

6. δ wave suggestive of WPW

7. Right bundle branch block + ST elevation in V1 to V3 (Brugada)

8. Negative T waves in right precordial leads and ε waves suggestive of arrhythmogenic right ventricular cardiomyopathy

9. Q waves suggesting myocardial infarction, HCM

undiagnosed IEM, and a delicate scrutiny for NAT. Questions regarding abdominal pain, vomiting, and character of stool are also important when evaluating an older infant for intussusception.

As the patient gets older, encephalitides becomes a more common possibility. Again, toxicologic causes of AMS are beyond the scope of this article but should be considered. Infectious symptoms should be elicited, as previously described in infants, and special care should be taken to elicit clues that suggest a diagnosis of PRES, nonclinical status epilepticus, DKA, or hypoglycemia. Recent history of head trauma or headaches should alert the clinician that a space-occupying lesion may be present in the brain, whether blood, mass, or excessive CSF.

Physical Examination

The most critical portion of the physical examination in a patient with AMS is careful evaluation of the vital signs. Primarily, the clinician needs to focus on adequate respirations (with normal respiratory rate and oxygen saturations) and perfusion (evaluation of pulses, heart rate, and BP). Fever can be a marker of both infectious cause as well as intracranial disease. Hypertension is concerning for PRES or increased intracranial pressure and tachypnea can indicate profound hyperglycemia. Once the patient has been stabilized, a careful neurologic, cardiovascular, and respiratory examination should be performed. The neurologic examination may be limited with an uncooperative, altered or comatose patient, and small focal neurologic deficits can be missed. Once airway, breathing, and circulation are established to be stable, the physician should consider the diagnostic workup while examining the patient. A change in mental status requires prompt and efficient assessment and evaluation, rather than a standard linear approach to history taking and physical examination, with subsequent testing.

Imaging and Additional Testing

Although the clinician obtains many clues in the history and physical examination, these patients usually require extensive diagnostic testing as well as admission to the hospital. Blood glucose must be measured. All abnormalities should be addressed before moving on to the next stage of the evaluation. If an infectious cause is on the differential, especially in a young infant, cultures should be obtained quickly, such that IV antibiotics can be administered as quickly as possible. Thus, blood counts, blood cultures, urinalysis, urine cultures, and CSF for cell count, Gram stain, protein, glucose, and culture should all be obtained. Timely administration of antibiotics should not await successful lumbar puncture.

Unlike patients with t-AMS, all patients who present with p-AMS should have emergent imaging of the head. Unless the AMS clears with the administration of glucose, even a hypoglycemic patient should receive imaging because one never knows if the patient sustained an injury while altered. Whether the lumbar puncture should await normal head CT is controversial and outside the scope of this article.

If there is concern for an inborn error of metabolism, blood for a serum ammonia, amino acid levels as well as urine for organic acids need to be obtained before the administration of dextrose, because this may alter the results. If intussusception is on the differential, the evaluation can include a plain film radiograph series, ultrasonography of the abdomen, or in cases of high pretest probability, a prompt enema by a radiologist that is both diagnostic and therapeutic. To evaluate for nonclinical status epilepticus, an EEG is required.

SUMMARY

Although AMS, transient or persistent, can cause a great deal of anxiety for patients and providers, a rational approach to these patients is essential to avoid underuse or excessive use of testing. An age-based approach is important, because the various diseases are common in different age groups. In patients with t-AMS, differentiating true syncope from other causes is the first step; a stepwise approach, guided by the history and physical examination can then proceed. p-AMS, on the other hand, is a life-threatening presentation, and time is of the essence. The differential diagnosis is broad and, rather than trying to recall long lists of highly specific causes, it is more helpful to consider broad categories of disease: structural lesions, insufficient delivery of appropriate substrate to the brain, metabolic imbalance, inflammation, infection, and abnormal electrical activity. Maintaining a broad differential and evaluating for multiple diseases simultaneously is critical in the care of these patients.

REFERENCES

1. McGovern MC, Smith MB. Causes of apparent life-threatening events in infants: a systematic review. Arch Dis Child 2004;89:1043–8.
2. Altman RL, Brand DA, Forman S, et al. Abusive head injury as a cause of apparent life-threatening events in infancy. Arch Pediatr Adolesc Med 2003; 157:1011–5.
3. DiMario FJ Jr. Breath-holding spells in childhood. Am J Dis Child 1992;146: 125–31.
4. Breningstall GN. Breath-holding spells. Pediatr Neurol 1996;14:91–7.
5. Walsh M, Knilans TK, Anderson JB, et al. Successful treatment of pallid breath-holding spells with fluoxetine. Pediatrics 2012;130:e685–9.
6. Russ SA, Larson K, Halfon N. A national profile of childhood epilepsy and seizure disorder. Pediatrics 2012;129:256–64.
7. Huff JS, Morris DL. Emergency department management of patients with seizures: a multicenter study. Acad Emerg Med 2001;8:622–8.
8. Covanis A. Panayiotopoulos syndrome: a benign childhood autonomic epilepsy frequently imitating encephalitis, syncope, migraine, sleep disorder or gastroenteritis. Pediatrics 2006;118:e1237–43.
9. Moya A, Sutton R, Ammirati F, et al. Guidelines for the diagnosis and management of syncope (version 2009). Eur Heart J 2009;30:2631–71.
10. Anderson JB, Czosek RJ, Cnota J, et al. Pediatric syncope: National Hospital Ambulatory Medical Care Survey results. J Emerg Med 2012;43:575–83.
11. Colman N, Nahm K, Ganzeboom KS, et al. Epidemiology of reflex syncope. Clin Auton Res 2004;14:i9–17.
12. Drezner JA, Fudge J, Harmon KG, et al. Warning symptoms and family history in children and young adults with sudden cardiac arrest. J Am Board Fam Med 2012;25:408–15.
13. Driscoll DJ, Jacobsen SJ, Porter CJ, et al. Syncope in children and adolescents. J Am Coll Cardiol 1997;29:1039–45.
14. Maron BJ, Shirani LC, Poliac LC. Sudden death in young competitive athletes: clinical, demographic, and pathologic profiles. JAMA 1996;276:199–204.
15. Colivicchi F, Ammirati F, Santini F. Epidemiology and prognostic implications of syncope in young competing athletes. Eur Heart J 2004;25:1749–53.
16. Maron BJ, Doerer JJ, Haas TS, et al. Sudden deaths in young competitive athletes: analysis of 1866 deaths in the United States, 1980-2006. Circulation 2009; 119:1085–92.

17. Davis JA, Cecchin F, Jones TK, et al. Major coronary artery anomalies in a pediatric population: incidence and clinical importance. J Am Coll Cardiol 2001; 37:593–7.
18. Basso C, Maron BJ, Corrado D, et al. Clinical profile of congenital coronary artery anomalies with origin from the wrong aortic sinus leading to sudden death in young competitive athletes. J Am Coll Cardiol 2000;35:1493–501.
19. Puranik R, Chow CK, Duflou JA, et al. Sudden death in the young. Heart Rhythm 2005;2:1277–82.
20. Corrado D, Basso C, Pavei A, et al. Trends in sudden cardiovascular death in young competitive athletes after implementation of a preparticipation screening program. JAMA 2006;296:1593–600.
21. Maron BJ, Doerer JJ, Haas TS, et al. Profile and frequency of sudden death in 1463 young competitive athletes: from a 25 year US national registry: 1980-2005. Circulation 2006;114:830.
22. Zipes DP, Ackerman MJ, Estes NA III, et al. Task Force 7: arrhythmias. J Am Coll Cardiol 2005;45:1354–63.
23. Van Dorn CS, Johnson JN, Taggart NW, et al. QTc values among children and adolescents presenting to the emergency department. Pediatrics 2011;128:1395–401.
24. Shalem T, Goldman M, Breitbart R, et al. Orthostatic hypotension in children with acute febrile illness. J Emerg Med 2013;44:23–7.
25. Napolitano C, Priori SG. Diagnosis and treatment of catecholaminergic polymorphic ventricular tachycardia. Heart Rhythm 2007;4:675–8.
26. Corrado D, Basso C, Thiene G. Arrhythmogenic right ventricular cardiomyopathy: an update. Heart 2009;95:766–73.
27. Maron BJ, Pelliccia A, Spirito P. Cardiac disease in young trained athletes. Circulation 1995;91:1596–601.
28. Cohen MI, Triedman JK, Cannon BC, et al. PACES/HRS expert consensus statement on the management of the asymptomatic young patient with a Wolff-Parkinson-White (WPW, ventricular preexcitation) electrocardiographic pattern. Heart Rhythm 2012;9:1006–24.
29. Lee LH, Olness KN. Clinical and demographic characteristics of migraine in urban children. Headache 1997;37:269–76.
30. Pacheva I, Ivanov I. Acute confusional migraine: is it a distinct form of migraine? Int J Clin Pract 2013;67:250–6.
31. Khatri R, Hershey AD, Wong B. Prochlorperazine treatment for acute confusional migraine. Headache 2009;49:477–80.
32. Grubb BP, Gerard G, Wolfe DA, et al. Syncope and seizures of psychogenic origin: identification with head-upright tilt table testing. Clin Cardiol 1992;15:839–42.
33. Hindley D, Ali A, Robson C. Diagnoses made in a secondary care "fits, faints, and funny turns" clinic. Arch Dis Child 2006;91:214–8.
34. Benditt DG, Sutton R. Tilt-table testing in the evaluation of syncope. J Cardiovasc Electrophysiol 2005;16:356–8.
35. Burton BK. Inborn errors of metabolism in infancy: a guide to diagnosis. Pediatrics 1998;102:e69.
36. Gerber P, Coffman K. Nonaccidental head trauma in infants. Childs Nerv Syst 2007;23:499–507.
37. Newton AW, Vandeven AM. Update on child maltreatment. Curr Opin Pediatr 2008;20:205–12.
38. Luks FI, Yazbeck S, Perreault G, et al. Changes in the presentation of intussusception. Am J Emerg Med 1992;10:574–6.

39. Tenenbein M, Wiseman NE. Early coma in intussusception: endogenous opioid induced. Pediatr Emerg Care 1987;3:22–3.
40. Mandeville K, Chien M, Willyerd FA, et al. Intussusception: clinical presentations and imaging characteristics. Pediatr Emerg Care 2012;28:842–4.
41. Khan WA, Dhar U, Salam MA, et al. Central nervous system manifestations of childhood shigellosis: prevalence, risk factors, and outcome. Pediatrics 1999; 103:E18.
42. Goldberg EM, Balamuth F, Desrochers CR, et al. Seizure and altered mental status in a 12-year-old child with *Shigella sonnei* gastroenteritis. Pediatr Emerg Care 2011;27:135–7.
43. Shigella. In: Pickering LK, Baker C, Kimberlin DW, et al, editors. Red Book: 2012 Report of the Committee on Infectious Disease. Elk Grove Village (IL): American Academy of Pediatrics; 2012. p. 645–6.
44. Falchek SJ. Encephalitis in the pediatric population. Pediatr Rev 2012;33: 122–33.
45. Slattery DE, Pollack CV. Seizures as a cause of altered mental status. Emerg Med Clin North Am 2010;28:517–34.
46. Wilkes T, Tasker RC. Pediatric intensive care of uncontrolled status epilepticus. Crit Care Clin 2013;29(2):239–57.
47. Biton V, Gates J, DaPadua Sussman L. Prolonged post-ictal encephalopathy. Neurology 1990;40:963.
48. Krauss G, Theodore WH. Treatment strategies in the postictal state. Epilepsy Behav 2010;19:188–90.
49. Brown TB. Cerebral oedema in childhood diabetic ketoacidosis: is treatment a factor. Emerg Med J 2004;21:141–4.
50. Nyenwe EZ, Razavi LN. Acidosis: the prime determinant of depressed sensorium in diabetic ketoacidosis. Diabetes Care 2010;33:1837–9.
51. Levin DL. Cerebral edema in diabetic ketoacidosis. Pediatr Crit Care Med 2009; 10:429.
52. Moritz ML, Ayus JC. The pathophysiology and treatment of hyponatraemic encephalopathy: an update. Nephrol Dial Transplant 2003;18:2486–91.
53. Snyder H, Robinson K, Shah D, et al. Signs and symptoms of patients with brain tumors presenting to the emergency department. J Emerg Med 1993;11:253–8.
54. Jordan LC, Hillis AE. Hemorrhagic stroke in children. Pediatr Neurol 2007;36: 73–80.
55. Yock-Corrales A, Mackay MT, Mosley I, et al. Acute childhood arterial ischemic and hemorrhagic stroke in the emergency department. Ann Emerg Med 2011; 58:156–63.
56. Endo A, Fuchigami T, Hasegawa M, et al. Posterior reversible encephalopathy syndrome in children: report of four cases and review of the literature. Pediatr Emerg Care 2012;28:153–7.
57. Ritter S, Tani LY, Etheridge SP. What is the yield of screening echocardiography in pediatric syncope? Pediatrics 2000;105:e58.

Updates in the General Approach to Pediatric Head Trauma and Concussion

Shireen M. Atabaki, MD, MPH

KEYWORDS

- Traumatic brain injury • Prediction rules • Computed tomography
- Intracranial hemorrhage • Concussion

KEY POINTS

- Head trauma and concussion are the cause of significant morbidity and mortality in childhood and are an important public health concern, increasing in incidence worldwide.
- Acute recognition and management of traumatic brain injury along the spectrum from mild to severe is essential in optimizing neurocognitive outcomes and preventing long-term sequelae in children.
- A thorough history and physical examination is the foundation for the acute diagnosis of head trauma, and has recently been incorporated into validated risk stratification to reduce unnecessary imaging and associated radiation and costs.
- Knowledge translation and widespread dissemination of these prediction rules for pediatric head trauma is the next step to obviate unnecessary computed tomography (CT) scans in children.
- Children with blunt head trauma and normal cranial CT results generally do not require hospitalization for neurologic observation.

INTRODUCTION

A 12-year-old boy is brought into the Emergency Department (ED) of the local community hospital by ambulance, following a rollover motor vehicle collision. The patient had a brief loss of consciousness and presents with mild headache and amnesia for the event. Emergency physicians order a computed tomography (CT) scan of the head. The head CT is normal, and the patient is discharged home and told to follow up with his pediatrician. One week later the child returns to school and complains of headache while playing basketball; he is removed from the field and brought to the ED by his parents, where a decision is made to obtain a head CT to rule out intracranial

Division of Emergency Medicine, Department of Pediatrics and Emergency Medicine, Children's National Medical Center, 111 Michigan Avenue Northwest, Washington, DC 20010-1970, USA
E-mail address: satabaki@cnmc.org

Pediatr Clin N Am 60 (2013) 1107–1122
http://dx.doi.org/10.1016/j.pcl.2013.06.001
0031-3955/13/$ – see front matter © 2013 Elsevier Inc. All rights reserved.

hemorrhage. The scenario described is not uncommon, despite emerging evidence and guidelines for imaging and concussion management for children with head trauma.

Traumatic brain injury (TBI) is an important public health concern in children. There are 1.4 million patients with TBI evaluated and discharged from EDs annually in the United States.[1] Of these, nearly half are children or young adults younger than 19 years.[1] This figure may represent the tip of the iceberg, as it is believed that up to 5 million patients incur TBI that is often neither recognized nor treated. The head is the most frequently injured area in a child, and the most common causes of TBI in the pediatric population are falls and motor vehicle collisions.[1,2] TBI is also the most common cause of death following childhood injury. Football is the most common sport associated with TBI and with more than 1 million football players in the United States, many of whom are high school and collegiate players, it has evolved into an important area of national focus.[3] Emergency physicians have become astute in the diagnosis of severe and moderate TBI. However, as described in the vignette for the 12-year-old patient, the evaluation and management of mild TBI (mTBI) is an area in need of knowledge translation.

This article discusses the general approach to pediatric head trauma, skull fracture, and TBI along the continuum from mild to severe. The focus is on updates to diagnostic and management modalities, including some of the most recent evidence-based medicine guidelines and research. The article begins with mTBI, as this is the area harboring the most advances in recognition and management.

CONCUSSION/MILD TBI
Description

The Centers for Disease Control and Prevention (CDC) use the term mTBI, which accounts for 88% to 92% of cases of TBI, interchangeably with the term concussion.

> mTBI or concussion is defined as a complex pathophysiologic process affecting the brain, induced by traumatic biomechanical forces secondary to direct or indirect forces to the head. mTBI is caused by a blow or jolt to the head that disrupts the function of the brain. mTBI results in a constellation of physical, cognitive, emotional and sleep-related symptoms. Duration of symptoms is variable and may last as long as several days, weeks, months or even longer in some cases.[4]

This disturbance of brain function is typically associated with neurometabolic dysfunction with normal structural anatomy. The neurometabolic cascade following concussion consists of calcium influx, increase in glucose consumption, and increased metabolic demand.[5]

Concussion can result in a variety of physical, cognitive, emotional, and sleep-related symptoms lasting from days to months. **Table 1** lists these symptoms, including those most concerning, such as depression and anxiety. Unrecognized and poorly managed concussion can result in postconcussion syndrome, with duration of symptoms lasting beyond 2 weeks and up to several months.[6] Research has demonstrated promise in early intervention and a program of graduated return to play, sport, and school work for youth with concussion.[7–9]

Evaluation

The history and physical examination is the cornerstone of the diagnosis of concussion. Psychometrically validated concussion-screening tools based on the history and physical examination such as the Acute Concussion Evaluation (ACE) are effective, and have been coupled with management or "concussion care plans" available

Table 1			
Concussion symptom checklist			
Physical	**Cognitive**	**Emotional**	**Sleep**
Headache	Feeling mentally foggy	Irritability	Drowsiness
Nausea	Feeling slowed down	Sadness	Sleeping less than usual
Vomiting	Difficulty concentrating	More emotional	Sleeping more than usual
Balance problems	Difficulty remembering	Nervousness	Trouble falling asleep
Dizziness			
Visual problems			
Fatigue			
Sensitivity to light			
Sensitivity to noise			
Numbness			
Tingling			

Adapted from Centers for Disease Control and Prevention. Heads up: brain injury in your practice. Available at: http://www.cdc.gov/concussion/HeadsUp/physicians_tool_kit.html.

as head injury toolkits on the CDC Web site at http://www.cdc.gov/concussion/ HeadsUp/physicians_tool_kit.html.[4] A recent study found that very few EDs use any form of concussion screening in the evaluation of pediatric head trauma.[10] It was noted that very few of the EDs surveyed had adequate patient education for the management of concussion. The CDC has established an effective Web site to make these concussion toolkits available to physicians, patients, parents, school personnel, and coaches,[4] and has supported the work of investigators to adapt a previously psychometrically validated concussion-screening tool (the ACE) for use in the ED as the ACE-ED.[10] Current work is ongoing to incorporate these concussion-screening tools into the electronic health record and normal workflow to initiate assessment of children with head trauma at the time of triage.

Sports Concussion

There are 1.1 million high school football players in the United States each year, of whom nearly 70,000 are diagnosed with concussion.[11] However, it is widely believed that concussion is more prevalent in high school football. McCrea and colleagues[12] found that although 30% of high school football players stated that they had a previous history of concussion, fewer than half had reported the injury. Reasons for failure to report concussions included lack of awareness that a concussion had been sustained and lack of understanding of the potentially serious nature of injury.

Recent media attention has focused on the fact that high school football players may be reluctant to report concussion because of fear of being removed from competition[13] and loss of athletic scholarships http://www.npr.org/2012/08/07/158361384/ love-of-sports-can-start-early-so-can-injuries.

Education of student athletes and parents on the impact of unrecognized and poorly managed concussion is extremely valuable, and should be a discussion the medical provider initiates at the time of the acute evaluation in the ED, at school, or on the field.

Legislation and Return-to-Play

Since 2009, 43 states and the District of Columbia have implemented legislation for concussion management in youth athletics with established return-to-play guidelines. If a student athlete is suspected to have a concussion, the athlete is removed from play and requires clearance, in most cases from a licensed medical professional, to return to play. The recommendation is for those on the sidelines such as coaches and athletic trainers to pull a child from the field when concussion is suspected and to have the player "sit it out, if in doubt." The reasons for this proactive removal from play are to:

- Allow for healing
- Prevent "second-impact syndrome," a serious diffuse axonal injury resulting in uncal herniation[14]
- Prevent neurocognitive sequelae of reinjury[15]

In addition to restrictions on physical activity, both the American Academy of Pediatrics and Zurich Consensus Statement on Concussion in Sport recommend limitation of scholastic and other cognitive activities for athletes following concussion (**Table 2**).[16,17]

In addition, concussed players who continue to play are at increased risk of reinjury, have delayed symptom onset, and neuropsychological deficits.[18,19]

Whereas prior return-to-play guidelines for concussion were based on static measures such as duration of loss of consciousness, current stepwise recommendations for return to play are individualized and include[17]:

- Resolution of symptoms
- Return to baseline neurocognitive function

Subconcussive Injury

Talavage and colleagues[19] were the first to present evidence of subconcussive injury in a cohort of high school football players. This prospective study using head-impact telemetry, neurocognitive testing, and functional magnetic resonance imaging uncovered functionally detected cognitive impairment in high school football players with repetitive head trauma, without clinically diagnosed concussion. This finding raises concern for athletes who suffer subconcussive impact, and highlights the need for safety regulations in high-impact sports.

Table 2
Return-to-play guidelines for pediatric sport concussion

	Restrictions	Return to Play
Physical rest	No sports No weight training No cardiovascular training No Physical Education No bike riding	Clearance by Licensed Independent Practitioner (LIP) or concussion expert If symptom-free at rest and exertion Pass neurocognitive and balance assessment
Cognitive rest	No homework Shortened school day No reading No video games, computers, cell phones, or texting No television No travel Increased rest and sleep	Able to complete symptom-limited exercise program No same-day return to play!

Immediate removal of athlete from play recommended if any sign or symptom of concussion is witnessed.

Adapted from The Zurich Consensus Statement, an international conference of concussion experts, McCrory P, Meeuwisse, Aubry M, et al. Consensus statement on concussion in sport: the 4th International Conference on Concussion in Sport held in Zurich, November 2012. Br J Sports Med 2013;47:250–8; with permission.

Changes in Sports Regulation and Techniques

Student athletes participating in collision sports such as football may have as many as 2000 impacts to the head during the course of an athletic season. This fact is of particular concern, as high school football players appear to be more vulnerable and perform worse than collegiate athletes following concussion. Protracted recovery in high school players with concussion included prolonged memory dysfunction and worse performance on neuropsychological testing when compared with controls.[20]

Helmets and mouth guards have not been shown to decrease rates of concussion, although helmets are effective in preventing skull fracture and more severe TBI.[21] Ongoing research is aimed at understanding the mechanisms of injury and types of play most likely to result in head trauma during sport. Improving techniques for play and establishing regulation can decrease the rates of both head impact and concussion.

Chronic Traumatic Encephalopathy

The postmortem neuropathologic studies of McKee and colleagues[22] on chronic traumatic encephalopathy (CTE) resulting from repetitive head trauma have gained widespread media attention. Blinded to the patient's clinical history, McKee and colleagues[22] have documented CTE and associated neuropathologic changes with tau-immunoreactive neurofibrillary tangles in the cortex, resulting in a progressive motor neuron disease. These changes have been noted in a series of professional and youth athletes and a host of others who have suffered repetitive head trauma. **Table 3** lists some of the neuropathologic findings and symptoms associated with CTE.[23]

Imaging

Nearly 700,000 children visit the ED for head trauma in the United States each year, most with mTBI.[1] More than 300,000 cranial CTs are obtained to evaluate these children. Overall, a great deal of variation in practice exists in evaluation of mTBI with cranial CT. In addition, CT is not without associated cost and risk. Research on CT-radiation risk and extrapolated data from World War II atomic bomb survivors estimates that lifetime-attributable mortality from a single CT of the head in childhood is as high as 1 in 1200.[24] More recently, Pearce and colleagues[25] discovered a 3-fold increase in the risk of brain tumors following head CT (cumulative doses of 50–60 mGy to the brain). The study linked CT records for patients (birth to 22 years of age) in the

Table 3	
Neuropathologic findings and symptoms associated with chronic traumatic encephalopathy	
Neuropathologic Changes	**Symptoms**
Decreased brain mass	Depression/apathy
Enlarged lateral and third ventricles	Suicidal behavior
Brain atrophy	Problems with executive function
Neurofibrillary tangles	Problems with short term memory
β-Amyloid deposits	Emotionally labile
Pallor	Problems with impulse control

Adapted from Stern RA, Riley DO, Daneshvar DH, et al. Long-term consequences of repetitive brain trauma: chronic traumatic encephalopathy. Phys Med Rehabil 2011;3:S460–7; with permission.

British National Health Service to cancer registry data, and also found head CT to be the most common scan obtained in this cohort.

More than a decade ago, the National Cancer Institute and Food and Drug Administration disseminated a guide to physicians to minimize unnecessary CT scans in children.[26,27] Despite this work, there was a dramatic increase in the use of CT scans for children over the past 2 decades.[28]

Prediction Rules for Cranial CT after Head Trauma

In 2009, the Pediatric Emergency Care Applied Research Network (PECARN)[29] published 2 validated prediction rules to identify children at very low risk of clinically important TBI (ciTBI), not in need of a CT scan.[30] More than 40,000 children 0 to 18 years of age were prospectively enrolled in the PECARN study. **Table 4** lists the two prediction rules, one for preverbal children (<2 years) and the other for verbal children (≥2 years). The PECARN prediction rules have excellent performance characteristics, and were derived by incorporating clinical findings that were readily available and had good interobserver reliability.[31] If none of the 6 predictors in either prediction rule is present, the child is at very low risk of ciTBI, and CT can be avoided.

For children younger than 2 years the prediction rule had:

- Negative predictive value of 100% (95% confidence interval [CI] 99.7–100.0)
- Sensitivity of 100% (95% CI 86.3–100.0)

For children 2 years and older the prediction rule had:

- Negative predictive value of 99.95% (95%CI 99.81–99.99)
- Sensitivity of 96.8% (95% CI 89.0–99.6)

ciTBI, the outcome of interest, was defined as:

- Death from TBI
- Neurosurgical intervention for TBI

Table 4
PECARN prediction rule for clinically important TBI (ciTBI) in children younger than 2 and in those 2 years and older

PECARN Prediction Rule for <2 y	PECARN Prediction Rule for ≥2 y
GCS <15	GCS <15
Sign of altered mental status	Signs of altered mental status
Palpable skull fracture	Signs of basilar skull fracture
Occipital, parietal, or temporal scalp hematoma	Severe headache
History of LOC ≥5 s	History of LOC
Severe mechanism of injury[a]	Severe mechanism of injury[a]
Not acting normally per parent	History of vomiting

If patients have no sign or symptom in the prediction rule, CT scan is not recommended as they are at very low risk of ciTBI.

Abbreviations: GCS, Glasgow Coma Scale score; LOC, loss of consciousness.

[a] Severe mechanism of injury: motor vehicle crash with patient ejection, death of another passenger, or rollover; pedestrian or bicyclist without helmet struck by a motorized vehicle; falls more than 0.9 m (3 feet) for <2 years or more than 1.5 m (5 feet) for ≥2 years; head struck by a high-impact object.

Data from Kuppermann N, Holmes JF, Dayan PS, et al, for the Pediatric Emergency Care Applied Research Network (PECARN). Identification of children at very low risk of clinically-important brain injuries after head trauma: a prospective cohort study. Lancet 2009;374:1160–70.

- Intubation longer than 24 hours
- Hospitalization 2 nights or longer for TBI; with TBI on CT

The PECARN study risk stratifies children with minor head trauma into high risk, intermediate risk, and low risk, for clinically important TBI (**Fig. 1**). This risk stratification provides the Emergency Physician with easy-to-use recommendations for CT

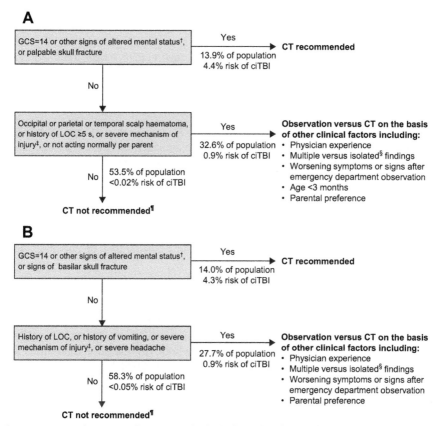

Fig. 1. Suggested computed tomography (CT) algorithm for children younger than 2 years (*A*) and for those aged 2 years and older (*B*) with Glasgow Coma Scale (GCS) scores of 14 to 15 after head trauma (Data are from the combined derivation and validation populations). ciTBI, clinically important traumatic brain injury; LOC, loss of consciousness. [†] Other signs of altered mental status: agitation, somnolence, repetitive questioning, or slow response to verbal communication; [‡] Severe mechanism of injury: motor vehicle crash with patient ejection, death of another passenger, or rollover; pedestrian or bicyclist without helmet struck by a motorised vehicle; falls of more than 0.9 m (3 feet) (or more than 1.5 m [5 feet] for panel B); or head struck by a high-impact object; [§] Patients with certain isolated findings (ie, with no other findings suggestive of traumatic brain injury), such as isolated LOC, isolated headache, isolated vomiting, and certain types of isolated scalp haematomas in infants older than 3 months, have a risk of ciTBI substantially lower than 1%; [¶] Risk of ciTBI exceedingly low, generally lower than risk of CT-induced malignancies. Therefore, CT scans are not indicated for most patients in this group. (*From* Kuppermann N, Holmes JF, Dayan PS, et al, for the Pediatric Emergency Care Applied Research Network (PECARN). Identification of children at very low risk of clinically-important brain injuries after head trauma: a prospective cohort study. Lancet 2009;374:1160–70; with permission.)

decision making. For the low-risk group CT is not recommended, and for the high-risk group (those with altered mental status, Glasgow Coma Scale [GCS] <15 or signs of skull fracture) CT is recommended. For the intermediate-risk group, for whom observation is recommended versus CT scan, observation often provides a reasonable alternative to cranial CT in the evaluation of the child with minor TBI. This finding holds particularly true for children with isolated predictors, such as isolated loss of consciousness,[32] isolated headache, or vomiting,[33,34] who have a low risk of ciTBI. In a secondary analysis of the PECARN cohort, with clinical observation periods documented to be 3 to 6 hours, investigators found that clinical observation was associated with reduced CT use.

Application of the PECARN prediction rules in general EDs, where the majority of children with head trauma are evaluated and CT scan rates are close to 50%, could result in a significant reduction in unnecessary scans.

Hospitalization

Children with minor blunt head trauma seen in the ED frequently undergo CT, and are hospitalized for observation and serial neurologic examinations. These children may at times also receive subsequent CT scans. Children with blunt head trauma and normal cranial CT results generally do not require hospitalization for neurologic observation. Holmes and colleagues[35] found that of approximately 14,000 children with minor blunt head trauma (GCS 14 or 15) and normal ED CT scans, nearly one-fifth were hospitalized and 2% had subsequent neuroimaging, although none required neurosurgical intervention.

Table 5 summarizes new developments in the management of pediatric head trauma.

MODERATE AND SEVERE TBI

TBI is the leading cause of morbidity and mortality in children. The incidence of TBI has increased worldwide, most likely as a result of increased automobile use. The World Health Organization (WHO) projects that mortality from TBI related to road traffic accidents will double over a 2-decade period from 2000 to 2020.[36]

Table 5 What's new in the management of pediatric head trauma		
Issue	Recommendation	Reference
CT	Validated PECARN prediction rules based on signs and symptoms can identify children with head trauma at very low risk of clinically important TBI in whom CT is not recommended	Kuppermann et al,[30] 2009
Repeat CT	Children with minor blunt head trauma and initial normal cranial CT generally do not warrant subsequent CT	Holmes et al,[35] 2011
Hospitalization	Children with minor blunt head trauma and normal cranial CT results generally do not require hospitalization for neurologic observation	Holmes et al,[35] 2011

From Kuppermann N, Holmes JF, Dayan PS, et al, for the Pediatric Emergency Care Applied Research Network (PECARN). Identification of children at very low risk of clinically-important brain injuries after head trauma: a prospective cohort study. Lancet 2009;374:1160–70; with permission.

It is essential to assess the pedestrian struck by an automobile for head trauma, as demonstrated in Waddell's triad (**Fig. 2**).[38]

Head trauma resulting in neuronal injury in moderate or severe TBI follows a biphasic pattern:

- Primary injury
  - Acute
- Secondary injury
  - May occur hours to days after head trauma
  - Indirect injury resulting from
    - Hypoxemia
    - Hypotension
    - Cerebral edema
    - Hypoglycemia

Early initiation of therapy and the use of standardized guidelines in the management of moderate and severe TBI are essential to improve outcomes in children. However, randomized controlled trials in children with moderate and severe TBI are rare and children and are often excluded from large randomized controlled trials in adults.

Prehospital care for severe TBI has not changed in the past decade, and focuses on:

- The management of ABCs (Airway, Breathing, Circulation)
  - Patient with GCS less than 9 should be intubated via rapid-sequence intubation
  - Ketamine is contraindicated, as it can increase intracranial pressure (ICP)
- Triage to a trauma center
  - Based on GCS
  - Signs of ICP, Cushing's triad, unequal pupils
  - Higher survival in severe TBI for patients directly transported by emergency medical services to a pediatric trauma center[39]
  - Reduced mortality in subdural hematoma if operated within 4 hours after injury[40]

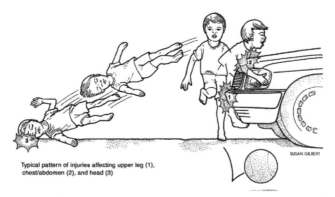

Typical pattern of injuries affecting upper leg (1), chest/abdomen (2), and head (3)

SUSAN GILBERT

Fig. 2. Waddell's triad[37] demonstrates a pedestrian child struck by an automobile. The child is hit on the left side with bumper impact to the femur and fender impact to the abdomen, then is thrown to the ground with impact to the head. (*From* Atabaki SM. Prehospital evaluation and management of traumatic brain injury in children. Clin Pediatr Emerg Med 2006;7:94–104; with permission.)

- Prevention and treatment of hypoxemia[41]
  - Brain injury can lead to respiratory depression and failure
- Treatment of hypotension
  - Fluid resuscitation
  - Maintain systolic blood pressure higher than 70 + (2 × age in years)
    - Prehospital initiation of treatment of hypotension improves outcomes[42]
    - Hypotension is a sensitive indicator of mortality[43]
  - Treatment of hypoglycemia[44]
    - Glucose should be checked
    - TBI induces increased energy demands and hyperglycolysis

In 2012, the Brain Trauma Foundation published guidelines for the acute medical management of severe TBI in children, based on a review of the literature. Levels were given on a scale of I (highest) to III (lowest) for recommendations based on the strength of the underlying research (**Table 6**).[45]

Indications for hypertonic saline or mannitol and hyperventilation include signs of increased ICP or cerebral herniation such as:

- Cushing's triad
  - Triad of hypertension, bradycardia, and irregular respirations
- Abnormal pupil examination
  - Asymmetric, fixed, or dilated pupils
- Neurologic deterioration
  - Drop in GCS greater than 2 points for patients with GCS less than 9[53]
- Posturing
  - Extensor posturing

Table 6 Select therapies for moderate or severe TBI	
	Reference
Therapy Recommended	

Hyperosmolar therapy
  Effective to control increased ICP in severe TBI
    Hypertonic 3% saline 0.1–1 mL/kg/h
    Mannitol 0.25–1 g/kg
  Level III recommendation
	Peterson et al,[46] 2000
	Simma et al,[47] 1998
	Fisher et al,[48] 1992

Temperature control
  Hyperthermia should be avoided in severe TBI
  Moderate hypothermia (32–33°C) may be considered
    in severe TBI
  Level III recommendation
	Adelson et al,[49] 2005
	Hutchison et al,[50] 2008

Therapy Not Recommended	

Hyperventilation
  Prophylactic hyperventilation to be avoided
  Level III recommendation
	Curry et al,[51] 2008

Corticosteroids
  Corticosteroids should be avoided in severe TBI
  Level III recommendation
	Fanconi et al,[52] 1988

Adapted from Kochanek PM, Carney N, Adelson PD, et al. Guidelines for the acute medical management of severe traumatic brain injury in infants, children and adolescents-second edition. Pediatr Crit Care Med 2012;13:S1–82; with permission.

Prophylaxis of Posttraumatic Seizure

Head trauma is the cause of 5% of epilepsy in children and is the cause of 20,000 new cases of epilepsy each year.[54] Nearly 20% of patients with severe TBI will develop posttraumatic epilepsy (PTE).[54,55] Prior trials of phenytoin, carbamazepine, and valproate to prevent PTE in animal models and humans have not been successful.[56,57] However, prophylaxis with phenytoin to prevent early posttraumatic seizure may be considered.

Levetiracetam has emerged as a promising therapy to prevent PTE. Levetiracetam has been effective in animal models in preventing PTE and is used in humans to treat nontraumatic epilepsy.[58] Recently published studies on the safety and pharmacokinetics of levetiracetam in children with severe TBI and intracranial hemorrhages pave the way for future randomized controlled trials.[59,60]

Intraventricular Hemorrhage

Children with isolated intraventricular hemorrhage (IVH) have better outcomes than those with combination of IVH and other intracranial injury on CT (nonisolated IVH). Lichenstein and colleagues[61] report that of approximately 15,000 children with CT for head trauma, 7% had intracranial injury and 0.9% had isolated IVH. This isolated IVH group had good outcomes; none required neurosurgery or died. By contrast, of 37% of patients with nonisolated IVH, 37% died and 42% required neurosurgery.

Skull Fractures

Head trauma in younger children often results in skull fracture, which may also be associated with an underlying intracranial injury. If skull fracture is suspected to result from a hematoma in the presence of underlying bony step-off or significant tenderness of the skull, and intracranial injury is also suspected, a cranial CT scan is warranted. Signs of skull fracture place children at higher risk of ciTBI, and a CT scan is often recommended in this population to uncover underlying intracranial disorder. In general, the majority of skull fractures are linear and are associated with good outcomes.

Basilar Skull Fracture

If a basilar skull fracture is suspected a CT scan should be obtained, owing to the poor sensitivity of plain radiography in detecting these injuries. Patients with identified

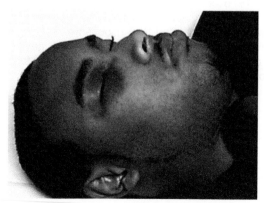

Fig. 3. Signs of a basilar skull fracture in a patient with head trauma include raccoon eyes and Battle sign. (*From* Atabaki SM. Prehospital evaluation and management of traumatic brain injury in children. Clin Pediatr Emerg Med 2006;7:94–104; with permission.)

basilar skull fractures are no longer routinely hospitalized, and can be closely observed by guardians as outpatients. The routine administration of prophylactic anti-biotic is also no longer recommended. However, these children should be closely observed for signs of intracranial infection, and told to return for immediate medical attention if they develop a fever or neurologic deficit, especially within the first few weeks following head trauma (**Fig. 3**).

SUMMARY

Head trauma and concussion are the cause of significant morbidity and mortality in childhood and are an important public health concern, increasing in incidence worldwide. Acute recognition and management of TBI along the spectrum from mild to severe is essential to optimize neurocognitive outcomes and prevent long-term sequelae in children. A thorough history and physical examination is the foundation for the acute diagnosis of head trauma, and has recently been incorporated into validated risk stratification to reduce unnecessary imaging and associated radiation and costs. Knowledge translation and widespread dissemination of these prediction rules for pediatric head trauma is the next step to obviate unnecessary CT scans in children. In addition, children with blunt head trauma and normal cranial CT results generally do not require hospitalization for neurologic observation.

Concussion is common following head trauma in children, and resulting symptoms can last for months if not diagnosed and managed properly. Postconcussive symptoms such as depression, anxiety, and difficulty with executive function can have a profound impact during vulnerable periods in a child's life. Emerging evidence and expert consensus demonstrate a program of cognitive and physical-activity management with a graduated program of return to play, sport, and school to be effective in improving outcomes following concussion. Over the last decade, "Return to Play" legislation for youth has been adopted by most states. There has also been an increased awareness of the long-term neurocognitive effects of concussion among professional and collegiate athletes. Now more than ever it is essential for health care providers to expand the latest research in concussion to the acute care of pediatric head trauma.

Outcomes of patients with head trauma have improved greatly, with a 20% drop in mortality rates from TBI over the last 30 years. The management of moderate and severe TBI in children is still an area of many unknowns; however, appropriate triage and systemic resuscitation to prevent and treat hypoxemia and hypotension have been effective in improving outcomes. Following standardized guidelines for the triage and management of children with severe TBI will pave the way for future trials of therapeutic interventions for moderate and severe pediatric TBI.

REFERENCES

1. Faul M, Xu L, Wald MM, et al. Traumatic brain injury in the United States: emergency department visits, hospitalizations and deaths 2002-2006. Atlanta (GA): Centers for Disease Control and Prevention, National Center for Injury Prevention and Control; 2010.
2. Langlois JA, Rutland-Brown W, Wald MM. The epidemiology and impact of traumatic brain injury. J Head Trauma Rehabil 2006;21:375–8.
3. Gilchrist J, Thomas KE, Xu L, et al. Nonfatal sports and recreation related traumatic brain injuries among children and adolescents treated in emergency

departments in the United States, 2001-2009. MMWR Morb Mortal Wkly Rep 2011;60:1337–42.

4. Centers for Disease Control and Prevention. National center for injury prevention and control. Facts for physicians. In: Heads up: brain injury in your practice. Atlanta (GA): Center for Disease Control and Prevention; 2007. Available at: http://www.cdc.gov/ncipc/tbi/Physicians_Tool_Kit.htm.

5. Giza CC, Hovda DA. The neurometabolic cascade of concussion. J Athl Train 2001;36:228–35.

6. Bazarian JJ, Atabaki S. Predicting postconcussion syndrome after minor traumatic brain injury. Acad Emerg Med 2001;8:788–95.

7. Ponsford J, Wilmott C, Rothwell A, et al. Impact of early intervention on outcome after mild traumatic brain injury in children. Pediatrics 2001;108:1297–303.

8. Moser RS, Glatts C, Schatz P. Efficacy of immediate and delayed cognitive and physical rest for treatment of sport related concussion. J Pediatr 2012. http://dx.doi.org/10.1016/j.jpeds.2012.04.012.

9. Majerske CW, Mihalik JP, Ren D, et al. Concussion in sports: postconcussive activity, levels, symptoms, and neurocognitive performance. J Athl Train 2008;43:265–74.

10. Atabaki S, Gioia G, Zuckerbraun N, et al. Practice patterns in emergency department management and follow-up of pediatric mild traumatic brain injury. Accepted abstracts from the International Brain Injury Association's Eighth World Congress on Brain Injuries. Brain Inj 2010;24:115–463.

11. Broglio SP, Sosnoff JJ, Shin S, et al. Head impacts during high school football: a biomechanical assessment. J Athl Train 2009;44:342–9.

12. McCrea M, Hammeke T, Olsen G, et al. Unreported concussion in high school football players: implications for prevention. Clin J Sport Med 2004;14(1):13–7.

13. "Love of sports can start early, so can injuries", tell me more with Michel Martin, National Public Radio. 2012. Available at: http://www.npr.org/2012/08/07/158361384/love-of-sports-can-start-early-so-can-injuries.

14. Cantu RC. Second-impact syndrome. Clin Sports Med 2002;1:7–11.

15. Iverson GL, Gaetz M, Lovell MR, et al. Cumulative effects of concussion in amateur athletes. Brain Inj 2004;18:433–43.

16. Halstead ME, Walter KD, Council on Sports Medicine and Fitness. American Academy of Pediatrics. Clinical report—sport-related concussion in children and adolescents. Pediatrics 2010;126(3):597–615.

17. McCrory P, Meeuwisse WH, Aubry M, et al. Consensus statement on concussion in sport: the 4th International Conference on Concussion in Sport held in Zurich, November 2012. Br J Sports Med 2013;47:250–8.

18. Guskiewicz KM, McCrea M, Marshall SW, et al. Cumulative effects associated with recurrent concussion in collegiate football players. JAMA 2003;290(19):2549–55.

19. Talavage TM, Nauman E, Breedlove EL, et al. Functionally detected cognitive impairment in high school football players without clinically-diagnosed concussion. J Neurotrauma 2013. [Epub ahead of print]. http://dx.doi.org/10.1089/neu.2010.1512.

20. Field M, Collins MW, Lovell MR, et al. Does age play a role in recovery from sports-related concussion? A comparison of high school and collegiate athletes. J Pediatr 2003;142(5):546–53.

21. Daneshvar DH, Nowinski CJ, McKee AC, et al. The epidemiology of sport-related concussion. Clin Sports Med 2011;30(1):1–17.

22. McKee AC, Cantu RC, Nowinski CJ, et al. Chronic traumatic encephalopathy in athletes: progressive tauopathy after repetitive head injury. J Neuropathol Exp Neurol 2009;68:709–53.

23. Stern RA, Riley DO, Daneshvar DH, et al. Long-term consequences of repetitive brain trauma: chronic traumatic encephalopathy. PM R 2011;3:S460–7.

24. Brenner DJ, Elliston CD, Hall EJ, et al. Estimated risks of radiation-induced fatal cancer from pediatric CT. Am J Roentgenol 2001;176:289–96.

25. Pearce MS, Salotti JA, Little MP, et al. Radiation exposure from CT scans in childhood and subsequent risk of leukaemia and brain tumours: a retrospective cohort study. Lancet 2012;380(9840):499–505.

26. National Cancer Institute Web site. Radiation risks and pediatric computed tomography (CT): a guide for health care providers. Available at: http://cancer.gov/cancerinfo/causes/radiation-risks-pediatric-ct. Accessed January 17, 2012.

27. Food and Drug Administration. FDA public health notification. Pediatr Radiol 2002;32(4):314–6.

28. Blackwell CD, Gorelick M, Holmes JF, et al. Pediatric head trauma: changes in use of computed tomography in emergency departments in the United States over time. Ann Emerg Med 2007;49(3):320–4.

29. The Pediatric Emergency Care Applied Research Network. The Pediatric Emergency Care Applied Research Network (PECARN): rationale, development, and first steps. Pediatr Emerg Care 2003;19:185–93.

30. Kuppermann N, Holmes JF, Dayan PS, et al, for the Pediatric Emergency Care Applied Research Network (PECARN). Identification of children at very low risk of clinically-important brain injuries after head trauma: a prospective cohort study. Lancet 2009;374:1160–70.

31. Gorelick MH, Atabaki SM, Hoyle J, et al. Interobserver agreement in assessment of clinical variables in children with blunt head trauma. Acad Emerg Med 2008; 15:812–8.

32. Kuppermann N, Holmes JF, Dayan P, et al. Does isolated loss of consciousness predict traumatic brain injury in children after blunt head trauma? Acad Emerg Med 2008;15:S82.

33. Dayan P, Holmes JF, Atabaki S, et al. Association of traumatic brain injuries (TBI) in children after blunt head trauma with degree of isolated headache or isolated vomiting. Acad Emerg Med 2008;15:S82.

34. Nigrovic LE, Schunk JE, Forester A, et al, Traumatic Brain Injury (TBI) group for the Pediatric Emergency Care Applied Research Network (PECARN). The effect of observation on head computed tomography (CT) utilization for children after blunt head trauma. Pediatrics 2011;127(6):1067–73.

35. Holmes JF, Borigalli DA, Nadel FM, et al, for the Traumatic Brain Injury Study Group of the Pediatric Emergency Care Applied Research Nework (PECARN). Do children with blunt head trauma and normal cranial computed tomography scan results require hospitalization for neurologic observation? Ann Emerg Med 2011;58(4):315–22.

36. WHO/OMS. Global status report on road safety: time for action. Geneva (Switzerland): World Health Organisation; 2009. Available at: http://whqlibdoc.who.int/publications/2009/.

37. Atabaki SM. Prehospital evaluation and management of traumatic brain injury in children. Clin Pediatr Emerg Med 2006;7:94–104.

38. Guidelines for the pre-hospital management of severe traumatic brain injury, 2nd edition. Brain Trauma Foundation Writing Team. Prehosp Emerg Care 2008;12(Suppl 1):S1–52.

39. Johnson D, Krishnamurthy S. Send severely head-injured children to a pediatric trauma center. Pediatr Neurosurg 1998;28(4):167–72.
40. Seelig JM, Becker DP, Miller JD, et al. Traumatic acute subdural hematoma. Major mortality reduction in comatose patients treated within four hours. N Engl J Med 1981;304:1511–8.
41. Pigula FA, Wald SL, Shackford SR, et al. The effect of hypotension and hypoxia on children with severe head injuries. J Pediatr Surg 1993;28:310–4.
42. Chestnut RM, Marshall LF, Kluber MR. The role of secondary brain injury in determining outcome from severe head injury. J Trauma 1993;34:216–22.
43. Vavilala MS, Bowen A, Lam AM, et al. Blood pressure and outcome after severe pediatric traumatic brain injury. J Trauma 2003;55(6):1039–44.
44. Luber S, Brady W, Brand A, et al. Acute hypoglycemia masquerading as head trauma: a report of four cases. Am J Emerg Med 1996;14:543–7.
45. Kochanek PM, Carney N, Adelson PD, et al. Guidelines for the acute medical management of severe traumatic brain injury in infants, children and adolescents-second edition. Pediatr Crit Care Med 2012;13:S1–82.
46. Peterson B, Khanna S, Fisher B, et al. Prolonged hypernatremia controls elevated intracranial pressure in head-injured pediatric patients. Crit Care Med 2000;28:1136–43.
47. Simma B, Burger R, Falk M, et al. A prospective randomized controlled study of fluid management in children with severe head injury: lactated Ringer's solution versus hypertonic saline. Crit Care Med 1998;26:1265–70.
48. Fisher B, Thomas D, Peterson B. Hypertonic saline lowers raised intracranial pressure in children after head trauma. J Neurosurg Anesthesiol 1992;4:4–10.
49. Adelson PD, Ragheb J, Kanev P, et al. Phase II clinical trial of moderate hypothermia after severe traumatic brain injury in children. Neurosurgery 2005;56:740–54.
50. Hutchison JS, Ward RE, Lacroix J, et al. Hypothermia therapy after traumatic brain injury in children. N Engl J Med 2008;358:2447–56.
51. Curry R, Hollingworth W, Ellenbogen RG, et al. Incidence of hypo- and hypercarbia in severe traumatic brain injury before and after 2003 pediatric guidelines. Pediatr Crit Care Med 2008;9:141–6.
52. Fanconi S, Kloti J, Meuli M, et al. Dexamethasone therapy and endogenous cortisol production in severe pediatric head injury. Intensive Care Med 1988;14:163–6.
53. Servadei F, Nasi MT, Cremonini AM, et al. Importance of a reliable admission Glasgow Coma Scale score for determining the need for evacuation of posttraumatic subdural hematomas: a prospective study of 65 patients. J Trauma 1998;44(5):868–73.
54. Temkin NR. Risk factors for posttraumatic seizures in adults. Epilepsia 2003;44(Suppl 10):18–20.
55. Statler KD. Pediatric posttraumatic seizures: epidemiology, putative mechanisms of epileptogenesis and promising investigational progress. Dev Neurosci 2006;28:354–63.
56. Silver JM, Shin C, McNamara JO. Antiepileptogenic effects of conventional anticonvulsants in the kindling model of epilepsy. Ann Neurol 1991;29:356–63.
57. Temkin NR. Preventing and treating posttraumatic seizures: the human experience. Epilepsia 2009;50(Suppl 2):10–3.
58. Loscher W, Brandt C. Prevention or modification of epileptogenesis after brain insults. Pharmacol Rev 2010;62(4):668–700.

59. Klein P, Herr D, Pearl PL, et al. Safety of levetiracetam administration to adults and children with traumatic brain injury and high risk for post traumatic epilepsy. Arch Neurol 2012;69(10):1290–5. http://dx.doi.org/10.1001/archneurol.2012.445.

60. Klein P, Herr D, Pearl PL, et al. Results of phase II pharmacokinetic study of levetiracetam for prevention of post-traumatic epilepsy. Epilepsy Behav 2012; 24(4):457–61.

61. Lichenstein R, Glass TF, Quayle KS, et al, for the Traumatic Brain Injury Study Group of the Pediatric Emergency Care Applied Research Nework (PECARN). Presentations and outcomes of children with intraventricular hemorrhages after blunt head trauma. Arch Pediatr Adolesc Med 2012;166(8):725–31.

Cervical Spine Injury

Julie C. Leonard, MD, MPH

KEYWORDS

- Pediatric • Children • Cervical spine injury

KEY POINTS

- Cervical spine injury is rare, especially in children younger than 8 years.
- Motor vehicle crashes are the most common cause of blunt cervical spine injury in children, although sports-related injuries and falls are also important.
- Violence, including penetrating trauma, is the third leading cause of spinal cord injury in children.
- Altered mental status, focal neurologic deficit, neck pain, torticollis, substantial torso trauma, high-risk motor vehicle crash, diving, and predisposing conditions are factors associated with blunt cervical spine injury in children, and can be used to develop screening guidelines.
- Manual in-line cervical stabilization should be used during intubation of the victim of blunt trauma.
- A rigid collar is an adequate precaution for the cervical spine following blunt trauma.
- The rigid long board should be used as an out-of-hospital extrication and transfer device for those children who are significantly injured. Use of the rigid long board should be discontinued as soon as possible because of its associated risks.
- Three-view plain cervical radiographs are good for screening children who have normal mental status and no focal neurologic findings.
- Children younger than 8 years are more likely to injure their upper cervical spine.
- There is a wide variety of cervical spine injury patterns; the most common injury is atlanto-axial rotary subluxation.
- Spinal cord injury without radiographic association is also common, but may be overreported.
- Mortality in children who sustain cervical spine injury is high.

EPIDEMIOLOGY

Cervical spine injury is uncommon in children, occurring in less than 1% of those evaluated following blunt trauma.[1,2] Furthermore, the age distribution among children with cervical spine injury is skewed toward older children and teenagers, with less than 5%

Division of Emergency Medicine, Department of Pediatrics, School of Medicine, Washington University in St. Louis, One Children's Place, Campus Box 8116, St Louis, MO 63110, USA
E-mail address: Leonard_ju@kids.wustl.edu

Pediatr Clin N Am 60 (2013) 1123–1137
http://dx.doi.org/10.1016/j.pcl.2013.06.015
0031-3955/13/$ – see front matter © 2013 Elsevier Inc. All rights reserved.

of injuries occurring in children younger than 2 years.[3] Similar to other types of injury, boys are almost twice as likely to be injured as girls.[3]

Mechanisms of blunt cervical spine injury are diverse. Similar to adults, the most common cause of injury in children is a motor vehicle crash.[2–4] Another frequent mechanism in children, especially those at younger ages, is being hit by motor vehicles while walking or riding recreational equipment.[2–4] However, mechanisms with lower biomechanical forces, such as falls in younger children and sports and recreational impacts in older children, can also result in injury.[2–4] Of recreational activities, diving puts children at greatest risk for cervical spine injury.[3] Child abuse is a rare, but perhaps underreported cause of cervical spine injury.[2] When penetrating spine injury is considered, however, violence is the third most common cause of spinal cord injury among youth.[4]

Furthermore, one-third of outcomes following cervical spine injury are poor in general, with up to one-third of children sustaining neurologic injury.[2] Mortality is directly related to the level of injury, with upper cervical spine injuries carrying 23% mortality versus 4% mortality in the lower cervical spine.[2] The long-term prognosis for those children who sustain cervical spinal cord injury and survive the first 24 hours is poor; life expectancy is reduced by anywhere from 6 to 45 years depending on the level and completeness of injury.[4]

DEVELOPMENTAL ANATOMY

Anatomically, the cervical spine is divided into 2 distinct regions: the axial (occiput, C1 and C2) and subaxial (C3–C7). The developmental anatomy of the axial vertebrae is distinct from the subaxial anatomy. The atlas (C1) has 3 primary ossification centers (1 anterior and 2 neural arches), which are associated with cartilaginous joints (synchondroses).[5] The anterior center fuses by the age of 3 and the neural centers fuse by age 7 years, thus forming a solid, bony ring structure.[5] The body of the axis (C2) has the same 3 primary ossification centers as the atlas; however, there is a fourth ossification site at the base of the dens, which fuses by age 11 years.[5]

All of the vertebrae of the subaxial cervical spine (C3–C7) follow the same developmental pattern. Three primary ossification centers occur at each level: a centrum for the body (which fuses by age 6 years) and 2 neural arches (which fuse by age 3 years).[6,7] Understanding this anatomy helps clinicians to distinguish between pathologic fracture and lucency associated with a synchondrosis.

Secondary ossification centers in the transverse and spinous processes of all vertebrae are present by puberty.[6,7] Additional growth occurs along the epiphyseal plates of the vertebral bodies.[6,7] Secondary ossification sites fuse during early adulthood. Compared with those of adults, pediatric vertebrae have anterior wedging of the bodies, absent uncinate processes, and shallow, horizontally oriented facets.[6,7] Additional developmental considerations that influence the patterns of cervical spine injury in children are a relatively large head size in comparison with the remainder of the body, immature neck and paraspinal musculature, and underdeveloped ligaments.[6,7] These developmental characteristics result in hypermobility and a fulcrum of motion at the C2 to C3 level, which renders the upper cervical spine more prone to injury.[6,7] By age 14 years the spine has sufficient support, and soft tissues have sufficiently matured such that the fulcrum migrates to the C5 to C6 level; injuries sustained at this age are similar to those in adults.[6,7]

CLINICAL PRESENTATION

Cervical spine injury is a heterogeneous disease (see the section on injury patterns), therefore so are the clinical characteristics (**Fig. 1**). Presenting complaints range

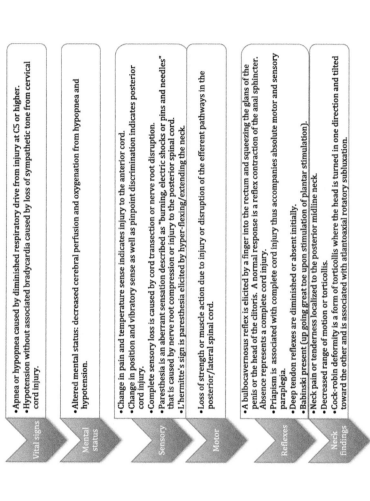

Vital signs
- Apnea or hypopnea caused by diminished respiratory drive from injury at C5 or higher.
- Hypotension without associated bradycardia caused by loss of sympathetic tone from cervical cord injury.

Mental status
- Altered mental status: decreased cerebral perfusion and oxygenation from hypopnea and hypotension.

Sensory
- Change in pain and temperature sense indicates injury to the anterior cord.
- Change in position and vibratory sense as well as pinpoint discrimination indicates posterior cord injury.
- Complete sensory loss is caused by cord transection or nerve root disruption.
- Paresthesia is an aberrant sensation described as "burning, electric shocks or pins and needles" that is caused by nerve root compression or injury to the posterior spinal cord.
- L'hermitte's sign is paresthesia elicited by hyper-flexing/extending the neck.

Motor
- Loss of strength or muscle action due to injury or disruption of the efferent pathways in the posterior/lateral spinal cord.

Reflexes
- A bulbocavernosus reflex is elicited by a finger into the rectum and squeezing the glans of the penis or the head of the clitoris. A normal response is a reflex contraction of the anal sphincter. Absence represents a complete cord injury.
- Priapism is associated with complete cord injury thus accompanies absolute motor and sensory paraplegia.
- Deep tendon reflexes are diminished or absent initially.
- Babinski present (up going great toe upon stimulation of plantar stimulation).

Neck findings
- Neck pain or tenderness localized to the posterior midline neck.
- Decreased range of motion or torticollis.
- Cock-robin deformity is a form of torticollis where the head is turned in one direction and tilted toward the other and is associated with atlantoaxial rotatory subluxation.

Fig. 1. Clinical signs and symptoms of acute cervical spine injury.

from cervicalgia to respiratory arrest. The findings at presentation help localize the level of injury and degree of spinal cord involvement. In general, findings that are localized to a dermatome indicate injury to a nerve root, whereas sensory and motor loss involving a cervical level and lower indicate injury to the spinal cord. In addition, there are characteristic spinal cord syndromes (**Fig. 2**).

CLINICAL SCREENING CRITERIA

Given that neck irradiation in childhood leads to tumors in adulthood, especially thyroid cancer, clinicians should limit radiographic imaging to those children at risk for cervical spine injury.[3] The following factors have been identified as being associated with cervical spine injury in children: altered mental status, focal neurologic deficit, neck pain, torticollis, substantial torso trauma, high-risk motor vehicle crash, diving, and predisposing conditions.[3] Although not prospectively validated, these factors are highly sensitive for cervical spine injury and, along with validated adult screening criteria, should serve as the basis for developing clinical guidelines for children.[3,8,9] **Fig. 3** is a suggested guideline for determining which children warrant diagnostic testing for cervical spine injury following blunt trauma.

INITIAL MANAGEMENT

Those children presenting in traumatic cardiopulmonary arrest should be managed according to Advanced Trauma Life Support (ATLS) guidelines, with prompt attention to gaining control of the airway while observing cervical precautions by maintaining in-line manual cervical stabilization.[10] Once the airway is secured, a rigid cervical collar should be placed. Use of a rigid long board for ease of extrication and transition is appropriate for the immobile or unconscious child in the out-of-hospital setting; however the child should be removed from the board as soon as possible to avoid adverse effects such as decubitus ulcers.[11,12] For children who are alert and have more subtle signs of cervical spine injury, a rigid cervical collar alone is sufficient for providing protection against potential worsening of injury.[13] Immobilization of alert and stable children on rigid long boards may cause pain that leads to unnecessary testing.[14]

Use of corticosteroids in the management of pediatric cervical spinal cord injury remains controversial. Although a large, randomized controlled trial in adults found that a regimen of high-dose methylprednisone (30 mg/kg) over 1 hour followed by a 23-hour infusion (5.4 mg/kg/h) improved neurologic outcome when initiated within 8 hours of injury, this finding has not been replicated and no comparable studies have been conducted in children younger than 13 years.[15] Corticosteroid therapy for spinal cord injury is a therapeutic option, but is not without risk and should be initiated only after consultation with a spine surgeon.

DIAGNOSTIC TESTING

The approach to diagnostic evaluation should take into consideration the clinical presentation (see **Fig. 3**). Plain radiographs, computed tomography (CT), and magnetic resonance imaging (MRI) are the mainstays of diagnostic evaluation for cervical spine injury. Routine plain radiographs alone are greater than 90% sensitive for bony cervical spine injury and are usually sufficient for screening the alert patient who has a normal neurologic examination.[16,17] Flexion-extension plain radiography plays a role in evaluating ligamentous stability, but is not useful in screening for acute injury.[18] CT is nearly 100% sensitive for bony cervical spine injury, and is the imaging modality of choice for critically injured children.[19–21] However, CT may miss up to 4% of

Syndrome	Features
Anterior Cord Syndrome	Complete motor paralysis
	Loss of pain and temperature sensation
	Preservation of position and vibration sensation
	Associated with severe flexion injury
Central Cord Syndrome	Diminished or absent upper extremity function
	Preserved lower extremity function
	Associated with extension injury
Posterior Cord Syndrome	Very rare
	Associated with spinal artery injury
	Loss of position and vibratory sensation only
Brown-Séquard Syndrome	Hemisection of the spinal cord
	Ipsilateral loss of motor function and position and vibratory sensation
	Contralateral loss of pain and temperature sensation
Spinal Shock	Flaccid below level of lesion
	Absent reflexes
	Autonomic dysfunction including hypotension and bradycardia
	Sensation may not be preserved; if absent indicates total cord transection

Fig. 2. Spinal cord syndromes.

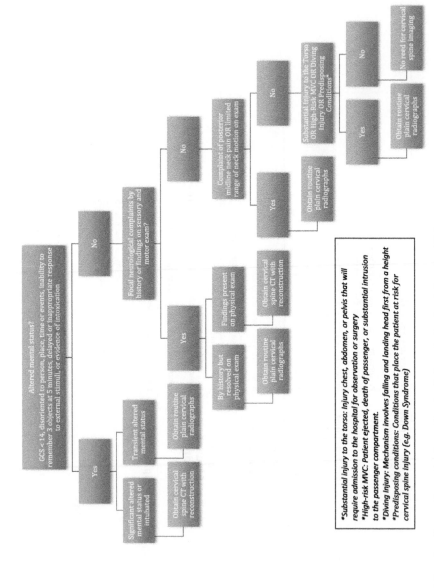

Fig. 3. Guideline for diagnostic evaluation of potential cervical spine injury in children.

ligamentous injuries, some of which are clinically relevant.[18–20] MRI is nearly 100% sensitive for acute cervical spine injury, including bony, ligamentous, and cord injuries.[19–21]

Clinicians who routinely evaluate children following blunt trauma should become familiar with plain cervical radiographs. **Fig. 4** presents the 3-view series. The lateral view is the most important single view, as it picks up nearly 80% of injuries (see **Fig. 4**).[22] The anterior-posterior (AP) view allows additional assessment of the overall alignment, the alignment of the spinous processes, and evaluation of the lateral masses, as well as evaluation for subtle signs of fracture and subluxation. The open-mouth view allows evaluation of the dens, and the alignment of the lateral masses of C1 to C2. There are several common pediatric variants that can be mistaken for injury on a plain radiograph. The most common of these are pseudosubluxation and physiologic wedging of the vertebrae (**Fig. 5**). In addition, given the aforementioned developmental anatomy of the cervical spine, a normal synchondrosis can be mistaken for fracture (**Fig. 6A**).

INJURY PATTERNS

Because of developmental and structural differences, injuries of the cervical spine are best described by axial and subaxial regions. Young children (less than 8 years) are more prone to injury in the axial region in comparison with older children and adults.[2] The most fatal of these, atlanto-occipital and atlantoaxial dislocations, occur from high-energy mechanisms that induce acceleration-deceleration motion, which results in excessive motion of the head relative to the cervical spine (**Fig. 7**).[2]

The most common injury involving the axial region is atlantoaxial rotatory subluxation (**Fig. 8**), which was first described in the setting of upper respiratory and pharyngeal infections (Grisel syndrome) and later in the settings of trauma and head and neck surgery.[23,24] "Cock robin" torticollis, characterized by chin rotation to the contralateral side and flexion of the neck, is the characteristic physical examination finding in atlantoaxial rotatory subluxation. Children are in a good deal of discomfort and may have C2 radiculopathy or myelopathy. The ligamentous laxity and robust synovium that are inherent in the pediatric spine predisposes children to these injuries. Because atlantoaxial rotatory subluxation is usually self-limiting, a conservative approach can be taken to evaluating these injuries.[25] For children in whom injury is suspected, screening with plain radiographs is appropriate. If these are normal aside from asymmetric positioning of the dens relative to the lateral masses, and the child does not have focal neurologic findings, a trial of rigid collar, analgesia, and muscle relaxant is warranted. For those children whose symptoms do not spontaneously resolve within 2 weeks, evaluation for atlantoaxial rotatory subluxation requires referral to a spine specialist and dynamic CT (images taken in 3 positions: at rest, in neutral position, and rotated to the opposite side).

Fractures to the atlas (C1) are usually the result of axial-loading compressive force, which causes a burst fracture (typically 4 fracture lines), otherwise known as a Jefferson fracture. Neurologic injury is uncommon with these injuries because the diameter of the spinal canal is large at this level, and burst fragments tend to project outward away from the spinal cord.[26,27] These fractures are usually stable unless the axis is also fractured or the transverse ligament is disrupted.[28,29] These injuries are usually detectable on plain radiographs by noting the atlanto-dens interval (ADI) on lateral view. The ADI is normally 5 mm or less in pediatric patients; ADI values in excess of 5 mm indicate disruption and instability of the transverse ligament. The open-mouth view can also be used to assess stability of the transverse ligament: a lateral mass

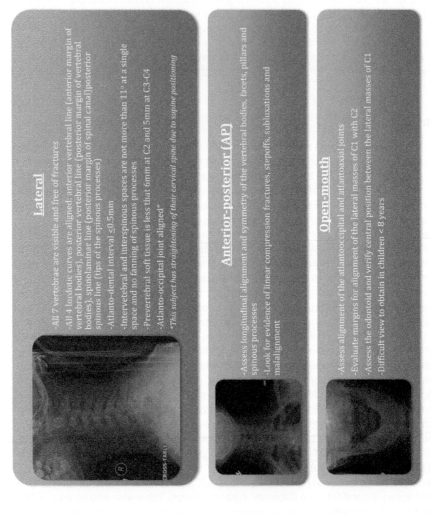

Lateral

- All 7 vertebrae are visible and free of fractures
- All 4 lordotic curves are aligned; anterior vertebral line (anterior margin of vertebral bodies), posterior vertebral line (posterior margin of vertebral bodies), spinolaminar line (posterior margin of spinal canal) posterior spinous line (tips of the spinous processes)
- Atlanto-dental interval ≤0.5mm
- Intervertebral and interspinous spaces are not more than 11° at a single space and no fanning of spinous processes
- Prevertebral soft tissue is less than 6mm at C2 and 5mm at C3-C4
- Atlanto-occipital joint aligned*

*This subject has straightening of their cervical spine due to supine positioning

Anterior-posterior (AP)

- Assess longitudinal alignment and symmetry of the vertebral bodies, facets, pillars and spinous processes
- Look for evidence of linear compression fractures, stepoffs, subluxations and malalignment

Open-mouth

- Assess alignment of the atlantooccipital and atlantoaxial joints
- Evaluate margins for alignment of the lateral masses of C1 with C2
- Assess the odontoid and verify central position between the lateral masses of C1
- Difficult view to obtain in children <8 years

Fig. 4. Evaluation of routine 3-view plain radiographs.

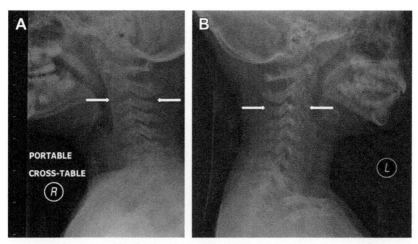

Fig. 5. Pseudosubuxation (*A*) Child with straightening of the cervical spine from supine positioning, which can exaggerate C2-C3 pseudosubluxation. The left arrow shows the C2 body overriding the body of C3. The right arrow shows normal alignment of the posterior elements. (*B*) A lateral radiograph taken with the child in upright positioning. The pseudosubluxation of C2-C3 is subtle, but present. In this image, the right arrow shows the C2 body overriding the body of C3, while the left arrow shows the normally aligned posterior elements. Also note the normal physiologic wedging of the vertebral bodies in both children.

overhang of C1 over C2 greater than 6.9 mm indicates disruption of the transverse ligament (the rule of Spence).[26,27]

The weakest point in the axis (C2) is the cartilaginous subdental epiphysis, which is present until the age of 7 years.[26,27] These fractures are infrequently displaced and may be difficult to distinguish from normal anatomy; anterior angulation with fracture helps distinguish the two (see **Fig. 6**B). Significant displacement of the fractured dens can result in neurologic deficit. True fractures of the odontoid process are seen in older children and adolescents, and are usually caused by mechanisms that cause forceful head and neck flexion.[26,27] True dens fractures are classified by their location: type I involve the superior portion of the dens as a result of avulsion of the alar ligament; type II involve the base of the neck, and are rarer and usually associated with C1 fracture (see **Fig. 6**C); and type III odontoid fractures extend into the body of C2.[26,27] Hyperextension of C2 can result in pars interarticularis fractures or "hangman's fracture."[26,27]

Subluxation of C2 on C3 can occur; however, this must be distinguished from pseudosubluxation in this region, which is a common physiologic variant in children (see **Fig. 5**). In addition, os odontoideum, a congenital anomaly that results in a bony fragment with smooth cortical margins located cranially to the body of the axis with associated small or hypoplastic dens, may be confused with healed type I or type II dens fracture (see **Fig. 6**D).[28] Os odontoideum can be unstable if the cruciate ligaments are disrupted.[28]

Subaxial injuries are less common until the age of 8 years.[2] The structure and biomechanics at these levels (C3–C7) are similar. Compression or burst fractures of the vertebral body are usually the result of axial load mechanisms (**Fig. 9**).[26,27] Compression fractures are usually stable and heal without surgical intervention (see **Fig. 9**A).[26,27] Burst fractures, however, involve retropulsion of bone into the spinal canal, and more frequently require surgical intervention (see **Fig. 9**B).[26,27] Teardrop fractures are avulsion fractures involving the anteroinferior aspect of the vertebral

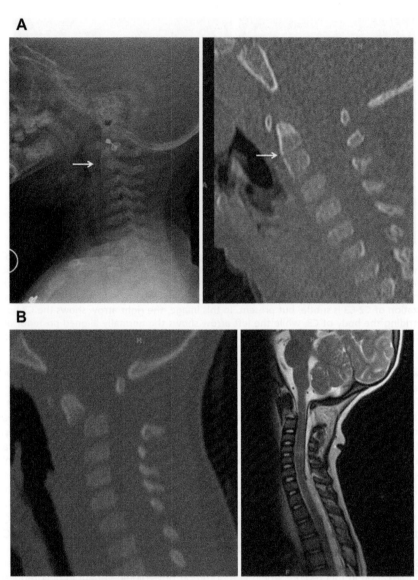

Fig. 6. (*A*) Normal synchondrosis shown on lateral plain radiograph (*left arrow*) and sagittal CT image (*right arrow*). (*B*) C2 subdental synchondrosis fracture seen on sagittal CT (*left*) and MR (*right*) images. Note the anterior angulation and dislocation of the dens relative to the body of C2. There are also subtle T2 changes in spinal cord. (*C*) Type 2 odontoid fracture illustrated by coronal (*left arrow*) and sagittal (*right arrow*) CT images. (*D*) Os odontoideum demonstrated on lateral plain radiograph (*left arrow*) and sagittal CT image (*right arrow*). Note the normal synchodrosis, hypoplastic dens and os fragment.

body,[26,27] which result from hyperflexion and involve disruption of the facet joints, the anterior and posterior longitudinal ligaments, and the disk. When identified on radiographs, these injuries should be evaluated for stability using flexion-extension radiographs and/or MRI to assess ligamentous integrity.[6,7,20] Hyperflexion/extension can result in a variety of other fractures including spinous process, lateral mass,

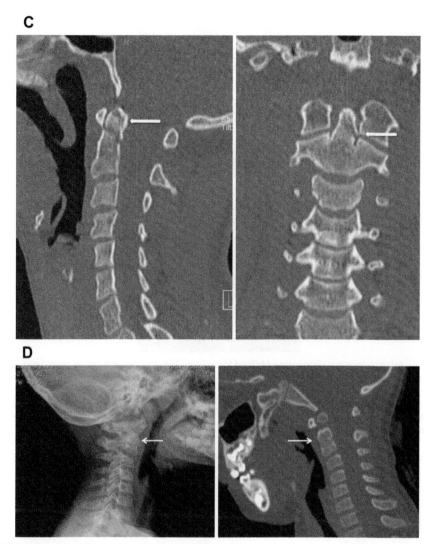

Fig. 6. (*continued*)

transverse process, and uncinate, laminar, and pedicle fractures.[26,27] Physeal fractures or separation of the vertebral body from the end plate through the epiphysis is an injury unique to children, and may require surgical intervention depending on the Salter-Harris type.[26,27]

Hyperflexion with or without distraction and rotation may result in unilateral or bilateral facet dislocation.[26,27] Occult ligamentous injury can also occur in the subaxial cervical spine as a result of ligamentous disruption without fracture. Plain radiograph findings suggestive of posterior ligamentous disruption include subluxation movement on flexion-extension views and increased interspinous distance on lateral radiograph.[6,7] In the acute setting, it may be difficult to distinguish ligamentous injury. For patients with persistent posterior neck pain, it is appropriate to continue cervical precautions for 2 weeks and then reassess.

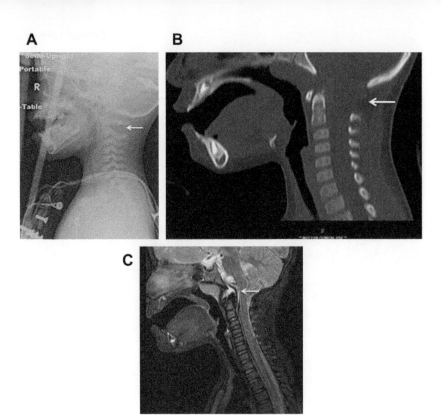

Fig. 7. Atlantooccipital dislocation (AOD) (*A*) Lateral plain radiograph status-post emergent halo placement and (*B*) Sagittal CT image. These images (*see arrows*) illustrate findings consistent with AOD including displacement of C1 anterior and inferior to the clivus and occipital condyle; and widening of the Occiput-C1-C2 spinous process interspaces. (*C*) Sagittal T2 MRI demonstrates (*see arrow*) prevertebral edema, epidural hemorrhage, and disruption of the apical odontoid and transverse ligaments.

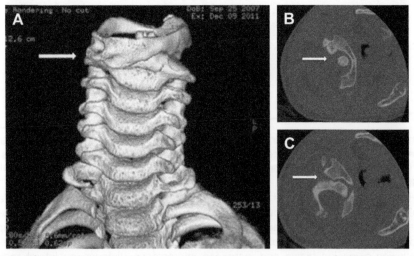

Fig. 8. Atlantoaxial rotatory subluxation (AARS) (*A*) CT reconstruction of a child with AARS involving the right lateral mass; C1 is subluxed anterior to C2 (*see arrow*). (*B*) Axial image through the C1-C2 complex illustrating the dens of C2 (*see arrow*) malaligned posterior and lateral. (*C*) Axial image caudal to prior image illustrating the arch of C1 (*see arrow*) subluxed anterior to C2.

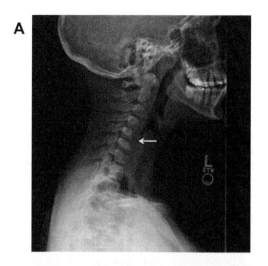

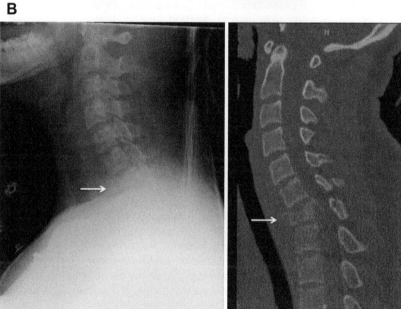

Fig. 9. (A) The arrow identifies compression fractures of C5 and C6. Important findings on this lateral plain radiograph include loss of contour and height of the vertebral body and subtle anterior subluxation with preservation of the posterior elements indicating with no retropulsion of fracture fragments into the spinal canal. (B) Burst fracture of C7 illustrated on lateral plain radiograph (*left arrow*) and sagittal CT image (*right arrow*). Important findings on the lateral plain radiograph include decreased contour and height of the vertebral body and loss of alignment indicating compromise of the anterior and posterior elements. This also demonstrates the importance of clear visualization of C7 on plain radiographs. The sagittal CT image shows retropulsion of the fracture fragments with clear spinal canal compromise.

Spinal cord injury without radiographic abnormality (SCIWORA) was originally used to describe traumatic myelopathy in individuals with evidence of vertebral injury on plain radiography (including flexion-extension views), myelography, or CT. It is speculated that SCIWORA occurs because the inherent hypermobility of the pediatric spine allows for transient deformation of the spinal column without fracture or ligamentous disruption at the expense of the spinal cord.[29] The reported incidence of SCIWORA ranges from 4% to 66% among all children with spinal cord injuries.[29–31] Emerging evidence suggests that clinicians may inappropriately label patients who have very transient neurologic complaints as SCIWORA, thus resulting in overreporting.[30,31] As MRI has improved and become universally available, clinicians have been able to identify spinal cord injuries that correlate to the neurologic findings. Nonetheless, SCIWORA is a diagnosis of exclusion, and clinicians must be vigilant to rule out persistent ligamentous incompetence that may place the patient at risk for further injury.

SUMMARY

Cervical spine injury is an uncommon and heterogeneous disease in children. Mechanisms of injury, clinical presentation, and injury patterns are diverse, and an understanding of this diversity aids clinical decision making. Previously identified risk factors for cervical spine injury in children can be used to create a sensible clinical guideline that meets the dual aims of prompt recognition, stabilization, and diagnosis for those children who are at greatest risk of cervical spine injury, while avoiding unnecessary and potentially harmful interventions for those at negligible risk.

REFERENCES

1. Viccellio P, Simon H, Pressman BD, et al. A prospective multicenter study of cervical spine injury in children. Pediatrics 2001;108(2):E20.
2. Patel JC, Tepas DL III, Mollitt DL, et al. Pediatric cervical spine injuries: defining the disease. J Pediatr Surg 2001;36(2):373–6.
3. Leonard JC, Kuppermann N, Olsen C, et al. Factors associated with cervical spine injury in children after blunt trauma. Ann Emerg Med 2011;58:145–55.
4. National Spinal Cord Injury Statistical Center. 2011 NSCISC annual statistical report - complete public version. Birmingham (AL): University of Alabama; 2011.
5. Ogden JA. Radiology of postnatal skeletal development-XI: the first cervical vertebra, XII: the second cervical vertebra. Skeletal Radiol 1984;12:12.
6. Harris JH Jr, Mirvis SE. The radiology of acute cervical spine trauma. In: Mitchell CW, editor. The radiographic examination. 3rd edition. Baltimore (MD): Williams & Wilkins; 1996. p. 180–211.
7. Swischuk LE. Emergency imaging of the acutely ill or injured child. The spine and the spinal cord. 4th edition. Philadelphia: Lippincott Williams & Wilkins; 2000. p. 532–87.
8. Hoffman JR, Mower WR, Wolfson AB, et al. Validity of a set of clinical criteria to rule out injury to the cervical spine in patients with blunt trauma. N Engl J Med 2000;343:94.
9. Stiell IG, Wells GA, Vandemheen K, et al. The Canadian C-spine rule for radiography in alert and stable trauma patients. J Am Med Assoc 2001;286:1841.
10. Committee on Trauma, American College of Surgeons. ATLS: advanced trauma life support program for doctors. 8th edition. Chicago: American College of Surgeons; 2008.
11. Linares H, Mawson A, Suarez E, et al. Association between pressure sores and immobilization in the immediate post-injury period. Orthopedics 1987;10(4):571.

12. Mawson AR, Biundo JJ, Neville P, et al. Risk factors for early occurring pressure ulcers following spinal cord injury. Am J Phys Med Rehabil 1988;67(3):123.
13. Position statement: EMS spinal precautions and the use of the long backboard. National Association of EMS Physicians and American College of Surgeons Committee on Trauma. Prehosp Emerg Care 2013;17(3):392–3.
14. Leonard JC, Mao J, Jaffe DM. Potential adverse effects of spinal immobilization in children. Prehosp Emerg Care 2012;16(4):513.
15. Bracken MB, Shepard MJ, Collins WF, et al. A randomised controlled trial of methylprednisolone or naloxone in the treatment of acute spinal cord injury. N Engl J Med 1990;322:1405–11.
16. Nigrovic LE, Rogers AJ, Adelgais KM, et al. Utility of plain radiographs in detecting traumatic injuries of the cervical spine in children. Pediatr Emerg Care 2012; 28(5):426.
17. Mower WR, Hoffman JR, Pollack CV, et al. Use of plain radiography to screen for cervical spine injuries. Ann Emerg Med 2001;38(1):1–7.
18. Pollack CV Jr, Hendey GW, Martin DR, et al. Use of flexion-extension radiographs of the cervical spine in blunt trauma. Ann Emerg Med 2001;38(1):8–11.
19. Rozycki GS, Tremblay L, Feliciano DV, et al. Prospective comparison of admission CT scan and plain film of the upper cervical spine in trauma patients with altered LOC. J Trauma 2001;51(4):663.
20. Flynn JM, Closkey RF, Soroosh M, et al. Role of magnetic imaging in the assessment of pediatric cervical spine injuries. J Pediatr Orthop 2002;22(5):573.
21. Kaiser ML, Whealon MD, Barrios C, et al. The current role of magnetic resonance imaging for diagnosing cervical spine injury in blunt trauma patients with negative computed tomography scan. Am Surg 2012;78(10):1156–60.
22. Baker C, Kadish H, Schunk JE. Evaluation of pediatric cervical spine injuries. Am J Emerg Med 1999;17:230–4.
23. Grisel P. Enucleation des atlas et torticollis nasopharyngien. Presse Med 1930; 38:50.
24. Fielding JW, Hawkins RJ, Hensinger RN, et al. Atlanto-axial rotatory deformities. Orthop Clin North Am 1978;9:955.
25. Phillips WA, Hensinger RN. The management of rotatory atlanto-axial subluxation in children. J Bone Joint Surg Am 1989;71:664–8.
26. Roche C, Carty H. Spinal trauma in children. Pediatr Radiol 2001;31:677.
27. Lebwohl NH, Eismont FJ. Cervical spine injuries in children. In: Weinstein S, editor. The pediatric spine: principles and practice. 2nd edition. Philadelphia: Lippincott Williams & Wilkins; 2001. p. 553.
28. Menezes A. Os odontoideum: pathogenesis, dynamics and management. In: Marlin A, editor. Concepts in pediatric neurosurgery. Basel (Switzerland): Karger; 1988.
29. Pang D. Spinal cord injury without radiographic abnormality in children, 2 decades later. Neurosurgery 2004;55(6):1325.
30. Trigylidas T, Yuh SJ, Vassilyadi M, et al. Spinal cord injuries without radiographic abnormality at two pediatric trauma centers in Ontario. Pediatr Neurosurg 2010; 46(4):283.
31. Yucesoy K, Yuksel KZ. SCIWORA in MRI era. Clin Neurol Neurosurg 2008; 110(5):429.

Emerging Concepts in Pediatric Emergency Radiology

Nicola Baker, MD*, Dale Woolridge, MD, PhD

KEYWORDS

• Pediatric • Radiology • Emergency • Imaging • Ionizing radiation

KEY POINTS

- Radiologic studies are an important adjunct in the diagnosis of disease in children, and multiple imaging modalities are available.
- Computed tomography (CT) exposes children to large doses of ionizing radiation, and its effect on the incidence of malignancy is under heated debate.
- Current trends in pediatric imaging support the increased use of ultrasound (US) and magnetic resonance imaging (MRI) to decrease radiation exposure.
- Clinical decision rules can be used to predict which child does not need imaging.

INTRODUCTION

Radiologic studies are a vital component in the workup and diagnosis of disease. Although an indispensable adjunct, they should not be used as a substitute for a thorough history and physical examination. Multiple imaging modalities are available for use. Each has its own advantages, disadvantages, and safety profile, and practitioners should be versed in these when selecting how to work up disease.

An appropriate radiographic study will accurately rule in or rule out disease with the least possible harm. Harm is often thought of as pain or physical injury, but broader definitions can include time, cost, radiation, and psychological stress to the patient. When compared with outpatient diagnostics, imaging choices within the emergency setting favor sensitivity over specificity to rule out diseases that require emergent intervention. A stepwise radiological approach may be used to identify illness. Accordingly, the time, cost, and potential harm of imaging studies may increase over time as a specific diagnosis is pursued.

Special considerations are necessary for the imaging of children. Sedation or anxiolysis may be required for either computed tomography (CT) or magnetic resonance imaging (MRI). The pediatric emergency provider should be trained in techniques for

Department of Emergency Medicine, University of Arizona, 1501 North Campbell Avenue, Tucson, AZ 85724, USA
* Corresponding author.
E-mail address: nbaker@aemrc.arizona.edu

Pediatr Clin N Am 60 (2013) 1139–1151
http://dx.doi.org/10.1016/j.pcl.2013.06.004
0031-3955/13/$ – see front matter © 2013 Elsevier Inc. All rights reserved.

the sedation of children for imaging. The availability of various imaging modalities will vary between facilities. If delay to diagnosis will place the child at imminent risk, transfer to a higher level of care should be initiated.

In this review, we highlight some of the emerging concepts in the radiographic workup of pediatric disease, with a focus on decreasing ionizing radiation, increasing ultrasound (US) use, and using clinical decision rules to identify children who do not need imaging.

IMAGING MODALITIES
Plain-Film Radiograph (X-Ray)

Radiographs emit ionizing radiation through a body part and project a 2-dimensional image. The effective dose of ionizing radiation from a single radiograph is negligible. Radiographs are nearly universally available, even in outpatient settings, and can be readily shared between providers using digital platforms. Major benefits of radiographs include low cost, accessibility, and speed. Radiographs are most commonly used in the evaluation of pediatric fracture and chest imaging, but they have multiple other uses.

Ultrasound

US uses high-frequency sound waves to project digital images of organs and tissues within the body. Its frequencies are generally between 2 MHz and 14 MHz. Lower frequencies penetrate deeper within the body, allowing for visualization of deep structures, but they do so at the expense of image resolution and/or quality. High frequencies allow for better resolution of superficial structures. In real time, US allows for dynamic observation of pathology and underlying physiology. The major advantages of US are low cost, noninvasive, lack of ionizing radiation, and minimal preparation. US can be limited in obese patients, and cannot easily visualize structures deep to overlying bone, air, or gas. It is operator dependent, and requires skill of the technician or physician.

Computed Tomography

CT uses x-ray technology to create digital representations of the body. The device rotates around a fixed access, creating multiple "slices" that are then put together to generate a 3-dimensional image. The major advantage of CT is its high sensitivity/specificity in working up disease. CT is rapid and has less operator dependence; however, it delivers ionizing radiation to the patient, which may increase their risk of malignancy in the future.[1] A single chest radiograph exposes a patient to a dose of 0.02 millisievert (mSv), whereas a CT of the chest or abdomen exposes the patient to roughly 8 mSv of ionizing radiation.[2] Its use in children is particularly controversial.[3,4] Also, contrast is often given intravenously to enhance the CT. Contrast-induced nephropathy occurs roughly 5% to 10% of the time in those with normal kidney function,[5] with much higher incidence in those with underlying renal dysfunction.[6] Oral contrast does not cause nephrotoxicity and can enhance the utility of CT for certain diagnoses, but requires time to fill hollow structures and may delay imaging.

Magnetic Resonance Imaging

MRI uses an electromagnetic field to align protons within water contained in body tissues, and then captures decay back to their inherent state. Complex images are produced based on the density and properties of body tissues. MRI produces remarkably detailed images of soft tissues, and uses gadolinium for contrast, which is not believed to cause nephrotoxicity in those with normal baseline function.[7] Disadvantages of MRI include high cost and the amount of time required to obtain the study. In children, MRI can be difficult to obtain because of noise, fear, claustrophobia, and inability to remain still. Sedation or general anesthesia is often required to obtain quality images. Rapid MRI protocols, particularly in neuroimaging and abdominal imaging, are being used with increased frequency and will likely change the face of MRI in the future (**Table 1**).[8–10]

THE AGE OF ALARA

Pediatric CT use has increased precipitously in the past few decades, because of increased availability, declining costs, and improved resolution of machines.[11,12] The impact of ionizing radiation on the incidence of childhood cancers is in the spotlight. Children are more prone to radiation-induced cancers and have a longer expected life span. The practice of ALARA (As Low As Reasonably Achievable) refers to a campaign to reduce the amount of ionizing radiation exposure by using specialized pediatric protocols and using alternate modalities when possible.[13]

Pearce and colleagues[14] recently published retrospective data suggesting that radiation doses of 50 to 60 mGy (2–3 head CTs) in children could triple their risk of brain tumors. Brenner and colleagues[3] estimated that of 600,000 CT scans performed in children per year, 500 may die from cancer related to their radiation exposure. Most data come from risk projection models, although cohort studies are currently in progress. Although the exact risk of ionizing radiation on children is still unknown, we are certainly now practicing in a culture that expects practitioners to be mindful of the potential risk.

CT will frequently be necessary despite the higher exposure to ionizing radiation. Its fast and accurate diagnostic capabilities will often outweigh the potential harm to a child. The concept of ALARA should never be used to withhold a gold standard diagnostic test from a sick child. Rather, it is a culture shift emphasizing efforts to decrease use of ionizing radiation whenever possible. The practice encourages providers to

Table 1
Advantages/disadvantages of imaging modalities

Imaging Modality	Advantages	Disadvantages
X-ray	• Very accessible • Rapid • Low cost	• 2-dimensional images • Artifact from superimposed structures • Limited use for soft tissues • Ionizing radiation (negligible dose)
Ultrasound	• Generally accessible • No ionizing radiation • Low cost • Dynamic image capture • Procedural guidance • Bedside test	• Operator dependence • Limited by body habitus • Potentially painful • Inconclusive results
Computed tomography	• Generally accessible • Rapid • High specificity/sensitivity • 3-dimensional images	• Ionizing radiation • Contrast-induced nephropathy • Intermediate cost • Contrast allergy
Magnetic resonance imaging	• No ionizing radiation • High sensitivity/specificity • No contrast nephropathy	• High cost • Limited availability • Long study duration • May require sedation for children or claustrophobia

consider alternatives, such as US, MRI, or observation periods. It has also facilitated the development of clinical decision rules that can guide imaging practices.

Clinical Decision Rules

To develop a clinical decision rule, researchers first identify a population of patients at risk for having a disease or outcome. The key features of their history, physical examination, and laboratory studies are identified to create highly sensitive criteria that most accurately predict the outcome in question (eg, diagnosis, prognosis, response to treatment). In the case of imaging, decision rules are typically designed to predict who *will not* have the disease in question, and therefore do not need imaging. Once derived, clinical decision rules are externally validated and ultimately incorporated into clinical practice.[15] They can then be used to support and inform practitioners' decisions.

HEAD TRAUMA

The role of imaging in head trauma is to identify injuries that may require observation, neurosurgical intervention, or invasive monitoring. Serious injuries include epidural hematoma, subdural hematoma, and subarachnoid hemorrhage. In children, neuroimaging is also often used to identify skull fracture.

Noncontrast CT remains the gold standard for the imaging of trauma patients with acute head injury. It identifies intracranial bleeds and skull fractures with excellent sensitivity. In clinically significant pediatric head trauma (low Glasgow Coma Scale [GCS], significant mechanism, obvious skull fracture), CT should be obtained without delay.

Children with less severe head injury represent a unique problem. They embody a key subgroup in which ionizing radiation may be avoided. Clinical decision rules can be helpful to identify children who are unlikely to have clinically significant injury. Extrapolation of adult prediction rules to the pediatric population is difficult, but multiple pediatric rules are now available to providers (outlined later in this article).

The CATCH (Canadian Assessment of CT for Childhood Injury) rule was derived from 3866 pediatric patients enrolled who had witnessed loss of consciousness, amnesia, disorientation, persistent irritability (younger than age 2), or persistent vomiting; 52% of the enrolled patients had a head CT performed. This study identified the following high-risk features:

- Failure to reach GCS 15 within 2 hours
- Suspicion of open skull fracture
- Worsening headache
- Irritability

Medium-risk features included the following:

- Boggy hematoma of scalp
- Signs of basal skull fracture
- Dangerous mechanism of injury

The 4 high-risk features had 100% sensitivity for neurosurgical intervention. Using the high-risk features would result in 30.2% of patients with minor head trauma having a CT. When the medium-risk features were included, the rule had 98.1% sensitivity for identifying brain injury, which was defined as any traumatic injury identified on CT, excluding nondepressed skull fracture or basilar skull fracture.[16]

The PECARN (Pediatric Emergency Care Applied Research Network) group published a validated clinical decision rule (2009) to guide neuroimaging in low-risk pediatric trauma. They prospectively enrolled 42,412 children for analysis. Children younger than 2 years who met the following 6 criteria were considered low risk and did not require neuroimaging (negative predictive value [NPV] 100%, Sensitivity 100%, n = 1176):

- Normal mental status
- No scalp hematoma (except frontal)
- No loss of consciousness/loss of consciousness less than 5 seconds
- Nonsevere injury mechanism
- No palpable skull fracture
- Acting normally according to patients

Children between 2 and 18 years of age with the following 6 criteria were low risk (NPV 99.95%, Sensitivity 96.8%, n = 3800):

- Normal mental status
- No loss of consciousness
- No vomiting
- Nonsevere injury mechanism
- No signs of basilar skull fracture
- No severe headache

In children older than 2 years, the rule missed 2 clinically important brain injuries, neither of which required neurosurgery, but did require observation. Children younger than 2 who satisfied all the criteria had less than 0.02% risk of clinically significant injury, and those older than 2 had less than 0.05% risk. Use of this rule could significantly reduce head CT use in pediatric head trauma (**Table 2**).[17]

For cases that are not straightforward, the clinician can consider a period of observation. In a subgroup analysis of PECARN patients, use of observation before deciding whether to perform CT resulted in a small but significant reduction in CT use (31.1% vs 35.0%) without missing any injury.[18]

BLUNT ABDOMINAL TRAUMA

Blunt abdominal trauma can result in life-threatening surgical emergencies, including liver/spleen lacerations, perforated viscous, ruptured diaphragm, and intra-abdominal hematoma. The age and demeanor of the child can limit the abdominal examination in pediatric trauma. Contrast CT of the abdomen is the diagnostic gold standard for assessing blunt abdominal trauma. It possesses high specificity and sensitivity for injury to blunt and hollow organs.[19] Not all traumatic intra-abdominal injuries identified on CT require surgery. Spleen and liver lacerations are being observed nonoperatively with increased frequency.[20]

Table 2	
Decision rule to avoid head computed tomography in mild pediatric head trauma (PECARN rule)	
Younger than 2 y Old	**2 to 18 y Old**
• Normal mental status	• Normal mental status
• No scalp hematoma (except frontal)	• No loss of consciousness
• No loss of consciousness (LOC) or LOC <5 s	• No vomiting
• Nonsevere injury mechanism	• Nonsevere injury mechanism
• No palpable skull fracture	• No signs of basilar skull fracture
• Acting normal per parents	• No severe headache

Which Child Does Not Need an Abdominal CT?

The PECARN network (Holmes and colleagues)[21] recently published a large multi-center prospective study with the goal to develop a clinical decision rule to identify children at very low risk of clinically significant injury to the abdomen, in an effort to decrease unnecessary CT imaging. The researchers included 12,044 children evaluated with blunt trauma to the torso (chest or abdomen). Children without clinically significant intra-abdominal injury met all 7 of the following criteria:

- No evidence of abdominal wall trauma or seat belt sign
- GCS >13
- No abdominal tenderness
- No evidence of thoracic wall trauma
- No complaint of abdominal pain
- No decreased breath sounds
- No vomiting

The rule had a sensitivity of 97.0%, specificity of 42.5%, NPV of 99.9%, and positive predictive value (PPV) of 2.8%. Use of the prediction rule could have prevented 23% of the CT scans performed in this study group. The results of this large study have not yet been externally validated.[21]

Focused Assessment with Sonography for Trauma

The Focused Assessment with Sonography for Trauma (FAST) examination is a rapid point-of-care US performed at the bedside for evaluation of blunt abdominal trauma. It involves imaging of 4 main locations (right upper quadrant, left upper quadrant, pericardial, pelvic) to assess for free fluid. The sensitivity of the FAST examination in children for identifying hemoperitoneum is 66% by meta-analysis.[22] The specificity for identification of clinically important intraperitoneal fluid was 96% in a prospective cohort study.[23] Accordingly, a "positive" FAST (free fluid seen) in a child with blunt abdominal trauma is useful, whereas a negative FAST has limited utility (**Fig. 1**).

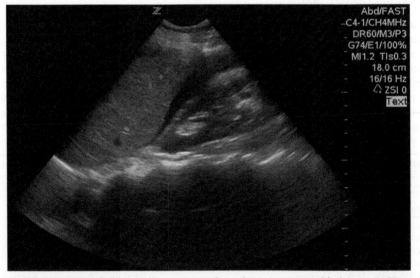

Fig. 1. Free peritoneal fluid in right upper quadrant (Morrison's pouch) view on FAST examination. (*Courtesy of* Srikar Adhikari, MD, University of Arizona, Tucson, AZ.)

A FAST that is positive for intraperitoneal fluid in a pediatric trauma patient should prompt immediate intervention, with surgical consultation and CT imaging (in the stable patient) or exploratory laparotomy (in the unstable patient). Holmes and colleagues[24] demonstrated that the sensitivity and specificity of the FAST examination is highest in the subgroup of patients presenting with hypotension. However, given marginal sensitivity of FAST to detect intraperitoneal fluid, a negative FAST examination alone should not be used as the sole screening tool for clinically significant injury.[22] Physical examination, laboratory studies (particularly aspartate aminotransferase/alanine aminotransferase), serial examinations, and/or CT scan can be used to approach improved sensitivity.[25]

The FAST examination was incorporated into the most recent ATLS (Advanced Trauma Life Support) recommendations as an adjunct to the primary survey. Routine use of FAST in all patients with blunt abdominal or multisystem trauma has become more common, but should be used with caution and kept in the context of current literature.

APPENDICITIS

The diagnosis of pediatric appendicitis can be difficult. Missed diagnosis can lead to increased morbidity and mortality from perforation and abdominal abscess. Either US or CT can be used to establish a diagnosis, but the utility of CT has increased because of its sensitivity and specificity for the disease. Diagnosis with physical examination alone has a reported negative appendectomy rate of 12%.[26]

The major benefits of US for appendicitis are lack of radiation and low cost. US can show the appendix dynamically through graded compression. It is limited, though, by operator dependence and the size of the child. Overlying bowel gas and adipose tissue affect the penetration of sound waves and can affect the quality of images. Often the appendix is not visualized on abdominal US. Also, it cannot reliably show complications of appendicitis, such as perforation.

Doria and colleagues[27] published a meta-analysis of studies evaluating use of US, CT, or both for the diagnosis of pediatric appendicitis, and demonstrated a pooled sensitivity for US of 88% and for CT of 94%. Specificity for US was 94% and CT was 95%. There was a significant difference in the sensitivity of US versus CT, favoring CT usage to reduce false-negatives. However, with similar specificities, and in light of radiation risks, an US-first versus an US-alone strategy makes sense (**Fig. 2**).

The Stanford radiology department instituted a protocol in 2003 of staged US and CT use for diagnosis of pediatric appendicitis. US was used first, and CT performed if US had equivocal findings. They performed a retrospective study of 631 patients in whom this protocol was used. The staged protocol resulted in a reduction of CT use in 52.0% of patients and had a sensitivity of 98.6%. There was no significant difference between the staged protocol versus CT alone in diagnostic capabilities.[28]

BEDSIDE US

US is becoming more accessible and affordable. Machines are more compact and user-friendly. Availability in the emergency department setting is becoming near ubiquitous, although individual practitioner use and training are variable. Given the current trajectory, it is reasonable to believe that US will have a role even in the outpatient setting in the near future.

Dramatic improvements have been made in the size of US machines, such that many facilities have machines that are portable enough to be taken to the bedside of a patient. Internationally, US may be the only advanced imaging modality available,

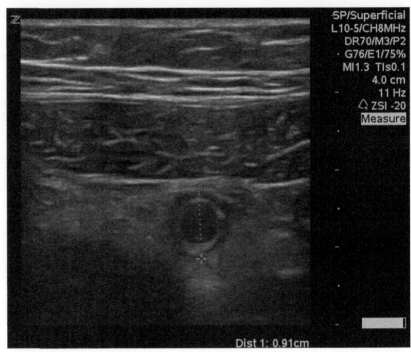

Fig. 2. US finding of appendicitis (enlarged, noncompressible). (*Courtesy of* Srikar Adhikari, MD, University of Arizona, Tucson, AZ.)

and its use can facilitate more specific diagnosis of disease. The cost of basic US machines continues to decrease and has made bedside US a more affordable adjunct.

Skin and Soft Tissue Infections

Soft tissue infections in children are increasing in incidence, particularly community-acquired MRSA. Abscess and cellulitis can be difficult to differentiate, and physical examination alone does not reliably predict the presence or absence of pus (sensitivity 78.7%, specificity 66.7%).[29] The standard of care for abscess is incision and drainage, whereas cellulitis can be managed with antibiotics and observation.

Bedside US can reliably distinguish between abscess and cellulitis, and requires only basic US knowledge. US has been shown in prospective studies to change the management in soft tissue infection, although the magnitude of effect has varied. Tayal and colleagues[30] demonstrated that US changed management in roughly 50% of patients, either by detecting occult abscess and prompting drainage, or by preventing incision and drainage or procedural sedations that would have proved unnecessary. Iverson and colleagues[29] recently demonstrated that US changed management in 13.8% of patients (**Figs. 3** and **4**).

Peritonsillar Abscess

Peritonsillar abscess (PTA) is the most common complication of strep pharyngitis. As in other purulent infections, management is generally with incision and drainage, usually by bedside needle aspiration. Conventional approach is done using anatomic

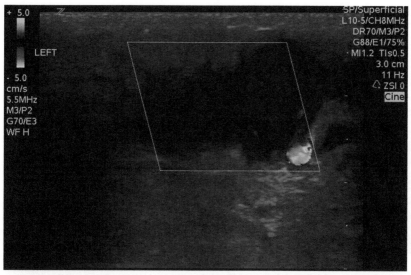

Fig. 3. Abscess cavity. (*Courtesy of* Srikar Adhikari, MD, University of Arizona, Tucson, AZ.)

landmarks. Intraoral US with an endocavitary probe can be used to visualize the area and identify if it is a true abscess or if it is peritonsillar cellulitis (**Fig. 5**).

Costantino and colleagues[31] recently published a prospective randomized controlled trial in which those with suspected PTA were randomized to US or conventional landmark technique. In this small study (n = 28), US had 100% diagnostic

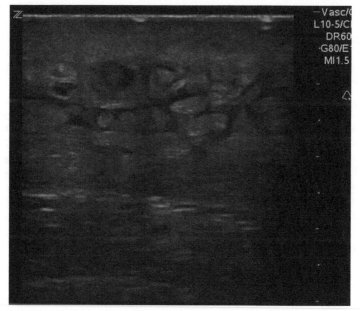

Fig. 4. Soft tissue cellulitis without abscess. (*Courtesy of* Srikar Adhikari, MD, University of Arizona, Tucson, AZ.)

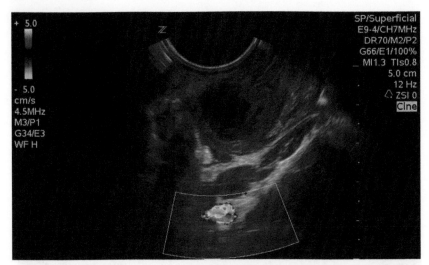

Fig. 5. Peritonsillar abscess seen on endocavitary US with carotid artery identified using Doppler. (*Courtesy of* Srikar Adhikari, MD, University of Arizona, Tucson, AZ.)

accuracy for distinguishing abscess from cellulitis, and the provider was able to effectively drain an abscess 100% of the time when US was used. Patients noted to have cellulitis alone on US did not have attempted aspiration.

Long-Bone Fractures

The diagnosis of long-bone fracture on US is simple, albeit unconventional. Long bones are imaged using a high-frequency (5–10 MHz) linear probe, with bone appearing as a bright hyperechoic line. Fracture is diagnosed by identifying cortical discontinuity. US can guide reduction of fractures in real time. This could have particular significance in the international or austere setting, where the availability or cost of plain-film radiograph can be a limitation.[32] Even in developed nations, the availability of C-arm fluoroscopy to guide reductions is limited, and US can be useful to ensure adequate alignment before splinting (**Fig. 6**).

Echocardiography

Pediatric echocardiography is a complex task, traditionally performed by trained ultrasonographers, and interpreted by pediatric cardiologists. However, focused point-of-care echocardiography can be performed accurately by an emergency provider,[33] and is being done with increasing frequency in the emergency and intensive care unit (ICU) setting. Bedside echocardiogram aids in the diagnosis of pericardial effusion, which is readily seem on limited examination. In this way, it can also be used to evaluate for the etiology of shock and hypotension, and to assess response to fluid resuscitation.

THE FUTURE OF PEDIATRIC IMAGING

In this age of ALARA, emphasis will continue to shift toward imaging modalities that do not use ionizing radiation, particularly US and MRI. Bedside US has been embraced in the emergency and ICU setting, and should be used in a point-of-care fashion to answer targeted questions about a patient. Practitioners should be taught basic US skills during their training. Rapid MRI protocols are being used with increased

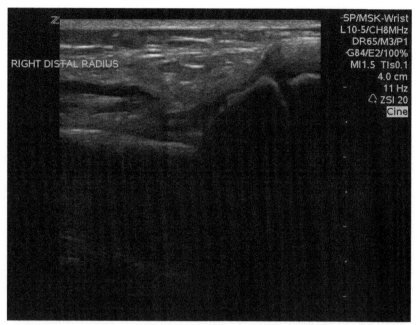

Fig. 6. Distal radius fracture diagnosed on US. (*Courtesy of* Srikar Adhikari, MD, University of Arizona, Tucson, AZ.)

frequency, and possess great potential to change the current face of imaging. For instance, the use of single-shot fast spin-echo, or "one-bang" MRI has been shown to be useful in evaluation for shunt malfunction,[8] and could significantly decrease CT use in this frequently radiated population of patients. Rapid protocols can also be used to diagnose appendicitis without the need for CT imaging.[10] Validated clinical decision rules can be incorporated into routine practice and will help select pediatric patients who do not require imaging.

REFERENCES

1. Berrington de Gonzalez A, Mahesh M, Kim KP, et al. Projected cancer risks from computed tomographic scans performed in the United States in 2007. Arch Intern Med 2009;169(22):2071–7.
2. Mettler FA Jr, Huda W, Yoshizumi TT, et al. Effective doses in radiology and diagnostic nuclear medicine: a catalog. Radiology 2008;248(1):254–63.
3. Brenner D, Elliston C, Hall E, et al. Estimated risks of radiation-induced fatal cancer from pediatric CT. American Journal Roentgenology 2001;176(2):289–96.
4. Baysson H, Etard C, Brisse HJ, et al. Diagnostic radiation exposure in children and cancer risk: current knowledge and perspectives. Arch Pediatr 2012;19(1): 64–73.
5. Kooiman J, Pasha SM, Zondag W, et al. Meta-analysis: serum creatinine changes following contrast enhanced CT imaging. Eur J Radiol 2012;81(10):2554–61.
6. Morcos SK, Thomsen HS, Webb JA. Contrast-media-induced nephrotoxicity: a consensus report. Contrast Media Safety Committee, European Society of Urogenital Radiology (ESUR). Eur Radiol 1999;9(8):1602–13.

7. Swan SK, Lambrecht LJ, Townsend R, et al. Safety and pharmacokinetic profile of gadobenate dimeglumine in subjects with renal impairment. Invest Radiol 1999; 34(7):443–8.
8. Moore MA, Wallace EC, Westra SJ. The imaging of paediatric thoracic trauma. Pediatr Radiol 2009;39(5):485–96.
9. Moore MM, Gustas CN, Choudhary AK, et al. MRI for clinically suspected pediatric appendicitis: an implemented program. Pediatr Radiol 2012;42(9):1056–63.
10. Cobben L, Groot I, Kingma L, et al. A simple MRI protocol in patients with clinically suspected appendicitis: results in 138 patients and effect on outcome of appendectomy. Eur Radiol 2009;19(5):1175–83.
11. Pearce MS. Patterns in paediatric CT use: an international and epidemiological perspective. J Med Imaging Radiat Oncol 2011;55(2):107–9.
12. Larson DB, Johnson LW, Schnell BM, et al. Rising use of CT in child visits to the emergency department in the United States, 1995-2008. Radiology 2011;259(3): 793–801.
13. Frush DP, Frush KS. The ALARA concept in pediatric imaging: building bridges between radiology and emergency medicine: consensus conference on imaging safety and quality for children in the emergency setting, Feb. 23-24, 2008, Orlando, FL—Executive Summary. Pediatr Radiol 2008;38(Suppl 4):S629–32.
14. Pearce MS, Salotti JA, Little MP, et al. Radiation exposure from CT scans in childhood and subsequent risk of leukaemia and brain tumours: a retrospective cohort study. Lancet 2012;380(9840):499–505.
15. McGinn TG, Guyatt GH, Wyer PC, et al. Users' guides to the medical literature: XXII: how to use articles about clinical decision rules. Evidence-Based Medicine Working Group. JAMA 2000;284(1):79–84.
16. Osmond MH, Klassen TP, Wells GA, et al. CATCH: a clinical decision rule for the use of computed tomography in children with minor head injury. CMAJ 2010; 182(4):341–8.
17. Kuppermann N, Holmes JF, Dayan PS, et al. Identification of children at very low risk of clinically-important brain injuries after head trauma: a prospective cohort study. Lancet 2009;374(9696):1160–70.
18. Nigrovic LE, Schunk JE, Foerster A, et al. The effect of observation on cranial computed tomography utilization for children after blunt head trauma. Pediatrics 2011;127(6):1067–73.
19. Sivit CJ. Contemporary imaging in abdominal emergencies. Pediatr Radiol 2008; 38(Suppl 4):S675–8.
20. Davies DA, Pearl RH, Ein SH, et al. Management of blunt splenic injury in children: evolution of the nonoperative approach. J Pediatr Surg 2009;44(5): 1005–8.
21. Holmes JF, Lillis K, Monroe D, et al. Identifying children at very low risk of clinically important blunt abdominal injuries. Ann Emerg Med 2013;62(2):107–16.
22. Holmes JF, Gladman A, Chang CH. Performance of abdominal ultrasonography in pediatric blunt trauma patients: a meta-analysis. J Pediatr Surg 2007;42(9):1588–94.
23. Fox JC, Boysen M, Gharahbaghian L, et al. Test characteristics of focused assessment of sonography for trauma for clinically significant abdominal free fluid in pediatric blunt abdominal trauma. Acad Emerg Med 2011;18(5):477–82.
24. Holmes JF, Brant WE, Bond WF, et al. Emergency department ultrasonography in the evaluation of hypotensive and normotensive children with blunt abdominal trauma. J Pediatr Surg 2001;36(7):968–73.
25. Schonfeld D, Lee LK. Blunt abdominal trauma in children. Curr Opin Pediatr 2012;24(3):314–8.

26. Park JS, Jeong JH, Lee JI, et al. Accuracies of diagnostic methods for acute appendicitis. Am Surg 2013;79(1):101–6.
27. Doria AS, Moineddin R, Kellenberger CJ, et al. US or CT for diagnosis of appendicitis in children and adults? A meta-analysis. Radiology 2006;241(1):83–94.
28. Krishnamoorthi R, Ramarajan N, Wang NE, et al. Effectiveness of a staged US and CT protocol for the diagnosis of pediatric appendicitis: reducing radiation exposure in the age of ALARA. Radiology 2011;259(1):231–9.
29. Iverson K, Haritos D, Thomas R, et al. The effect of bedside ultrasound on diagnosis and management of soft tissue infections in a pediatric ED. Am J Emerg Med 2012;30(8):1347–51.
30. Tayal VS, Hasan N, Norton HJ, et al. The effect of soft-tissue ultrasound on the management of cellulitis in the emergency department. Acad Emerg Med 2006;13(4):384–8.
31. Costantino TG, Satz WA, Dehnkamp W, et al. Randomized trial comparing intraoral ultrasound to landmark-based needle aspiration in patients with suspected peritonsillar abscess. Acad Emerg Med 2012;19(6):626–31.
32. McManus JG, Morton MJ, Crystal CS, et al. Use of ultrasound to assess acute fracture reduction in emergency care settings. Am J Disaster Med 2008;3(4):241–7.
33. Pershad J, Myers S, Plouman C, et al. Bedside limited echocardiography by the emergency physician is accurate during evaluation of the critically ill patient. Pediatrics 2004;114(6):e667–71.

Pediatric Office Emergencies

Susan Fuchs, MD

KEYWORDS

- Office emergencies • Office preparedness • Mock codes • Emergency information
- Disasters

KEY POINTS

- Pediatricians regularly see emergencies in the office, or children that require transfer to an emergency department, or hospitalization.
- An office self-assessment is the first step in determining how to prepare for an emergency.
- The use of mock codes and skills drills make office personnel feel less anxious about medical emergencies.
- Emergency information forms provide valuable, quick information about complex patients for emergency medical services and other physicians caring for patients.
- Disaster planning should be a part of an office preparedness plan.

Office preparedness for an emergency requires an office self-assessment, consisting of a review of personnel and skills, equipment, supplies, medications, and emergency medical services response; practice using mock codes or skill drills; and disaster planning.

A 15-month-old boy with a fever is in the office waiting room when he begins to have a seizure. A 3-year-old girl brought to the office for breathing problems is cyanotic and very lethargic. A patient with multiple medical problems is on vacation when he gets sick and is taken to a local hospital, where the emergency department needs to know some of his medical history. These scenarios are not uncommon for a pediatrician.

Important questions are whether the pediatrician and office staff are prepared; whether the office has the personnel with skills, appropriate equipment, medications, and emergency protocols to handle these problems until emergency medical services (EMS) arrive and are the capabilities of these services known; whether the patients with special health care needs carry an emergency information form (EIF) with them; and what happens when a disaster strikes the surrounding community.

Conflict of Interest: Dr Fuchs receives royalties for being an UpToDate Section author.
Division of Emergency Medicine, Ann & Robert H. Lurie Children's Hospital of Chicago, 225 East Chicago Avenue, Box 62, Chicago, IL 60611, USA
E-mail address: s-fuchs@northwestern.edu

This article reviews methods to optimize readiness for pediatric emergencies in the office setting, provides information about the EIF, and provides some insight into office preparedness for disasters.

Numerous surveys of offices have been conducted on local and national levels to assess pediatric preparedness.[1–8] Most of these studies showed that pediatricians do see emergencies in the office, or children that require transfer to an emergency department, or hospitalization, especially those with asthma and respiratory difficulties.[8,9] The good news is that more offices are now equipped with basic equipment, increasing from 42% of offices with oxygen and 35% with bag-valve masks in 1985 to 98% with oxygen and 96% with bag-valve masks in 2011.[1,8]

In 2007, the American Academy of Pediatrics (AAP) Committee on Pediatric Emergency Medicine developed a policy statement on Preparation for Emergencies in the Offices of Pediatricians and Pediatric Primary Care Providers.[9] This document provides a wonderful framework to review one's own office preparedness, and will be used, along with other references to help pediatricians adjust their current plan or develop one for their office.

OFFICE SELF-ASSESSMENT

One of the first steps in preparing for emergencies is to look at the office practice. What types of patients are seen (eg, newborns through adolescents)? Does the office care for children with chronic medical problems, children with special health care needs, and those who are technology-assisted (eg, ventilator-dependent, tracheostomies)? What emergencies are encountered in the office, and how often? The staffing patterns in the office should be considered: who opens the office and when do patients begin to arrive; whether a nurse or physician is always there, what happens at lunchtime, and what is the weekend staffing situation; whether the office is freestanding, part of a large multispecialty group, or hospital-based.

Further considerations are how far the office is from the local hospital, the nearest children's hospital with a pediatric intensive care unit, or the closest trauma center; whether contacting the EMS as easy as dialing 911 or does a private company need to be called, and is this number handy; what is the response time of these services to the office; what is their skill level: EMT or EMT-P (paramedic); do they provide a basic or an advanced life support ambulance; what medication can they provide en route; what pediatric equipment they carry; and will they bypass the local hospital and transport the patient to a children's hospital/medical home if not too far away.[9]

OFFICE PERSONNEL AND SKILLS

Factors to consider with regard to office personnel and skill are: who greets parents and children entering the office; whether this individual trained is to recognize a child in distress; whether the office has a quick assist/help button or does the staff have to go find someone; and, once a child is signed in, whether someone checks the waiting room to assure that the symptoms are not worsening if there will be delay in that child being seen.

Other considerations are whether the office staff include registered nurses, nurses' aides, medical assistants, and nurse practitioners. Each of these individuals is part of the "response team," and therefore their knowledge and capabilities must be understood so that appropriate roles can be assigned. Pediatricians should consider their own capabilities, such as when they last intubated a child, when they last inserted an intravenous or intraosseous line. All of these factors will play into what a pediatrician and the office staff can and should do in an emergency.

Education and training of staff can go a long way to improving an office's readiness. A simple list of worrisome signs and symptoms may help the person checking in patients understand when to alert a nurse or physician that someone in the waiting room needs immediate attention. Complaints or findings such as wheezing, stridor, cyanosis, seizures, altered mental status, or lethargy should prompt a help/assist call.[9,10]

Education of the entire staff, at a minimum, should include basic life support training, such as first aid/cardiopulmonary resuscitation (CPR)/automated external defibrillator (AED) training, which includes techniques used in CPR, such as chest compressions, rescue breathing, use of an AED, and foreign body airway maneuvers. This training can be accomplished through the American Red Cross or American Heart Association (AHA). Another option is Pediatric Emergency Assessment, Recognition, and Stabilization (PEARS) offered by the AHA and AAP, which covers additional topics such as recognition of respiratory distress and failure, shock, cardiac arrest, the team approach to resuscitation, and additional skills based on an individual's level of training. Education of nursing staff can include providing them time to take courses such as Pediatric Advanced Life Support (PALS) and PEARS from the AAP and AHA, Emergency Nursing Pediatric Course from the Emergency Nurses Association, or Advanced Pediatric Life Support from the AAP and American College of Emergency Physicians (ACEP), which all provide education and skills reviews. These courses also provide continuing medical/nursing education, which is required in most states for physicians, and is now required in many states for nurses. The important issue is that although these course do provide instruction and practice time in skills, none provides true competency in the skills taught, such as bag-mask ventilation, intubation, or intraosseous insertion, and therefore frequent "skill days" may be appropriate if the staff is expected to maintain these skills. Another excellent way to practice these skills and prepare for emergencies is through performing mock codes or drills in the office.

A specific plan, including who responds to the quick assist/help call from the receptionist, where the patient should go (eg, is there a larger room in the office that would allow more equipment and people than a standard examination room), and what everyone's roles are, must be defined beforehand. This plan should also be tailored to when staffing is at a minimum. Roles on the response team can include who will provide airway assistance/oxygen and bag-mask ventilation if needed; who will get vital signs and begin to chart; who will get intravenous/intraosseous access (if needed); who will get, prepare, and administer medications (if needed); who will do chest compressions (if needed); who will run the response (team leader); who will get the medical history from the parents and keep them informed; who will document any actions, drugs given, and response; and who will contact EMS.[9,10]

Documentation of the event is a critical part of the true event or mock code/drill. It provides EMS with information on transfer; a review of the response can provide the office staff with education about what went right or wrong and how to improve the response if a similar situation occurs again; and it also obviously represents legal documentation.

OFFICE EQUIPMENT

The decision about what equipment to purchase should be based on an analysis of office emergencies. Having a laryngoscope and blades in the office, when the last time the physician intubated an infant or child was 3 years ago, is asking for trouble. In fact, the key skill to maintain and practice is bag-mask ventilation, because studies have shown that the outcome of pediatric patients who received bag-mask ventilation was better than those who underwent endotracheal intubation by EMS personnel.[11] In addition, EMS providers' skill retention time for pediatric intubation is only 6 months,[12] and they also intubate adults, so this is likely to be less for a physician who does not practice this skill regularly. If a pediatrician is not comfortable with intubation, use of a laryngeal mask airway (LMA) can be considered. Although it is not a definitive airway, it can provide another option for ventilating an unconscious child. Because it is inserted in the mouth, no gag reflex should occur. However, many EMS agencies do not carry LMAs, and therefore providers have not been instructed on its use. They will likely have an alternative airway they use, and may switch to that device on transport.

Although a child's weight may be on record from a prior visit, one of the most important decisions involves choosing the correct size equipment for the child's age/length and the correct medication dose according to weight. Having length-based resuscitation tape (eg, Broselow Pediatric Emergency Tape, Armstrong Medical Industries, Lincolnshire, IL, USA) or a computer/phone application (eg, PALS Advisor 2012 Pediatric Advanced Life Support, PediSTAT, PediCalc, Epocrates, Pedi QuikCalc)[13] to determine the correct equipment and medication is critical.

Decisions about purchasing more-expensive equipment, such as a cardiac monitor, a monitor/defibrillator with pediatric pads/paddles, or an automated external defibrillator with pediatric capabilities, should be based on the office assessment. However, a sphygmomanometer (manual or electronic) and a pulse oximeter with sensors should be in every office.

Other equipment that can be helpful include a device to check serum glucose, urine test strips, extremity splints, and nasogastric tubes.

Whatever equipment is present, its location should be known by all staff. The decision whether to keep it in one room versus having it mobile should be based on the office configuration. The equipment should be well organized and labeled, and an inventory list should be kept and checked regularly to ensure that the equipment is working and, in some cases, not expired. A suggested list of equipment is provided in **Box 1**.

MEDICATIONS

One decision that should be made is what vascular access skills the pediatrician and staff should have. Some of the most important and even life-saving medications can be administered via a nonvenous route. Oxygen is given through mask or blow-by, and albuterol is given through a nebulizer or metered dose inhaler. Epinephrine 1:1000 should be delivered intramuscularly or subcutaneously for an allergic reaction/anaphylaxis, and via a nebulizer for croup. Diazepam and acetaminophen can be given rectally, whereas ceftriaxone, glucagon (for low blood sugar), and hydrocortisone (for a patient with congenital adrenal hyperplasia or panhypopituitarism/cortisol deficiency from other causes), and naloxone given intramuscularly. Oral medications include corticosteroids (methylprednisolone or dexamethasone), activated charcoal, acetaminophen, and ibuprofen.

Medications requiring vascular access include epinephrine 1:10,000, 25% dextrose, diphenhydramine, and other antiepileptic drugs (lorazepam). A list of suggested medications is provided in **Box 2**.

No matter which medications are kept in the office, they should be checked regularly for expiration dates and restocked as needed.

EMS RESPONSE AND EIF

When contacting EMS, it is important to provide them with key information, such as age and condition of child, current vital signs, complaint, and what has been done, so

Box 1
Recommended equipment

Airway management

Length-based resuscitation tape or computer/phone application to determine equipment size and medication dose

Oxygen and administration equipment

Self-inflating resuscitation bags with reservoir (450 and 100 mL) with clear masks (infant, child, adult sizes)

Face masks for oxygen delivery: simple or venture (adjustable flow), plus a partial/nonrebreather mask (infant, child, and adult sizes)

Mask for nebulized medication (metered-dose inhaler with spacer can also be used)

Suction (wall or machine) with tubing and catheter (Yankauer, plus suction catheters 8F, 10F, 14F)

Bulb syringe

Oral airways (infant to adult sizes: 00F–5F)

Nasopharyngeal airways (infant to adult sizes: 12F–30F)

Pulse oximeter and probes

Magill forceps (pediatric, adult)

Vascular access/intravenous supplies

Over-the-needle intravenous catheters (18–24 gauge)

Butterfly needles (21–25 gauge)

Intraosseous needles/device (15–18 gauge)

Intravenous tubing

Normal saline (0.9%)

Miscellaneous equipment and supplies

Sphygmomanometer (manual or electronic) with cuff (infant to large adult)

Syringes

Armboards

Tape

Tourniquet

Blood glucose device

Urine test strips

Splints

Nasogastric tubes (6F–14F)

Optional monitoring equipment

Cardiac monitor/defibrillator with pediatric pads/paddles or automatic external defibrillator with pediatric capabilities

Optional intubation/airway equipment

Laryngoscope with handle and batteries

Laryngoscope blades with bulbs: straight (Miller) 0–3, curved (Macintosh) 1–3

Endotracheal tubes: cuffed or uncuffed (2.5–8.0)

Stylets (pediatric, adult)

End-tidal carbon dioxide detector

Laryngeal mask airway (size 1–5)

Data from Refs.[7,9,10]

Box 2
Recommended medications

Nonintravenous medications

Oxygen[a]

Albuterol[a]

Epinephrine 1:1000[a] for IM or subcutaneous use

Hydrocortisone

Ceftriaxone

Diazepam rectal gel

Glucagon

Naloxone

Acetaminophen

Ibuprofen

Diphenydramine

Intravenous medications

Epinephrine 1:10,000

Lorazepam

25% Dextrose

[a] Required.

Data from Refs.[7,9,10]

---

that the appropriate level of team (basic life support vs advanced life support) will respond (if available). If the office is situated in a large complex, providing specific directions to the office or having someone from the office staff or building security meet the EMS team at the main entrance to show them the way can save valuable time.[9]

If complex patients are cared for in the office, providing EMS with names and addresses of those requiring electricity/generator backup for ventilators, who use oxygen in the home, or with critical illnesses (congenital adrenal hypoplasia, panhypopituitarism, complex seizures), may be beneficial. Visiting these families may also be beneficial, so that if EMS has to respond, the providers knows what to expect. The EIF is beneficial in this instance (accessible at https://www2.aap.org/advaocacy/eif.doc). This form was developed by the AAP and ACEP and provides EMS and any physician seeing the child with quick and vital information about the child.[14] It should be completed by the pediatrician and updated regularly. It provides a quick summary of underlying medical problems, clinical baseline, medications, allergies, immunizations, specialists seen, the family's location and phone numbers, and disaster planning needs.

MOCK CODES/SKILL DRILLS

The use of a mock code provides the office staff with a chance to practice their response to an emergency. One study used education followed by mock codes in primary care offices and found that the mock codes helped office personnel feel less anxious about medical emergencies.[15] A doll or just a piece of paper with presenting complaints and initial assessment can be used to start the process.[9] The receptionist/secretary can be given this information, call for help, and see who responds. The "patient" can then be taken to a room, and patient assessment and treatment begun. Appropriate equipment and medication should be found, and although not really used, drug doses should be determined and patient responses recorded (although the physicians act as the team leaders, they should have realistic responses predetermined and placed on new cards or communicated verbally). Someone must document the entire exercise on an evaluation form so that a critique/debriefing can be performed afterward to see what was done well, what did not go so well, and where improvements can be made.[9]

Because the mock code may not allow the staff to practice specific skills such as bag-mask ventilation unless a manikin is available, some skills drills may also be necessary. Vascular access can be performed on office personnel (as allowed) and intraosseous insertion can be performed on chicken legs. A manikin may be able to be borrowed from a local hospital, or local EMS providers and instructors can be invited to the office and, if they have the equipment, bag-mask ventilation and other skills can be practiced together. They can also be involved in the mock drill so staff can measure their response time and observe how they work as a team and with the office, and so the EMS team can similarly learn more about the office's capabilities.

WHEN DISASTER STRIKES

Recent events such as Hurricane Sandy, the Sandy Hook School shootings, and the Asiana airplane crash, have highlighted the need for disaster preparedness at an individual, community, and national level. It has also documented that children's needs are not being met adequately, and therefore pediatricians must be ready.[16] Pediatricians must discuss with families how to prepare an emergency kit and develop a family emergency plan. Pediatricians must think about their office staff and make sure they do the same. Considerations include whether the office uses paper medical records or an electronic system. If the former, wat happens if the office is destroyed by a tornado or a flood ruins the records; how will the records be accessed? If the latter, is a backup system in place to save the information, and can the information be accessed outside the office? If the office is not usable immediately or for weeks after a disaster, can patients be seen at another location (another physicians' office, local hospital, board of health, school), and how will patients be notified? If the office is functioning after a disaster, it could be a community asset, used to see other physicians' patients (and one's own) and provide immunizations and other care.[16] Therefore, an office disaster plan should be coordinated with the local hospital and community emergency response agencies so that office's expertise can be used during the response and recovery. Many references about disaster response are available from several agencies, including the AAP (http://www.aap.org/en-us/advocacy-and-policy/aap-health-initiatives/Children-and-Disasters/Pages/default.aspx).[16]

SUMMARY

Pediatricians care for children in their offices every day. The very sick children are the ones who make office staff nervous. Everyone's anxiety levels can be reduced and patient care improved through preparing the office and staff for those children; having the right equipment, supplies, and medication; having everyone know their roles and proper response; involving EMS; and practicing scenarios using mock codes or skill drills.

Useful Web sites

Emergency information form: https://www2.aap.org/advocacy/eif.doc.

American Academy of Pediatrics: Children & Disasters: http://www.aap.org/en-us/advocacy-and-policy/aap-health-initiatives/Children-and-Disasters/Pages/default.aspx

Emergency Medical Services for Children: National Resource Center: http://childrensnational.org/EMSC

REFERENCES

1. Fuchs S, Jaffe DM, Christoffel KK. Pediatric emergencies in the office: prevalence and office preparedness. Pediatrics 1989;83:931–9.
2. Altieri M, Bellet J, Scott H. Preparedness for pediatric emergencies encountered in the practitioners' office. Pediatrics 1990;85:710–4.
3. Schweich P, DeAngelis C, Duggan A. Preparedness of practicing pediatricians to manage emergencies in the office. Pediatrics 1991;88:223–9.
4. Flores G, Weinstock DJ. The preparedness of pediatricians for emergencies in the office: what is broken, should we care, and how can we fix it? Arch Pediatr Adolesc Med 1996;150:249–56 [correction published Arch Pediatr Adolesc Med 1996;150:592].
5. American Academy of Pediatrics. Periodic survey #27 emergency readiness of pediatric offices. Available at: http://www.aap.org/en-us/professional-resources/Research/Pages/PS27_Executive_Summary_EmergencyReadinessofPediatric Offices.aspx. Accessed February 11, 2013.
6. Santillanes G, Gausche-Hill M, Sosa B. Preparedness of selected offices to respond to critical emergencies in children. Pediatr Emerg Care 2006;22:694–8.
7. Toback SL. Medical emergency preparedness in office practice. Am Fam Physician 2007;75:1679–84.
8. Pendleton AL, Martin-Thompson MA, Stevenson MD. Outpatient emergency preparedness: a survey of pediatricians [abstract]. Pediatr Emerg Care 2012;28: 1095.
9. American Academy of Pediatrics, Committee on Pediatric Emergency Medicine. Preparation for emergencies in the office of pediatricians and pediatric primary care providers. Pediatrics 2007;120:200–12.
10. Frush K, Hohenhaus S, Bailey B, et al. Office preparedness for pediatric emergencies. 1997. Available at: http://www.ems.ohio.gov/emsc%20web%20site_11_04/pdf_doc%20files/provider%20manual.pdf. Accessed July 9, 2013.
11. Gausche M, Lewis RJ, Stratton SJ, et al. Effect of out-of-hospital pediatric endotracheal intubation on survival and neurologic outcome. JAMA 2000;283:783–90 [Erratum published J Am Med Assoc 2000;283:3204].
12. Henderson DP, Gausche M, Goodrich SM, et al. Education of paramedics in pediatric airway management: effects of different retraining methods on self-efficacy and skill retention. Acad Emerg Med 1998;5:429.
13. Blackmon LB. 10 useful apps for everyday pediatric use. Pediatr Ann 2012;41: 209–11.
14. American Academy of Pediatrics, Committee on Pediatric Emergency Medicine and Council on Clinical Technology, American College of Emergency Physicians, Pediatric Emergency Medicine Committee. Policy statement- emergency information forms and emergency preparedness for children with special health care needs. Pediatrics 2010;125:829–37.

15. Toback SL, Fiedor M, Kilpela B, et al. Impact of a pediatric primary care office-based mock code program on physician and skill confidence to perform life-saving skills. Pediatr Emerg Care 2006;22:415–22.
16. American Academy of Pediatrics, Committee on Pediatric Emergency Medicine, Committee on Medical Liability, Task Force on Terrorism. The pediatrician and disaster preparedness. Pediatrics 2006;117:560–5.

Common Office Procedures and Analgesia Considerations

Amy Baxter, MD[a,b],*

KEYWORDS

• Abscess • Analgesia • Laceration • Child life • Distraction • Anesthetic

KEY POINTS

• Time of onset of medications should coincide with procedural pain.
• Pain management requires preparation and intervention for the caregivers as well as patients.
• Untreated pain results in a negative template that complicates future procedures; attention to the fear and focus of pediatric patients, as well as pain, is essential.

INTRODUCTION

One of the most satisfying parts of medicine is improving an acute or painful problem. Procedures in the outpatient setting provide an opportunity for immediate resolution of the problem, such as reducing subluxed radial heads or repairing lacerations. When a painful procedure is not approached correctly, however, short-term and long-term consequences follow. Poorly controlled procedural pain can prolong treatment times, drain staff resources, dissatisfy parents, and leave patients with a lasting fear of medical treatment.[1] When anxiety or motion prevent successful completion, an additional trip to the emergency department may be necessary. With the correct approach to pediatric distress and proper pain management, many office procedures can be accomplished with minimal discomfort and distress, and improved office flow.

RATIONALE FOR PEDIATRIC PAIN MANAGEMENT

Before 1987, the prevailing teaching was that children were born incapable of experiencing pain in a meaningful way. Anand and colleagues[2] demonstrated that withholding analgesia for procedures resulted in poorer outcomes in preterm patent ductus arteriosus ligation patients, including bradycardia, hypotension, and even

[a] Pediatric Emergency Medicine Associates, Children's Healthcare of Atlanta Scottish Rite, 1001 Johnson Ferry Road North East, Atlanta, GA 30342, USA; [b] Department of Emergency Medicine, Medical College of Georgia at Georgia Regents University, 1120 15th Street, Augusta, GA 30912, USA
* 322 Sutherland Place Northeast, Atlanta, GA 30307.
E-mail address: abaxter@mmjlabs.com

Pediatr Clin N Am 60 (2013) 1163–1183
http://dx.doi.org/10.1016/j.pcl.2013.06.012
0031-3955/13/$ – see front matter © 2013 Elsevier Inc. All rights reserved.

intraventricular hemorrhage. An increased awareness of adverse long-term consequences from oligoanalgesia (whether in cases of circumcision,[3] venipuncture,[1,4–6] lumbar puncture [LP],[7] or acute multisystem trauma[8–11]) has led the American Academy of Pediatrics to recommend adequate procedural pain management, even for venipuncture.[12]

COMMON OBJECTIONS TO PAIN MANAGEMENT

A primary barrier to effective acute pain management in children includes the inability to assess pain in younger children, as well as a fear of overmedicating.[13–15] Parents, as well as clinicians, fear using opioid medication. In one postoperative tonsillectomy study, despite having access to acetaminophen with codeine, 99% of home doses were for acetaminophen alone.[16] Procedural pain control is limited by more operational issues, primarily perceived lack of time and inconvenient access to medications.[17] In addition, early experiences with lidocaine-prilocaine cream for intravenous (IV) access left the perception that topical pain relief decreases procedural success.[18] In fact, addressing IV pain has been found to significantly decrease time and increase first-attempt success.[19–21]

NATURE OF PEDIATRIC PROCEDURAL DISTRESS

Procedural distress in children and, to a lesser extent, adults, combines behavioral components (fear, lack of control, temperament) with physical pain and how focused they are on the procedure (**Fig. 1**). Patient and family assessment is critical to determine the amount and type of nonpharmacologic management to best support a family during procedures.

Fear

Lack of knowledge of what to expect, lack of control over the procedure, and physical vulnerability all contribute to a sense of fear. Fear is highly correlated with reported pain[22,23] and has implications for future memory of painful experiences.[7] Because

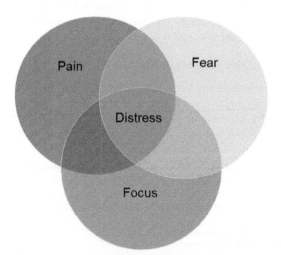

Fig. 1. Procedural distress for a child includes the level of fear, how much attention is focused on the procedure versus something comforting or neutral, and how much pain is involved. (Copyright © Baxter. Used with permission.)

the contribution of parental anxiety accounts for 50% of a child's distress[24] and is predictive of children's reported pain,[25,26] awareness and addressing the parent and child as a unit can improve procedural success.

Recent research evaluated serum beta-endorphin, a stress and pain biomarker. Higher preoperative levels in adults correlated with increased postoperative pain.[27] Compared with nonsurgical hospitalized patients, neonates had a moderate elevation and preschool children had an "explicitly high" elevation in endorphins, indicating a significant presence of presurgical anxiety ($P < .0005$).[28] Interestingly, before and after an operation, infants had low biomarker levels and did not differ from nonsurgical hospitalized patients. This suggests that the conditioned responses of neonates (who may have had more previous procedural interventions), and preschool children "who exhibit increased emotional perception" are more susceptible to the effects of fear. Preschool children may benefit the most from fear-reducing preparation and intraprocedural interventions.

Preparation

Preparation should include a brief age-appropriate explanation of the ensuing sequential procedural steps presented in a calm, confident manner. Ideally, incorporate gentle touch at a location distant to a painful area and include descriptions of any sounds, sights, or physical sensations that the patient may experience. Allowing patients and their parents to ask questions may alleviate any fears or inaccurate expectations. Preparation should include guidance toward appropriate coping skills, such as relaxation techniques (eg, deep breathing, muscle relaxation) or distraction. "A lot of kids find it helps when they blow out on a pinwheel, or find things in my picture book, or play on my iPad. Let's make a plan for what you would like to do." Although certain language increases fear and pain (**Table 1**),[29] focused mental and physical distraction provided by the parent can improve the experience. In addition, assigning both patient and parent a distraction or restraint responsibility during a procedure is an anchoring point to return to if either becomes distressed. "OK, remember, your job is to hold really still. We said you'd take a huge breath and hold it like a statue if you got nervous, so go ahead now and take that breath."

Sinha and colleagues[30] found distraction to be effective for all children by parent-report, although self-report only differed for older children. In contrast, a smaller study by Gursky and colleagues[31] found that extensive preparation and active distraction was extremely effective, even in a younger cohort. Gursky and colleagues used a 15-minute protocol that included modeling the procedure to the patient on dolls and allowing the patient to feel the suture material. Although this extensive level of

	Neutral or Reduces Distress	Increases Distress
Table 1		
Language and pediatric distress		
Language	Pressure, tight squeeze	Shot, sting, pinch
	Bother, uncomfortable	Hurt
	Push	"I'm sorry"
	Metal tube, squirter	Needle, syringe
Behaviors	Redirecting	Empathizing
	Nonprocedural discussion	Apologizing
	Talk before touch	Punishing
	Firm, warm confidence	Allowing the child to delay
	Humor	Multiple adults talking

preparation may be excessive for many primary care settings, explaining the procedure while a topical anesthetic is placed on the child may mitigate fear even without using anxiolytic medications.

A good resource incorporating multiple aspects of preparation can be found at http://www.youtube.com/watch?v=T2f7G6zMdXA.

Restraint

Lying supine is the most vulnerable position for humans, particularly when physically restrained with a papoose board or by adults. In contrast to preparation (tell-show-do) being the most helpful technique to allay anxiety for pediatric dentistry, the papoose board and physical restraint were the most detrimental.[32] Techniques to restrain without physical force or use of papoose boards include sheet wrapping[33] and insertion of a child's arms behind them into a pillowcase on which to recline (**Fig. 2**).[34] To reduce further the anxiety caused by lying supine, a parent can sit next to a child or sit on the table with the child in his or her lap (**Fig. 3**). Placing an arm around the child's shoulder, the parent can tuck one of the child's arms behind the parent's back, using a shoulder to restrain gently the child's other arm, or use one arm to control the forearm (**Figs. 4** and **5**). This position-of-comfort approach significantly reduced distress

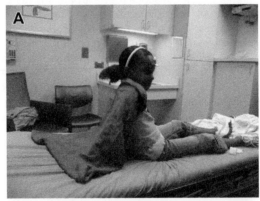

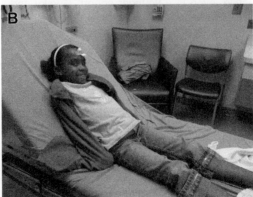

Fig. 2. To use the pillowcase restraint, have the child place arms into a pillowcase located behind their back (*A*), then lie down on the case (*B*). This allows limited movement of the arms without jeopardizing a sterile field. (*Courtesy of* Amy Baxter, MD, Augusta, GA.)

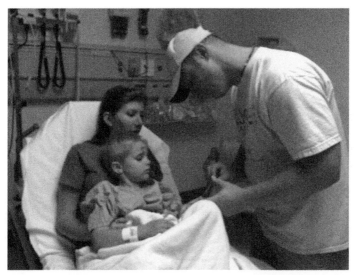

Fig. 3. Security is enhanced by having the child sit on the parent's lap for laceration repair. The mother is in a good position to control the patient's upper arm in case of forgetful movement or distress. The anxiety is further reduced before the procedure by the father's use of distraction cards. (*Courtesy of* Amy Baxter, MD, Augusta, GA.)

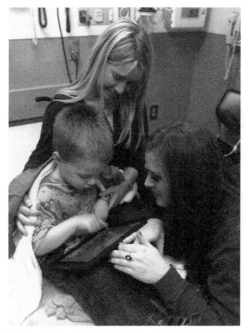

Fig. 4. The child is sitting upright, with the mother able to secure his arms from either side. He is engaged in active distraction with a tablet game. (*Courtesy of* Amy Baxter, MD, Augusta, GA.)

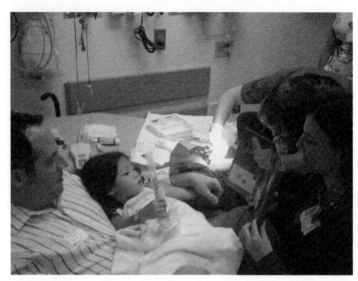

Fig. 5. Note that with a position of comfort, distraction, and a good digital block, the patient can be allowed to be distracted further and rewarded with a popsicle because eating is not a concern with nonpharmacologic interventions. The father's hand is in a position to restrain the forearm during this thumb nailbed repair. (*Courtesy of* Amy Baxter, MD, Augusta, GA.)

when used for IV placement (**Figs. 6** and **7**).[35] An excellent video demonstrating multiple examples is available at http://www.youtube.com/watch?v=VOqIVIFN5Bo. A PDF is available at http://ministryhealth.org/SaintJosephsChildrensHospital/ChildLife Program/Positioning_for_Comfort_2007.pdf.

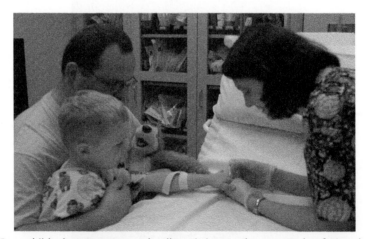

Fig. 6. For a child who wants to watch, allow sitting on the parent's lap facing the procedure. Note that the father's left hand should move up past the bear and gently secure the forearm during the procedure. (*Courtesy of* Heidi Giese, BS, CCLS, CTRS, CIMI, Child Life Manager, Saint Joseph's Children's Hospital, Marshfield Clinic Children's, Marshfield, Wisconsin.)

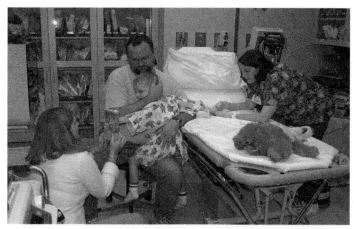

Fig. 7. To secure a child who is less cooperative, have them face their parent and secure the arm for an IV on a gurney at just below axilla height. Ideally, the father's left arm would be above the patient's shoulder to secure the arm further. (*Courtesy of* Heidi Giese, BS, CCLS, CTRS, CIMI, Child Life Manager, Saint Joseph's Children's Hospital, Marshfield Clinic Children's, Marshfield, Wisconsin.)

Focus of Attention–Active and Passive Distraction, Environment, One Voice

Passive distraction

Although the literature supports passive distraction (watching television, looking at a book) for IV access, in more painful procedures such as injection or LP, passive distraction may be inadequate.[36] Although ambient interventions, such as music or asking parents of toddlers to sing, are ineffective for shots,[37] for older children, choosing their own music has provided significant reduction in distress.

Active distraction

Offering a child a game (eg, blowing bubbles, playing video games)[22] or task (finding visual pictures) not only reduces fear but can improve the child's recollection of the procedure compared with previous experiences performed without distraction.[38] The use of active interventions is being revolutionized by smart phone or tablet computer applications, with strong anecdotal support and new applications daily (see **Fig. 4**).[39] Frequently recommended applications recommended by child life professionals are available at http://www.buzzy4shots.com/Pain-Managment-Ideas/ hi-tech-distraction.html. Beyond simple finding or hand-eye coordination tasks, cognitive distraction, such as asking a patient to recall, tell a story, or perform arithmetic, is not effective.[40] Letting the child choose their form of distraction helps mitigate the feeling of loss of control. Even without props, knowing available visual stimuli in the room that can be counted (eg, ceiling tiles, windowpanes) and having a plan to count or repeat ABCs are helpful, easily available options.

Environment

Although literature on environmental factors such as ambient temperature, light, and sound is scarce for in-office procedures, both preanesthesia and dental literature offer some support beyond a common sense approach to children. Without parental preparation, parental presence alone is the least effective way of decreasing anxiety.[41–43] In addition to preparation and a position of comfort, decreasing the amount of noise and chaos can lower the anxiety preprocedure.[44] One randomized, controlled trial of 70 children preanesthesia found significantly decreased anxiety with a three-pronged approach: dimming operating room lights, playing Bach's *Air on a G String*, and having only one person, the attending anesthesiologist, interact with the child.[45] Keeping lights low and using only the ceiling spotlight for suturing can minimize stimulation (**Fig. 8**).

Music and dimmed lights may be difficult to provide; however, "One Voice," which is only one person speaking during the intervention, is a simple technique available at http://www.onevoice4kids.com/learning.html. This method designates one person to provide information and distraction during the procedure to reduce chaos and give the child more control. A YouTube video is available at https://www.mededportal.org/icollaborative/resource/546.

Humor, normalizing discussion, and calm redirection are powerful tools to reduce anxiety. Often, when words such as pain, hurt, shot, or medical jargon are used, fear increases. Ironically, empathy and reassurance ("I know, honey, it's okay") also increase distress in children.[26,46]

PHARMACOLOGIC ANXIOLYSIS

The fast-acting benzodiazepine midazolam as a single agent is by far the most studied anxiolytic for procedural sedation (**Box 1**, **Table 2**).[47,48] Oral doses of 0.5 to 0.7 mg/kg, with a maximum of 15 mg, result in mild sedation within 15 to 30 minutes. Recently, Klein and colleagues[49] described 0.5 mg/kg aerosolized buccal administration of

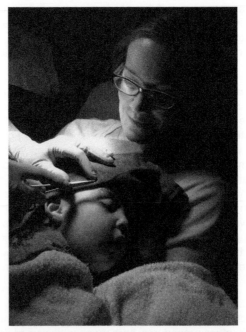

Fig. 8. With the use of LET and naptime, this child could be sutured completely without sedation. He was allowed to fall asleep on his mother. During the procedure, she restrained his head with her right arm under the drape and controlled his shoulders with her left hand. This also illustrates draping for retaining vision for an awake, anxious child.

Box 1
Recipe for LET

Lidocaine 20%100 mL (20 g lidocaine powder/100 mL normal saline)

Racemic epinephrine 2.25%50 mL

Tetracaine 2%125 mL

Sodium metabisulfite 315.4 mg

225 mL sterile H20

This mixture can be stored in refrigeration for up to 5 months. Maximum dose: 3 mL for children >17 kg, or 0.175 mL/kg. Leave in contact with the wound 20 minutes or until skin is locally blanched.

---

the IV formulation having improved efficacy to oral, with less distress than when administered intranasally.

The IV form of midazolam can be administered at a dose of 0.3 to 0.4 mg/kg intranasally, yielding effective sedation in 5 to 15 minutes.[50] To improve absorption, use a mucosal atomizer device (approximately $1.00) and divide the dose between the nares. Because the pH of the IV formulation is 3.3, pretreatment with lidocaine 10 mg per puff in the nares, or an oral drop of cherry syrup afterwards may make the administration more tolerated.[51] The duration of sedation from oral midazolam is between 20 and 40 minutes. Intranasal administration had an average of 23.1 minutes duration of sedation.

Paradoxic Reactions

Instead of sedation, midazolam can rarely cause a paradoxic tachycardia, inconsolability, and agitation. This has been documented 1.4% of the time with IV administration at 0.1 mg/kg, 6% with oral administration,[52] and up to 27% with 1 mg/kg rectal administration.[53] In a large IV series, onset occurred when sedation would have

---

Table 2
Medications to facilitate procedural anxiolysis or analgesia

	Route or Form	Dose	Maximum Dose	Onset	Duration
Midazolam	IV	.025–.05 mg/kg	2 mg	3–5 min	30–45 min
Midazolam	Oral	0.5–0.7 mg/kg	15 mg	20–30 min	40–70 min
Midazolam	Intranasal or IV form	0.3–0.5 mg/kg	10 mg	10–20 min	30 min
Midazolam	Buccal IV form	0.3–0.5 mg/kg	10 mg	20–30 min	40–70 min
Fentanyl	Intranasal	2–3 μg/kg	200 μg	5–10 min	30 min
Hydrocodone	Oral	0.13 mg/kg (0.2 mL/kg of 2.5 mg/kg elixir)	7.5 mg	60 min	3 h
Oxycodone	Oral	0.2–0.3 mg/kg	15 mg	30 min	3 h

Combined opioids and benzodiazepines is considered moderate sedation and should only be administered in adherence to the American Academy of Pediatrics sedation guidelines.

Data from Cote CJ, Wilson S. Guidelines for monitoring and management of pediatric patients during and after sedation for diagnostic and therapeutic procedures: an update. Pediatrics 2006;118(6):2587–602.

been expected (average 17 minutes) and resolved within a mean of 14 minutes when flumazenil was administered.[54] Although flumazenil can be administered intranasally, use by this route as a sedation-reversal agent has only been described in case reports. Agitation tends to wear off at approximately the duration of sedation.

ENTERAL PHARMACOLOGIC PAIN MANAGEMENT
Over-the-Counter Treatment

When a painful procedure is anticipated, dosing ibuprofen at least 30 minutes before initiation of the procedure can help. Ibuprofen has been shown to be more effective for initial management of pediatric fractures than acetaminophen with codeine[55] and is an important part of optimizing pain relief. Because a small study found ibuprofen alone not significantly different than oxycodone, or a combination of oxycodone and ibuprofen, the clinical effect of using both may not be advantageous.[56,57] This may be due to the delayed effect of the oral opioids, however, because both trials gave the doses simultaneously and may not have allowed for the optimum opioid level.

Oral Opioids

Oxycodone is typically dosed at 0.2 to 0.3 mg/kg and has peak plasma effects in 1 hour. Hydrocodone comes in a 2.5 mg/5 mL formulation dosed at 0.2 mL/kg formulation, or 1 teaspoon per 10 kg of body weight. Because its peak is delayed to between 60 and 90 minutes, for optimal use and safety, give this medication when postprocedural pain is anticipated and when time permits.

Intranasal Fentanyl

Intranasal fentanyl is commonly used for emergency department pain relief without IV access. When dosed at 1 to 2 μg/kg up to 200 μg, fentanyl offers rapid pain relief and mild euphoria within 10 minutes, with resolution of most of the effects by 30 minutes after administration. Unlike intranasal midazolam the IV formulation does not burn. It is also best delivered with a mucosal atomizer. The combination of oral fentanyl lollipops and oral midazolam led to increased vomiting without significant improvements in procedural success, but the edible formulation could be the problem.[58] Intranasal fentanyl and midazolam have not been studied, but effective preoperative pain relief in one study supports the concept.[59]

TOPICAL ANESTHETICS

Because lidocaine is hydrophilic, administration through intact skin presents a challenge. For a laceration, placing a mixture of lidocaine, tetracaine, and adrenaline (epinephrine), also known as LET or LAT (see **Table 2**), directly on the wound before cleaning and suturing is between 73% and 90% effective.[60] Ideally, saturate a wound-sized piece of cotton and pack into the wound for 20 minutes before cleaning. When the wound is blanched, cleaning may be initiated. LET's analgesic effects dissipate within 40 to 50 minutes, so timing of the procedure is important. Because only half of extremities are adequately anesthetized with topical LET alone, injecting lidocaine may still be needed.

When LET is not available, lidocaine-prilocaine cream, an eutectic mixture of local anesthetics, has been found moderately effective.[61] When lidocaine injection is needed, allow the syringe to be warmed or, at least, room temperature. Using 10:1 lidocaine to sodium bicarbonate to buffer the acidity[62] and injecting from within the wound rather than through intact skin also improves comfort.[63] The maximum dose of lidocaine is 4 mg/kg of plain, or 7 mg/kg of lidocaine with epinephrine.

For procedures on intact skin, options include lidocaine-prilocaine cream, 4% lidocaine in liposomes, and tetracaine. The eutectic mixture of prilocaine 2.5% and lidocaine 2.5% reduces pain from IV catheter insertion when applied for a minimum of 45 minutes,[64] although it can vasoconstrict for the first hour before a vasodilation after 2 hours of application.[21] In contrast to the other topical anesthetics, lidocaine-prilocaine cream can be left on up to 4 hours with a depth of penetration up to 5 mm.[65] Because of possible methemoglobinemia, lidocaine-prilocaine cream should be limited to infants of at least 37-weeks gestational age. A purpuric rash may occur with lidocaine-prilocaine cream in 1% to 2% of patients, particularly those with a history of atopic reactions.

Effective in 30 minutes, 4% lidocaine in liposomes works as well as lidocaine-prilocaine cream does in 45 minutes for venipuncture pain and meatotomy.[66,67] The rapid absorption correlates with a rapid dissipation of the drug, with diminishing anesthesia approximately 40 to 60 minutes after application. Compared with placebo, 4% lidocaine in liposomes improved cannulation success on the first attempt (74% vs 55%, $P = .03$) with decreased time of insertion and reported pain.[20] Tetracaine gel, formerly known as amethocaine is available alone and compounded with lidocaine. The 4% formulation works in 30 to 45 minutes, and lasts 4 to 6 hours with an efficacy similar to lidocaine-prilocaine cream.[68]

PHYSIOLOGIC PAIN MANAGEMENT—GATE CONTROL AND DESCENDING NOXIOUS INHIBITORY CONTROL

Pain is transmitted to a final common pathway in the dorsal column of the spinal cord with large, myelinated Aβ vibration reception and nonmyelinated C-fibers that transmit cold or chronic pain. Like rubbing a bumped elbow or placing a burned finger under water, overwhelming the Aβ vibration nerves or the C-fiber cold nerves can reduce sharp pain. Cold spray (vapocoolant, ethyl chloride) has been found effective for children older than the age of 12 years.[69] Although a vibrating, cold medical device that stimulates both Aβ and C-fibers has been shown to reduce IV pain in children,[19,70] simply scratching the same dermatome, or applying an ice pack proximally to it, may achieve the same effect.

Although gate control happens locally, another effective mechanism of pain control is called descending (or diffuse) noxious inhibitory control. This also works with cold stimuli, which ramps up C-fiber intensity. An almost unpleasant degree of cold can work anywhere on the body because intense cold activates a supraspinal modulation, raising the body's overall pain threshold, even away from the nerve. Using local cold spray and a vibration stimulus distant from the injection has been shown to decrease immunization pain.[71]

Sucrose Analgesia

For infants, a 24% sucrose and water solution on a pacifier provides procedural pain relief. The effectiveness of sucrose is most commonly cited for preterm infants and neonates younger than 2 months of age, although some literature supports pain relief in 6-month-old infants for less invasive procedures.[72,73]

IV and Phlebotomy

Preparation
Place topical anesthetic in a timely fashion. Before placing tourniquet, explain in developmentally appropriate terms, such as "We're going to use a small straw to take a sample that shows how healthy your blood is. You'll feel a tight squeeze on your

arm, and it will take about as much time as one commercial, then you'll get a sticker! Your job is to look at this [distraction] and, when I'm ready, [blow bubbles/pinwheel/see if you can find x]."

Patient positioning
Allow parent to put an arm around the patient if in a phlebotomy chair, or sit on parent's lap with arm secured on a gurney or table.

Approach
Explain what you are doing before touching the patient. If the child is engaged in distraction, just say, "You'll feel me touching you now."

Technique or procedure
Fein and Cohen[74,75] provide full resources specifically for IV access. Slifer and colleagues[76] offer suggestions for working with children with intellectual disabilities.

Catheterization

Preparation
For infant catheterization, prepare parents for the procedure. For older children, an age-appropriate explanation should include the coldness of cleaning and the feeling of pressure.

Patient position
Older children can be on a parent's lap with the parent holding the patient's legs.

Technique or procedure
Before catheterization, 2% lidocaine jelly (available in a prefilled syringe) can be applied to the urethra for 1 to 2 minutes. Although effective at reducing pain in adult males, research to date in children either has been underpowered or has shown equivocal results. One study found decreased crying in children during catheterization ($P = .036$) compared with children who did not have a lubricant instilled in urethra, but found no statistic change in observational pain scales or vital sign parameters.[77,78] Suprapubic aspiration is more painful than catheterization.[79]

Injections

Give parenteral analgesic and/or place topical anesthetic in a timely fashion. Before getting vaccinations, explain in developmentally appropriate terms, such as "We're going to give you three boosters today to help keep you healthy. I'm going to bring them on a little tray, with your sticker! We have some new things to make you more comfortable. While I get them, why don't you and [your parent] do [this distracting thing]." When ready, let the child know they will feel coldness first, and consider allowing them to feel the alcohol swab. "Your job is to look at [this distraction] and, when I'm ready, [blow bubbles/pinwheel/see if you can find x]."

Patient positioning
For infants, nonnutritive sucking and breastfeeding have been found to decrease immunization distress.[72] Patients over 18 months should receive shots in the deltoid. Allow parent to put an arm around the patient, or have the patient sit facing the parent on parent's lap. Promote patient's ability to look at distraction. If using a vibrating, cold medical device or contralateral vibration, allow patient to interact with the device while immunizations are being prepared.[23,71]

Approach
Have patient immediately ready to leave after immunizations to replace the stimulus of waiting in the room with the positive activity of cuddling, receiving a sticker, and changing the environment.

Technique or procedure
Extensive evidence-based guidelines for immunization pain relief are provided by Taddio and colleagues[80] and Schechter and colleagues.[81]

Stretch, vibrate, apply pressure or apply cold proximal to the site.[82]

Give the least painful injection first. Less subsequent reaction is caused by 23-gauge 25 mm needles compared with 25-gauge 16 mm needles.[83,84]

Data in infants and 4- to 6-year-olds support that faster completion of all vaccinations causes lower distress. Although parents prefer shots be given simultaneously, this has not been shown to reduce distress.[85]

Lacerations

Preparation
Explain the procedure in developmentally appropriate terms and let the child experience sensations of feeling the instruments and sutures before feeling them near the laceration. If LET is applied properly 20 minutes before procedure, reassure the child that the procedure will not hurt. Make a distraction plan.

Patient positioning
Use a position of comfort, such as restraining arms in a "superman" pillowcase or using a sheet to restrain, if necessary. Make sure patient can see distraction elements. For facial lacerations, drape patient so that at least one eye is uncovered to anticipate motion during procedure (see **Fig. 8**; **Fig. 9**).

Approach
Fear can be reduced by the practitioner moving slowly and deliberately while setting up the laceration tray.

Technique or procedure
Because the cleaning phase is often the most distressing, warming the irrigant under warm tap water, letting the child feel the temperature of it on his or her hand immediately before, and dripping the first few drops slowly can set the child's expectations and avoid the delay of having to calm a child midprocedure.

Alert the child before each touch and give an indication of duration. "Now you're going to feel some wetness" or "Now you might feel a little push" or "I'm going to be pushing two more times."

Debridement and Burn Cleaning

Preparation
For an area less than 1% of body weight, 30 minutes before the procedure, apply topical anesthetic under self-stick plastic wrap rather than under tightly adhering occlusive dressing. For burns, consider intranasal fentanyl 5 minutes before the procedure.

Patient positioning
Use a position of comfort, such as restraining arms in a "superman" pillowcase or, if necessary, use a sheet to restrain. Make sure patient can see distraction elements. For facial lacerations, drape patient so that at least one eye is uncovered to anticipate motion during procedure.

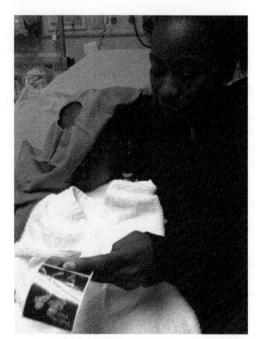

Fig. 9. For this anxious 6-year-old, providing distraction by asking seek and find questions around the stickers ("How many teeth does the alligator have?") and draping her head to allow for preservation of some vision enabled laceration repair without sedation.

Approach
Fear can be reduced by the practitioner moving slowly and deliberately while setting up the laceration tray.

Technique or procedure
Because the cleaning phase is often the most distressing, warming the irrigant under warm tap water, letting the child feel the temperature of it on his or her hand immediately before, and dripping the first few drops slowly can set the child's expectations and avoid the delay of having to calm a child midprocedure. For burns, consider vibration or cold in the same dermatome proximal to the site during the procedure.

Digital Blocks

Preparation
Give ibuprofen and apply liposomal lidocaine 4% over site of injection 30 minutes before the procedure. Explain the procedure in developmentally appropriate terms. Let the child know she or he will feel coldness with cleaning, and that you will let the child know when he or she will feel one or two big pushes and tight squeezes, but, after that, the procedure will not hurt. Make a distraction plan. If applying vibration and/or ice[86] proximal to the site of injection, explain the technique and allow child to experience the sensations at a location distant to the injury.

Patient positioning
Use a position of comfort, such as restraining arms in a "superman" pillowcase or using a sheet to restrain if necessary. If being held by a parent, ensure the parent is comfortable and knows to make sure that the extremity is secure. Make sure patient

can see distraction elements. Consider intranasal fentanyl 5 minutes before digital block.

Approach
Fear can be reduced by the practitioner moving slowly and deliberately while setting up the procedure tray. Prepare the lidocaine or bupivacaine syringe out of sight of the patient.

Technique or procedure
Options include bilateral subcutaneous injection on either side of the affected digit or a single transthecal digital nerve block on the palmar side at the base of the digit. Although transthecal options are effective in pediatric patients,[87] an adult crossover trial found the single injection technique more painful in the short-term and at follow-up, with patients preferring the double subcutaneous injections.[88] In addition, numbness took longer (186 seconds) for the transthecal approach compared with 100 seconds for the bilateral subcutaneous approach.

Abscesses

Preparation
Provide ibuprofen and opioid with sufficient time before procedure. Consider intranasal fentanyl 5 minutes before procedure. Research on local pain management for abscess drainage is scant. Because lidocaine-prilocaine cream can descend up to 0.5 cm when left in place up to 4 hours, this may at least dull the pain of an injected lidocaine ring block. For larger abscesses, adjunct sedation or, minimally, a combination nonsteroidal, antiinflammatory and opioid is likely necessary. One clinical pearl is to use self-stick plastic wrap, which pulls off painlessly, instead of tightly adhering occlusive dressing to occlude larger areas. Prepare patient and parent using developmentally appropriate language.

Positioning
Use a position of comfort, such as restraining arms in a "superman" pillowcase or, if necessary, using a sheet for restraint. Make sure patient can see distraction elements.

Technique or procedure
Prepare lidocaine for ring block out of sight of the patient. Prepare the tray using slow and deliberate movements. Using gate control stimulation simultaneously will help with lidocaine injection or when a small-needle aspiration is anticipated. Provide opioid analgesia and advise round-the-clock ibuprofen for the first 24 to 48 hours for pain management.

Packing Changes

Preparation
Provide ibuprofen with or without opioids orally at least 30 and 60 minutes before the procedure, respectively. When packing material has been left in place, a mix of LET and lidocaine-prilocaine cream or 4% lidocaine in liposomes for 30 minutes can wick into the wound to numb the interior and the intact skin edges while providing moisture to loosen the gauze. Provide age-appropriate explanations of the procedure, emphasizing that this should be much less uncomfortable than the initial procedure.

LP

Preparation
Pain control for infant LP has become commonplace, with more than 70% of pediatric residents reporting using some form of analgesia or anesthetic.[89,90] Topical anesthetics

improve success, and the rapid efficacy of 4% lidocaine in liposomes makes it a feasible option when placed before obtaining blood and urine for a septic work-up.[89,91] For older children, the trend is for procedural sedation. If this is not possible, providing optimal pain control (ibuprofen, opioid) before the procedure is an adjunct to help avoid hyperalgesia and increased pain response with subsequent LPs.

Lidocaine-prilocaine cream has been extensively demonstrated to decrease the pain of LPs in older children.

Patient positioning
For neonates and small infants, using a sitting, rather than a lateral recumbent position, may improve success and, statistically, results in less respiratory compromise. For older children, positioning the parent near the head with an arm around the shoulders but outside the field may help.

Approach
Procedural sedation is the standard of care for older children undergoing LP. Nitrous 50%-oxygen 50% may be used if access to a sedation service for propofol and fentanyl is not available. IV midazolam and IV fentanyl together result in moderate-to-deep sedation and cannot safely be used without clinicians trained in sedation in a setting prepared to rescue from the effects of general anesthesia.

Technique or procedure
By approximately 2 to 3 months, infants are large enough that topical anesthetics will not penetrate far enough past the epidermis for optimal pain control. Infiltrating a generous amount of buffered lidocaine (approximately 1 mL per 10 kg of body weight up to a maximum of 5 mL) into the predural space provides improved pain relief. Intranasal fentanyl can further improve comfort with the procedure.

SUMMARY

Always keep in mind the time of onset of medications so that it coincides with procedural pain.

To be effective, pain management in emergency and procedural settings requires preparation and intervention for the caregivers as well as patients. Because untreated pain can result in a template that complicates future procedures, attention to the fear and focus of pediatric patients, as well as to their pain, is essential.

REFERENCES

1. Kennedy RM, Luhmann J, Zempsky WT. Clinical implications of unmanaged needle-insertion pain and distress in children. Pediatrics 2008;122(Suppl 3): S130–3.
2. Anand KJ, Sippell WG, Aynsley-Green A. Randomised trial of fentanyl anaesthesia in preterm babies undergoing surgery: effects on the stress response. Lancet 1987;1(8524):62–6.
3. Taddio A, Katz J, Ilersich AL, et al. Effect of neonatal circumcision on pain response during subsequent routine vaccination. Lancet 1997;349(9052): 599–603.
4. Deacon B, Abramowitz J. Fear of needles and vasovagal reactions among phlebotomy patients. J Anxiety Disord 2006;20(7):946–60.
5. Hodgins MJ, Lander J. Children's coping with venipuncture. J Pain Symptom Manage 1997;13(5):274–85.

6. Kleinknecht RA. Acquisition of blood, injury, and needle fears and phobias. Behav Res Ther 1994;32(8):817–23.
7. Weisman SJ, Bernstein B, Schechter NL. Consequences of inadequate analgesia during painful procedures in children. Arch Pediatr Adolesc Med 1998; 152(2):147–9.
8. Holbrook TL, Galarneau MR, Dye JL, et al. Morphine use after combat injury in Iraq and post-traumatic stress disorder. N Engl J Med 2010;362(2):110–7.
9. Holmes A, Williamson O, Hogg M, et al. Predictors of pain 12 months after serious injury. Pain Med 2010;11(11):1599–611.
10. Nixon RD, Nehmy TJ, Ellis AA, et al. Predictors of posttraumatic stress in children following injury: the influence of appraisals, heart rate, and morphine use. Behav Res Ther 2010;48(8):810–5.
11. Stoddard FJ Jr, Sorrentino EA, Ceranoglu TA, et al. Preliminary evidence for the effects of morphine on posttraumatic stress disorder symptoms in one- to four-year-olds with burns. J Burn Care Res 2009;30(5):836–43.
12. American Academy of Pediatrics. Committee on Psychosocial Aspects of Child and Family Health, Task Force on Pain in Infants, Children, and Adolescents. The assessment and management of acute pain in infants, children, and adolescents (0793). Pediatrics 2001;108:793–7.
13. Rupp T, Delaney KA. Inadequate analgesia in emergency medicine. Ann Emerg Med 2004;43(4):494–503.
14. Dong L, Donaldson A, Metzger R, et al. Analgesic administration in the emergency department for children requiring hospitalization for long-bone fracture. Pediatr Emerg Care 2012;28(2):109–14.
15. Thompson RW, Krauss B, Kim YJ, et al. Extremity fracture pain after emergency department reduction and casting: predictors of pain after discharge. Ann Emerg Med 2012;60(3):269–77.
16. Wilson ME, Helgadottir HL. Patterns of pain and analgesic use in 3- to 7-year-old children after tonsillectomy. Pain Manag Nurs 2006;7(4):159–66.
17. Leahy S, Kennedy RM, Hesselgrave J, et al. On the front lines: lessons learned in implementing multidisciplinary peripheral venous access pain-management programs in pediatric hospitals. Pediatrics 2008;122(Suppl 3):S161–70.
18. Lander J, Hodgins M, Nazarali S, et al. Determinants of success and failure of EMLA. Pain 1996;64(1):89–97.
19. Baxter AL, Cohen LL, Lawson ML, et al. A randomized clinical trial of a novel vibrating tourniquet to decrease pediatric venipuncture pain. Pediatr Emerg Care 2011;27(12):1151–6.
20. Taddio A, Soin HK, Schuh S, et al. Liposomal lidocaine to improve procedural success rates and reduce procedural pain among children: a randomized controlled trial. CMAJ 2005;172(13):1691–5.
21. Baxter AL, Ewing PH, Young GB, et al. EMLA application exceeding two hours improves pediatric emergency department venipuncture success. Adv Emerg Nurs J 2013;35(1):67–75.
22. Windich-Biermeier A, Sjoberg I, Dale JC, et al. Effects of distraction on pain, fear, and distress during venous port access and venipuncture in children and adolescents with cancer. J Pediatr Oncol Nurs 2007;24(1):8–19.
23. Baxter AL, Cohen LL, Weisman SJ, et al. Does Buzzy decrease adolescent immunization pain? Poster Presentation, PAS meeting. Boston, April 29, 2012; 2915.209A.
24. Jay SM, Elliott CH. A stress inoculation program for parents whose children are undergoing painful medical procedures. J Consult Clin Psychol 1990;58(6): 799–804.

25. Bernard RS, Cohen LL, McClellan CB, et al. Pediatric procedural approach-avoidance coping and distress: a multitrait-multimethod analysis. J Pediatr Psychol 2004;29(2):131–41.

26. Cohen LL, Blount RL, Cohen RJ, et al. Dimensions of pediatric procedural distress: children's anxiety and pain during immunizations. J Clin Psychol Med Settings 2004;11:41–7.

27. Matejec R, Ruwoldt R, Bodeker RH, et al. Release of beta-endorphin immunoreactive material under perioperative conditions into blood or cerebrospinal fluid: significance for postoperative pain? Anesth Analg 2003;96(2):481–6 table of contents.

28. Mirilas P, Mentessidou A, Kontis E, et al. Serum beta-endorphin response to stress before and after operation under fentanyl anesthesia in neonates, infants and preschool children. Eur J Pediatr Surg 2010;20(2):106–10.

29. Langer DA, Chen E, Luhmann JD. Attributions and coping in children's pain experiences. J Pediatr Psychol 2005;30(7):615–22.

30. Sinha M, Christopher NC, Fenn R, et al. Evaluation of nonpharmacologic methods of pain and anxiety management for laceration repair in the pediatric emergency department. Pediatrics 2006;117(4):1162–8.

31. Gursky B, Kestler LP, Lewis M. Psychosocial intervention on procedure-related distress in children being treated for laceration repair. J Dev Behav Pediatr 2010;31(3):217–22.

32. Luis de Leon J, Guinot Jimeno F, Bellet Dalmau LJ. Acceptance by Spanish parents of behaviour-management techniques used in paediatric dentistry. Eur Arch Paediatr Dent 2010;11(4):175–8.

33. Raskin BI. A simple pediatric restraint. Cutis 2000;66(5):335–6.

34. Brown JC, Klein EJ. The "Superhero Cape Burrito": a simple and comfortable method of short-term procedural restraint. J Emerg Med 2011;41(1):74–6.

35. Sparks LA, Setlik J, Luhman J. Parental holding and positioning to decrease IV distress in young children: a randomized controlled trial. J Pediatr Nurs 2007;22(6):440–7.

36. Cassidy KL, Reid GJ, McGrath PJ, et al. Watch needle, watch TV: audiovisual distraction in preschool immunization. Pain Med 2002;3(2):108–18.

37. Sobieraj G, Bhatt M, LeMay S, et al. The effect of music on parental participation during pediatric laceration repair. Can J Nurs Res 2009;41(4):68–82.

38. Inal S, Kelleci M. Distracting children during blood draw: looking through distraction cards is effective in pain relief of children during blood draw. Int J Nurs Pract 2012;18(2):210–9.

39. McQueen A, Cress C, Tothy A. Using a tablet computer during pediatric procedures: a case series and review of the "apps". Pediatr Emerg Care 2012;28(7):712–4.

40. Mitchell LA, MacDonald RA, Brodie EE. A comparison of the effects of preferred music, arithmetic and humour on cold pressor pain. Eur J Pain 2006;10(4):343–51.

41. Kazak Z, Sezer GB, Yilmaz AA, et al. Premedication with oral midazolam with or without parental presence. Eur J Anaesthesiol 2010;27(4):347–52.

42. Yip P, Middleton P, Cyna AM, et al. Non-pharmacological interventions for assisting the induction of anaesthesia in children. Cochrane Database Syst Rev 2009;(3):CD006447.

43. Scully SM. Parental presence during pediatric anesthesia induction. AORN J 2012;96(1):26–33.

44. Kirby V. Less noise = less anxiety for children's perioperative experience. Nurs Qual Connect 1994;4(2):6.

45. Kain ZN, Wang SM, Mayes LC, et al. Sensory stimuli and anxiety in children undergoing surgery: a randomized, controlled trial. Anesth Analg 2001;92(4): 897–903.
46. Blount RL, Corbin SM, Sturges JW, et al. The relationship between adults behavior and child coping and distress during BMA/LP procedures: a sequential analysis. Behav Ther 1989;20:585–601.
47. Shane SA, Fuchs SM, Khine H. Efficacy of rectal midazolam for the sedation of preschool children undergoing laceration repair. Ann Emerg Med 1994;24(6): 1065–73.
48. Lane RD, Schunk JE. Atomized intranasal midazolam use for minor procedures in the pediatric emergency department. Pediatr Emerg Care 2008;24(5):300–3.
49. Klein EJ, Brown JC, Kobayashi A, et al. A randomized clinical trial comparing oral, aerosolized intranasal, and aerosolized buccal midazolam. Ann Emerg Med 2011;58(4):323–9.
50. Heden L, von Essen L, Frykholm P, et al. Low-dose oral midazolam reduces fear and distress during needle procedures in children with cancer. Pediatr Blood Cancer 2009;53(7):1200–4.
51. Chiaretti A, Barone G, Rigante D, et al. Intranasal lidocaine and midazolam for procedural sedation in children. Arch Dis Child 2011;96(2):160–3.
52. Davies FC, Waters M. Oral midazolam for conscious sedation of children during minor procedures. J Accid Emerg Med 1998;15(4):244–8.
53. Kanegaye JT, Favela JL, Acosta M, et al. High-dose rectal midazolam for pediatric procedures: a randomized trial of sedative efficacy and agitation. Pediatr Emerg Care 2003;19(5):329–36.
54. Massanari M, Novitsky J, Reinstein LJ. Paradoxical reactions in children associated with midazolam use during endoscopy. Clin Pediatr (Phila) 1997;36(12): 681–4.
55. Drendel AL, Gorelick MH, Weisman SJ, et al. A randomized clinical trial of ibuprofen versus acetaminophen with codeine for acute pediatric arm fracture pain. Ann Emerg Med 2009;54(4):553–60.
56. Koller DM, Myers AB, Lorenz D, et al. Effectiveness of oxycodone, ibuprofen, or the combination in the initial management of orthopedic injury-related pain in children. Pediatr Emerg Care 2007;23(9):627–33.
57. Clark E, Plint AC, Correll R, et al. A randomized, controlled trial of acetaminophen, ibuprofen, and codeine for acute pain relief in children with musculoskeletal trauma. Pediatrics 2007;119(3):460–7.
58. Klein EJ, Diekema DS, Paris CA, et al. A randomized, clinical trial of oral midazolam plus placebo versus oral midazolam plus oral transmucosal fentanyl for sedation during laceration repair. Pediatrics 2002;109(5):894–7.
59. Roelofse JA, Shipton EA, de la Harpe CJ, et al. Intranasal sufentanil/midazolam versus ketamine/midazolam for analgesia/sedation in the pediatric population prior to undergoing multiple dental extractions under general anesthesia: a prospective, double-blind, randomized comparison. Anesth Prog 2004;51(4):114–21.
60. Resch K, Schilling C, Borchert BD, et al. Topical anesthesia for pediatric lacerations: a randomized trial of lidocaine-epinephrine-tetracaine solution versus gel. Ann Emerg Med 1998;32(6):693–7.
61. Singer AJ, Stark MJ. LET versus EMLA for pretreating lacerations: a randomized trial. Acad Emerg Med 2001;8(3):223–30.
62. Bartfield JM, Crisafulli KM, Raccio-Robak N, et al. The effects of warming and buffering on pain of infiltration of lidocaine. Acad Emerg Med 1995;2(4): 254–8.

63. Bartfield JM, Sokaris SJ, Raccio-Robak N. Local anesthesia for lacerations: pain of infiltration inside vs outside the wound. Acad Emerg Med 1998;5(2):100–4.

64. Lander JA, Weltman BJ, So SS. EMLA and amethocaine for reduction of children's pain associated with needle insertion. Cochrane Database Syst Rev 2006;(3):CD004236.

65. Wahlgren CF, Quiding H. Depth of cutaneous analgesia after application of a eutectic mixture of the local anesthetics lidocaine and prilocaine (EMLA cream). J Am Acad Dermatol 2000;42(4):584–8.

66. Eichenfield LF, Funk A, Fallon-Friedlander S, et al. A clinical study to evaluate the efficacy of ELA-Max (4% liposomal lidocaine) as compared with eutectic mixture of local anesthetics cream for pain reduction of venipuncture in children. Pediatrics 2002;109(6):1093–9.

67. Smith DP, Gjellum M. The efficacy of LMX versus EMLA for pain relief in boys undergoing office meatotomy. J Urol 2004;172(4 Pt 2):1760–1.

68. O'Brien L, Taddio A, Lyszkiewicz DA, et al. A critical review of the topical local anesthetic amethocaine (Ametop) for pediatric pain. Paediatr Drugs 2005;7(1): 41–54.

69. Ramsook C, Kozinetz CA, Moro-Sutherland D. Efficacy of ethyl chloride as a local anesthetic for venipuncture and intravenous cannula insertion in a pediatric emergency department. Pediatr Emerg Care 2001;17(5):341–3.

70. Inal S, Kelleci M. Relief of pain during blood specimen collection in pediatric patients. MCN Am J Maternal Child Nurs 2012;37(5):339–45.

71. Berberich FR, Landman Z. Reducing immunization discomfort in 4- to 6-year-old children: a randomized clinical trial. Pediatrics 2009;124(2):e203–9.

72. Naughton KA. The combined use of sucrose and nonnutritive sucking for procedural pain in both term and preterm neonates: an integrative review of the literature. Adv Neonatal Care 2013;13(1):9–19 [quiz: 20–1].

73. Stevens B, Yamada J, Lee GY, et al. Sucrose for analgesia in newborn infants undergoing painful procedures. Cochrane Database Syst Rev 2013;(1): CD001069.

74. Fein JA, Zempsky WT, Cravero JP. Relief of pain and anxiety in pediatric patients in emergency medical systems. Pediatrics 2012;130(5):e1391–405.

75. Cohen LL. Behavioral approaches to anxiety and pain management for pediatric venous access. Pediatrics 2008;122(Suppl 3):S134–9.

76. Slifer KJ, Hankinson JC, Zettler MA, et al. Distraction, exposure therapy, counterconditioning, and topical anesthetic for acute pain management during needle sticks in children with intellectual and developmental disabilities. Clin Pediatr (Phila) 2011;50(8):688–97.

77. Gerard LL, Cooper CS, Duethman KS, et al. Effectiveness of lidocaine lubricant for discomfort during pediatric urethral catheterization. J Urol 2003;170(2 Pt 1): 564–7.

78. Mularoni PP, Cohen LL, DeGuzman M, et al. A randomized clinical trial of lidocaine gel for reducing infant distress during urethral catheterization. Pediatr Emerg Care 2009;25(7):439–43.

79. Kozer E, Rosenbloom E, Goldman D, et al. Pain in infants who are younger than 2 months during suprapubic aspiration and transurethral bladder catheterization: a randomized, controlled study. Pediatrics 2006;118(1):e51–6.

80. Taddio A, Ilersich AL, Ipp M, et al. Physical interventions and injection techniques for reducing injection pain during routine childhood immunizations: systematic review of randomized controlled trials and quasi-randomized controlled trials. Clin Ther 2009;31(Suppl 2):S48–76.

81. Schechter NL, Zempsky WT, Cohen LL, et al. Pain reduction during pediatric immunizations: evidence-based review and recommendations. Pediatrics 2007;119(5):e1184–98.
82. Barnhill BJ, Holbert MD, Jackson NM, et al. Using pressure to decrease the pain of intramuscular injections. J Pain Symptom Manage 1996;12(1):52–8.
83. Diggle L, Deeks J. Effect of needle length on incidence of local reactions to routine immunisation in infants aged 4 months: randomised controlled trial. BMJ 2000;321(7266):931–3.
84. Diggle L, Deeks JJ, Pollard AJ. Effect of needle size on immunogenicity and reactogenicity of vaccines in infants: randomised controlled trial. BMJ 2006; 333(7568):571.
85. Ipp M, Taddio AP, Sam JB, et al. Vaccine related pain: randomized controlled trial of two injection techniques. Arch Dis Child 2007;92(12):1105–8.
86. Aminabadi NA, Farahani RM. The effect of pre-cooling the injection site on pediatric pain perception during the administration of local anesthesia. J Contemp Dent Pract 2009;10(3):43–50.
87. Antevy PM, Zuckerbraun NS, Saladino RA, et al. Evaluation of a transthecal digital nerve block in the injured pediatric patient. Pediatr Emerg Care 2010;26(3): 177–80.
88. Keramidas EG, Rodopoulou SG, Tsoutsos D, et al. Comparison of transthecal digital block and traditional digital block for anesthesia of the finger. Plast Reconstr Surg 2004;114(5):1131–4 [discussion: 5–6].
89. Baxter AL, Fisher RG, Burke BL, et al. Local anesthetic and stylet styles: factors associated with resident lumbar puncture success. Pediatrics 2006;117(3): 876–81.
90. Bhargava R, Young KD. Procedural pain management patterns in academic pediatric emergency departments. Acad Emerg Med 2007;14(5):479–82.
91. Nigrovic LE, Kuppermann N, Neuman MI. Risk factors for traumatic or unsuccessful lumbar punctures in children. Ann Emerg Med 2007;49(6):762–71.

Pediatric Mental Health Emergencies and Special Health Care Needs

Thomas H. Chun, MD, MPH[a,b,*], Emily R. Katz, MD[c],
Susan J. Duffy, MD, MPH[a,b]

KEYWORDS

- Psychiatric emergency • Pediatric • Autism • Developmental disorders

KEY POINTS

- Patients with suicidal and homicidal ideation, as well as autism and/or developmental disability are commonly cared for in the emergency department.
- Evaluation for underlying medical condition, as well as a thorough risk and safety assessment should be performed for all these patients.
- A number of calming and distraction techniques may facilitate the care of children with autism and/or developmental disabilities.

INTRODUCTION

Visits for mental health problems to both pediatric primary care settings and pediatric emergency departments have increased markedly in recent decades, and now account for up to 25% to 50% of primary care and 5% of pediatric emergency department visits.[1–6] Both pediatricians[7] and pediatric emergency physicians[8,9] identify lack of training in and lack of confidence in their ability to care for mental health problems as barriers to caring for these patients. The focus of this article is the 2 most common pediatric mental health emergencies, both of which involve threats to safety: suicide, whereby there is risk of harm to the patient, and homicide or aggression, whereby

Conflict of Interest: The authors have no conflicts of interest to disclose.
Grant Support: Supported in part by "Teaching an Alcohol Intervention to Pediatric ER Staff," National Institute for Alcohol Abuse and Alcoholism, K23 AA014934 and "Teen Alcohol Screening in the Pediatric Emergency Care Applied Research Network," National Institute for Alcohol Abuse and Alcoholism, R01 AA021900 (T.H. Chun).
[a] Department of Emergency Medicine, Rhode Island Hospital, 593 Eddy Street, Providence, RI 02903, USA; [b] Department of Pediatrics, Rhode Island Hospital, 593 Eddy Street, Providence, RI 02903, USA; [c] Department of Child and Family Psychiatry, Rhode Island Hospital, 593 Eddy Street, Providence, RI 02903, USA
* Corresponding author. Department of Emergency Medicine, Rhode Island Hospital, Claverick 243, 593 Eddy Street, Providence, RI 02903.
E-mail address: Thomas_Chun@brown.edu

there is risk of harm to others. In addition, the challenges of caring for children with autism or other developmental disabilities are discussed.

SUICIDAL IDEATION AND SUICIDE ATTEMPTS
Key Points

- Suicide is one of the leading causes of death in pediatric patients.
- Constant observation is necessary to ensure patient safety during suicide evaluation and crisis stabilization.
- Evaluation includes assessment for potential underlying or associated medical conditions.
- Laboratory and/or imaging should be obtained on an as-needed basis.
- High-risk patients should be referred directly for inpatient psychiatric admission.
- Less intensive treatment options may be considered for patients who are able to maintain their safety in outpatient settings.
- Although there are no medications with which to directly treat suicidality, there are safe and effective treatments for the majority of the associated psychiatric conditions.
- All evaluations of patients in the setting of suicidal ideation or suicide attempts should include a thorough discussion of safety planning, including means restriction and indications for seeking emergency care.

Introduction

Suicide is the third leading cause of death among persons aged 10 to 24 years in the United States, accounting for more than 4000 deaths per year.[10] Approximately 16% of teenagers report having seriously considered suicide in the past year, 12.8% report having planned a suicide attempt, and 7.8% report having attempted suicide in the past year. Although only a small percentage of suicide attempts lead to medical attention,[11] suicide attempts still account for a significant number of emergency visits.[12]

Risk factors

Females are more likely to consider and attempt suicide, but males are more than 5 times more likely to complete suicide. This difference is primarily accounted for by the use of more lethal means: males are more likely to attempt suicide using firearms and hanging, whereas females are more likely to attempt suicide via a drug overdose.[11]

Other risk factors for attempting and/or completing suicide include[13–21]:

- History of previous suicide attempts
- Impulsivity, mood, or behavior disorders
- Recent psychiatric hospitalizations
- Substance abuse
- Family history of suicide
- History of physical or sexual abuse
- Homelessness/runaways
- Identification as lesbian, gay, bisexual, or transsexual

Evaluation

Identifying at-risk patients

Some patients will identify themselves as being suicidal, with suicidal ideation or suicide attempt as their chief complaint. However, many may not proactively report their suicidality to providers.[22] Given the prevalence of suicidal ideation and attempts as well as the morbidity and mortality associated with attempts, pediatric providers are encouraged to screen all of their teen patients for suicidality.[23–25] Screens may be brief and focused directly on suicide risk[26] or a more extensive part of a broader mental health screening tool, such as the Pediatric Symptom Checklist. Another clinical resource is the TeenScreen National Center for Mental Health Checkups.[27] All patients presenting with mood symptoms, substance abuse, ingestions, acute intoxication, single-car motor vehicle crashes, self-inflicted or accidental gunshot wounds, and falls from significant heights should be screened for the presence of suicidal ideation.

Ensuring safety
First and foremost, providers must ensure the safety of the patients, their family, and health care staff during the course of the evaluation. Whenever concern for suicidal ideation or attempt is present, patients should be constantly monitored. Patients should not be left unobserved, as they are at risk for further injuring themselves or eloping. Patients should undergo a search of their person and belongings, be asked to change into hospital attire or an examination gown, and be placed in as safe a setting as possible, ideally one without access to medical equipment that could be used for self-harm.

Confidentiality
When a physician is concerned that the patient may be at imminent risk for harm to self or others, confidentiality requirements no longer apply. Physicians may disclose information gathered by patients to caregivers and may obtain information from others (including friends, family members, school personnel, and other caregivers) without obtaining consent from the patient or guardians.

Interview
Patients and caregivers should be interviewed both together and alone. It is essential that providers obtain collateral information from caregivers, as patients frequently minimize the severity of their symptoms or the intention behind their acts. It is paramount to ask patients directly about suicidality. Asking patients about suicidal ideation and attempts does not increase suicidal behaviors. In fact, it may have the opposite effect, as having an open, honest conversation about their suicidal thoughts may provide patients with a sense of safety and relief. In turn, this may enable them to fully disclose their suicidality and engage in treatment.

In addition to obtaining routine historical data (both medical and mental health histories), clinicians should obtain thorough details of the events and symptoms leading up to presentation of patients. Specific attention should be paid to:

- Recent psychosocial stressors, for example:
  - Family conflict
  - Breakup of a romantic relationship
  - Bullying
  - Academic difficulties
  - Disciplinary actions/legal troubles
- Depression
- Mania
- Anxiety
- Psychosis
- Impulsivity
- Aggression
- Substance abuse
- Access to lethal means

- ○ Firearms
- ○ Knives
- ○ Medications
- Access to a responsible, supportive adult to whom they could turn if they had suicidal thoughts

Younger patients tend to be triggered more often by family conflict, whereas older adolescents are more likely to cite peer or romantic conflicts.[28]

When discussing suicidal ideation, clinicians should inquire about patients' reasons for considering/attempting suicide, and what, if any, are their reasons for living. Where were they, and what was happening immediately before the attempt? Was the attempt planned or impulsive? Did they do anything to avoid discovery? What was their expectation of the outcome would be? It should be noted that adolescents are typically poor judges of the dangerousness of their acts.[29,30] Although patients with low-lethality attempts may not be at significant medical risk, patients' understanding of the potential lethality of their actions should form the basis of the suicide risk assessment.

Patients may deny that their behaviors constituted a suicide attempt and instead report that they "did it without thinking" or that they were just trying to go to sleep or get high, or get a break from their feelings. Clinicians should be wary of accepting these explanations at face value, and should probe for any signs of ambiguity or ambivalence. For example, in the setting of an overdose it may be useful to ask patients if they questioned the safety of the ingestion beforehand. Was there any part of them that thought it might endanger their life? If so, it may be helpful to wonder out loud whether there was part of them that would not have cared if they did not wake up from the ingestion. If the patient acknowledges any ambivalence, the clinician should follow up by exploring what parts of the patient would not have cared. The clinician should also assess how, given the patient's awareness of the ingestion's potential lethality, he or she arrived at the decision to carry it out.

If patients respond by steadfastly denying any suicidal thoughts and/or maintaining that they did not consider the consequences of their actions, it may be that there truly was no intent for self-harm. However, there are some circumstances in which there is enough evidence supporting suicidal intent (such as statements to family and friends or postings on social media) that is concerning enough to overcome any potential reassurance from patients' denial of intent for self-harm. There may also be circumstances in which patients may not have had any intent to harm themselves, but their lack of judgment about the dangerousness of their actions could be considered life-threatening and still necessitate intensive psychiatric treatment.

Family interview

Parents should be questioned about recent signs, symptoms, and stressors as well as the details of the any events that may have led to their presentation. In addition, pediatricians should inquire about the patient's access to lethal means, the level of caregivers' knowledge of/concern for the patient's safety and well-being, their willingness/ability to monitor the patient, their level of openness to psychiatric treatment, and any barriers that might impede engagement in care. Clinicians should also work to identify areas of competence in both the patient and the family. These areas of strength form the basis for a successful treatment plan that enables the family to respond effectively to the crisis at hand.

Physical Examination

There are several purposes to the medical examination in suicidal patients. Clinicians should evaluate the patient for any evidence of injury or ingestion. Specific attention should be paid to the skin examination to look for evidence of cutting and also for signs suggestive of a toxidrome. Clinicians should examine the patient for any signs suggestive of an underlying medical cause for the patient's psychiatric symptoms or for any medical conditions that would require treatment beyond the initial medical evaluation.

Laboratory Testing

Many patients, particularly those with preexisting psychiatric diagnoses and who have normal vital signs, a normal physical examination, and no "red flags" for medical illness on history and review of systems, do not require routine laboratory or radiologic testing. Decisions to obtain laboratory testing should be based on the patient's presenting medical and mental health condition. Clinicians should have a low threshold, however, for obtaining toxicology screens and pregnancy screening. In addition, patients with an acute change in psychiatric symptoms typically require at least some laboratory evaluation.[31–33]

Pharmacologic Considerations

There are no medications whose primary indication is the prevention or treatment of suicide. Pediatricians may consider starting a selective serotonin reuptake inhibitor (SSRI) for patients with a significant depressive episode or an anxiety disorder. If SSRIs are initiated, these patients and their caregivers should receive extensive education about and be closely monitored for worsening suicidal ideation.[34] Pediatricians should be wary of prescribing disinhibiting medications such as benzodiazepines to suicidal patients, and use extreme caution in prescribing medications that could be lethal in overdose (eg, tricyclic antidepressants or narcotics). If such medications are necessary, special care should be taken to ensure the safety of their administration, such as dispensing a week's worth of medicine at a time and/or having a responsible caregiver lock up and directly administer the medication.

Nonpharmacologic Strategies

One of the primary roles of a pediatrician managing a suicidal patient and their family is to provide psychoeducation about the need and support for engaging in adequate treatment. Caregivers may need help in recognizing the seriousness of the child's symptoms, and may also harbor negative feelings and/or misunderstandings about mental health diagnoses and their management options. Pediatricians should try to impress on patients and families the many dangers of untreated mental illness and/ or unaddressed psychological stressors (including family discord) and that there are safe, confidential, and effective treatments available. It may be useful to inform caregivers that patients are at the highest risk of reattempting suicide in the months following the initial attempt[35–37] and that, while treatment may take time to help, they should do everything they can to help support the patient in adhering to recommended care.

Determining the Level of Care

There are no validated criteria available to guide a pediatrician in assessing the level of risk for subsequent suicide and determining the level of care needs. However, it is generally agreed that criteria for immediate referral for an inpatient psychiatric admission include any the following:

- Continued desire to die
- Severe hopelessness
- Ongoing agitation

- Inability to engage in a discussion around safety planning
- Inadequate support system/ability to adequate monitoring and follow-up
- High lethality attempt or an attempt with clear expectation of death

Under certain circumstances, pediatricians must insist on admission to a psychiatric inpatient unit over the objections of patients and/or their guardians. Every state in the United States has laws governing involuntary admission (ie, a "psychiatric hold") for inpatient psychiatric hospitalization. Laws vary from state to state, but in most cases physicians are able to admit a patient against his or her will for a brief period. Pediatricians should familiarize themselves with the relevant statutes and involuntary commitment procedures in the states where they practice.

Patients who do not meet criteria for inpatient psychiatric hospitalization should be referred for subsequent mental health intervention. Partial hospital programs, intensive outpatient services, or in-home treatment/crisis stabilization interventions should be considered when a patient needs treatment more intensive or urgent than weekly counseling. It should be noted that even patients who are deemed to be at relatively low risk of future suicidal or self-injurious acts still warrant at least some outpatient follow-up. Unfortunately, outpatient mental health providers are not always readily accessible. In such circumstances, primary care providers may need to play an ongoing treatment role, by providing frequent follow-up, bridging care, and/or in-office counseling.[38]

Safety Planning

Although having a patient sign a no-suicide contract has not been shown to prevent subsequent suicides,[39] pediatricians should still engage in a safety-planning discussion. Safety plans typically include elements such as identification of: (1) warning signs and potential triggers for recurrence of suicidal ideation; (2) coping strategies the patient could use; (3) healthy activities that could provide distraction or suppression of suicidal thoughts; (4) responsible social supports to which the patient could turn should suicidal urges return; (5) contact information for professional support, including instructions on how and when to reaccess emergency services; and (6) means restriction.[40]

Means restriction refers to counseling families about restricting access to potentially lethal methods. Because a large percentage of suicide attempts are impulsive in nature, educating caregivers about "suicide-proofing" their home is critical. One study of patients aged 13 to 34 years who had near-lethal attempts found that 24% of patients went from deciding to attempt suicide to implementing their plan within 0 to 5 minutes, and another 47% took between 6 minutes and 1 hour.[41] Several studies have demonstrated that patients usually misjudge the lethality of their attempts.[29,30,42] There is also a wide variation in the case-fatality rates of common methods of suicide attempt, ranging from 85% for gunshot wounds to 2% for ingestions and 1% for cutting.[43] It thus follows that interventions that decrease access to more lethal means and/or increase the amount of time and effort it would take for someone to carry out their suicidal plan are likely to have a positive effect.

Means restriction education should include recommendations for securing knives, locking up medicines, and removing firearms. Of importance is that parents often underestimate their children's abilities to locate and access firearms,[44] and that a gun in the home has been shown to double the risk of youth suicide.[45] Families who are reluctant to permanently remove firearms from the home may be open to temporarily relocating them until the child is in a better emotional state. If families insist on keeping firearms in the home, they should be counseled to secure them with trigger locks, to store them unloaded in a specialized or tamper-proof safe, to separately lock or temporarily remove ammunition, and ensure that minors do not have access to keys or lock combinations. Given the rates of drug and alcohol intoxication among attempters and completers, physicians may also want to recommend restricting access to alcohol and drugs, as well as referral for substance-abuse treatment.

Instill Hope

At the conclusion of the visit, pediatricians should review with patients their reasons for living. Many patients may need help in generating this list. Pediatricians should highlight any of the patient's stated goals for the future and the ways in which the recommended treatment plan is designed to help the patient to not only survive but thrive.

HOMICIDAL IDEATION, AGGRESSION, AND RESTRAINT

Key Points

- Aggression is the final common pathway for a variety of medical and mental health conditions.
- Similar to the approach to the suicidal patient, careful evaluation for potential medical causes that may be the underlying cause and/or may complicate treatment of the aggression is vital.
- Mandatory federal and regulatory standards should guide the use of restraints with children and adolescents, including using the least restrictive methods possible, frequent reassessment of the need for continued versus discontinuing restraint, and offering food, drink, and bathroom facilities.
- Physical and chemical restraint may have significant adverse effects, and require careful planning, administration, and monitoring.

Introduction

Aggressive, violent behavior is not a diagnosis unto itself but is the result of an underlying medical, toxicologic, or mental problem(s), or a combination of these conditions. Symptoms vary widely, depending on the patient's age, developmental level, and physical condition, and may include restlessness, hyperactivity, confusion, disorientation, and verbal threats to frank violence toward property, others, or oneself. It is a frequent cause of injury to both patients and medical staff.[46,47] As the evaluation of homicidal ideation and aggression share many of the priorities and strategies of the evaluation of the suicidal patient, this section focuses primarily on the management of aggressive patients.

Risk factors

Risk factors associated with aggression and violence are listed in **Box 1**.

Evaluation

Strategies and priorities for evaluating the aggressive patient are the same as those detailed for the evaluation of the suicidal patient. The first priority is ensuring the safety of the patient and the medical staff. One critical difference with these patients regards the potential victim(s) of future violence. If (a) potential victim(s) of an aggressive patient is/are identified, there is an established legal precedent and duty to warn the victim(s) of the possibility of future violence.[48] Similar to the situation with the suicidal patient, this duty supersedes patient confidentiality.

When interviewing an aggressive patient, one should use the same techniques as discussed with the suicidal patient. Asking directly about homicidal ideation, thoughts or plans of violence, probing ambiguous or ambivalent statements, obtaining a comprehensive medical, mental health, substance abuse, legal/law enforcement

---

Box 1
Aggression/violence risk factors

- History of violence (especially recent)
- Possession of weapons
- Intoxication
- Command hallucinations
- Impulse control disorders
- Concurrent psychosocial stressor(s)
- Verbal/physical threats
- Psychomotor agitation
- Paranoia
- Impaired executive functioning
- History of antisocial behavior
- Concrete plans to harm others

---

history, inquiring about past and current psychosocial stressors, and access to weapons, from both the patient and caregivers, should all be undertaken. The goal of the physical examination and any laboratory workup is to evaluate for potential medical causes of the patient's aggression, as well as to detect any potential injuries or illnesses.

Management Goals

In 1998 the *Hartford Courant* published a series of articles detailing deaths of psychiatric patients which, it believed, were attributed to the use of physical restraint.[49] In response to these articles, the Centers for Medicare and Medicaid, and subsequently the Joint Commission for the Accreditation of Hospital Organizations, adopted regulations governing the use of and monitoring requirements for restraint (CMS-3018-F [42 CFR Part 482, RIN 0938-AN30]).[50] Key features of these regulations are listed in **Box 2**.

Nonpharmacologic Strategies

Verbal restraint and staff training in restraint reduction and de-escalation strategies have both been shown to be effective at reducing the need for chemical and physical restraint. Common verbal restraint strategies are listed in **Box 3**.[51] The presence of family members, caregivers, and friends are usually calming to a patient, although in some situations they may escalate a patient's agitation. In these situations, asking the person(s) to temporarily leave the room is advisable.

Physical restraint has been associated with adverse outcomes, including death. Recommended approaches to physical restraint are listed in **Box 4**. Physical restraint should be applied with a minimum of 5 staff, 1 to control each limb and 1 for the patient's head. Restraints made of sturdy (eg, leather) materials should be used while those of less durable construction (eg, "soft restraints") should be avoided. Once a patient has calmed, removal of restraints should be considered. Restraint removal will be dictated by the severity of the patient's condition. In some cases they may be removed all at once; in others, they may need to removed one at a time with reassessment of the patient's agitation after the removal of each restraint. In every case, the same number

---

Box 2
CMS restraint regulations

- Regulations apply to both physical and chemical restraint
- Must document need for and monitoring of restraint on 100% of patients

Restraint Order Time Limit (Time to Renew)

- Younger than 9 years: every 1 hour
- 9 to 17 years: every 2 hours
- Older than 18 years: every 4 hours

Monitoring/Basic Care Requirements

- Visual check: every 15 minutes or constant observation
- Release a restraint: every 2 hours (may reapply if needed)
- Neurovascular check: every 2 hours
- Offer food/water/bathroom: every 2 hours
- Behavior check: every 2 hours
- Respiratory status check: every 2 hours
- Change physical position: every 2 hours

---

of personnel that were present during the placement of the restraints should be available during removal of restraints, in case the restraints need to be reapplied.

Pharmacologic Strategies

Whereas many first-generation and second-generation antipsychotics have been approved by the Food and Drug Administration for use in children with autistic,

---

Box 3
Verbal restraint strategies

- Introduce oneself, staff
- Prepare patient for what will happen
- Respect patient autonomy
- Offer food and liquids
- Empathetic listening
- Ask about patient requests/preferences
- Honor reasonable requests
- Nonpunitive limit setting
- Simple direct language, soft voice
- Decrease environmental stimulation
- Allow patient to walk/move in room
- Reassure patient that (s)he will be safe
- Offer distraction (eg, toy/books/movie)
- Nonthreatening movement/posture
- Remove breakable objects, equipment

1194 Chun et al

> **Box 4**
> **Physical restraint recommendations**
>
> - Supine position preferred
> - Avoid pressure on neck/back/chest
> - Mandatory staff training on restraint
> - Avoid covering patient's face/mouth/nose
> - Elevate head of bed, if possible

mood, psychotic, and tic disorders, none have been approved for use in agitation or aggression.[52] Despite a growing body of literature on the use of benzodiazepines and antipsychotics for agitated adults in emergency department and psychiatric settings,[53–56] very few children were included in these studies and there are no high-quality pediatric trials. These limitations aside, most psychiatric and emergency medicine experts believe that these medications are both efficacious and safe, with rare but easily treated adverse reactions.

Table 1 lists commonly used medications and starting doses for pediatric chemical restraint. If a patient is already on one of these medications, administering their usual or an increased dose of that medication is acceptable. Regarding which medication should be used as the first-line agent, most experts recommend tailoring the choice of medication to the severity and underlying cause of the agitation (**Table 2**).

The most common adverse effects of chemical restraint medications are cardiorespiratory and central nervous system depression, and extrapyramidal reactions. The former are usually easily treated with simple supportive measures, and the latter with anticholinergics (eg, diphenhydramine, benztropine, or trihexyphenidyl). Invasive or aggressive treatment measures are rarely needed. The most serious acute, adverse effects of antipsychotics are arrhythmias due to QT_c prolongation. These events are rare and are most likely to occur in patients receiving other QT_c-prolonging

Table 1
Medications for pediatric chemical restraint

Medication	Initial Dose	Onset (min)	Half-Life (h)
Diphenhydramine	1.25 mg/kg Teen: 50 mg	20–30 (PO) 5–15 (IM)	2–8
Lorazepam	0.05–0.1 mg/kg Teen: 2–4 mg	20–30 (PO) 5–15 (IM)	12
Midazolam	0.05–0.15 mg/kg Teen: 2–4 mg	20–30 (PO) 5–15 (IM)	3–4
Haloperidol	0.1 mg/kg Teen: 2–4 mg	30–60 (PO) 15–30 (IM)	21
Risperidone	<12 y: 0.5 mg Teen: 1 mg	45–60 (PO)	20
Olanzapine	<12 y: 2.5 mg Teen: 5–10 mg	45–60 (PO) 30–60 (IM)	30
Ziprasidone	<12 y: 5 mg Teen: 10–20 mg	60 (PO) 30–60 (IM)	2–7
Aripiprazole	<12 y: 1–2 mg Teen: 2–5 mg	60–180 (PO) 30–120 (IM)	75

Abbreviations: IM, intramuscular; PO, by mouth.

Table 2
Choice of initial chemical restraint agent

Etiology of Agitation	Symptom Severity	
	Mild/Moderate	Severe
Medical	Benzodiazepine	Benzodiazepine or antipsychotic
Psychiatric	Benzodiazepine or antipsychotic	Antipsychotic

medications and/or with underlying cardiac conditions. Continuous cardiorespiratory monitoring is thus recommended for patients receiving chemical restraint.

CARE OF CHILDREN WITH AUTISM AND DEVELOPMENTAL DISORDERS
Key points
- Children with autism and other developmental disorders span a wide range of symptoms of severities, ranging from very high functioning with minimal disabilities to profound impairment.
- Accordingly, such children may have unique and idiosyncratic communication methods, interaction styles, and responses to sensory stimuli.
- Parents and caregivers are the pediatrician's greatest allies in planning and delivering optimal treatment for their children.
- Several simple strategies, such as communication adjuncts, transition planning, sensory and environmental modification, and distraction techniques, may be useful in caring for these patients.

Introduction

The incidence of autism spectrum disorders (ASD) is increasing for a multitude of reasons, many of which are still unclear.[57] The 3 cardinal features of ASD are impaired communication and social interaction, and repetitive/restrictive areas of interest. The severity of these symptoms and the degree of impairment vary greatly, and include people who have obtained PhDs (eg, Temple Grandin) to people who are nonverbal, and cannot communicate nor care for themselves. In addition, each person may have specific and distinctive interaction patterns and response to stimuli. For all these reasons, caring for these children can be extremely challenging.

Children with other developmental disorders (DD) similarly span a wide range of symptoms, severity, and disabilities, too numerous to list and beyond the scope of this article. As the strategies for caring for these children are similar to those used in caring for children with ASD, for the purposes of this article the term ASD/DD will be used to collectively refer to all such children.

Evaluation

One of the most challenging aspects of caring for children with ASD/DD is interpreting the unique meaning of their behaviors, as well as discovering the optimal methods for interacting with and caring for the child. Fortunately, most of these children are accompanied by an expert in these areas, namely their parent(s) and/or caregiver(s). Time spent asking them about the child is likely to be time well spent, increasing the efficiency with which care is delivered and the patient's, family's, and clinician's satisfaction with the encounter. Suggested topics to discuss with the parent/caregiver are:

- What is your child's level of communication, cognitive, and psychosocial functioning?
- How does your child communicate?

- When your child does (behavior), what does it mean?
- What upsets or scares your child? What calms/soothes you child?
- Is your child sensitive to light, sound, or other stimuli?
- What is the best way to prepare your child for something new?
- Does your child like to be touched? If so, what types of tactile sensations does your child like?
- Are there things (eg, toys, a favorite object, electronic devices) that are good distractions for your child?

Transition Planning

Preparing children with ASD for what is about to happen is one of the most common strategies used by their caregivers. In ideal cases, the parent/caregiver begins talking to the child about what to expect while en route to the medical setting. Once there, it is worthwhile discussing what will occur during the visit and determining a plan for how to prepare the child for the visit.

Transition planning may also include planned breaks for the child. Some children with ASD/DD are able to stay on task or remain in one location for only brief periods of time. Building rest periods, distractions, bathroom breaks, and so forth into the visit may be an important component to a successful visit. Finally, a method for signaling transitions and/or new activities may also be helpful. A transition cue may be auditory (eg, certain words or phrases, ringing a bell), visual (eg, pointing to a picture, turning on a light, showing the child a certain object), or tactile (eg, a touching a specific object).

Sensory/Environmental Modification and Distraction

Some patients may be very sensitive to environmental stimuli such as light, noise, crowds of people, or complex/cluttered environments. If a child has such sensitivities, altering the environment and visit may be helpful. For example, instead of sitting in a busy, noisy waiting room, have the child wait in a quiet office or counseling area. Turning the lights in a room off or down, or lighting a room with a single lamp, may help a child who is sensitive to light. A rocking chair or rocking toy (with supervision) may soothe a child who prefers motion. For children who respond to tactile stimulation, a weighted blanket (available through occupational therapy vendors), a radiology leaded vest, or a "bean-bag" chair can all serve to provide the sensation of a heavy touch. Those who prefer the sensation of a light touch may respond to gentle massage (manual or mechanical devices) or stroking the skin with a soft object (eg, a cotton ball, gauze pad, soft blanket). Any toy or electronic device that holds the child's attention and forms a distraction may assist in caring for the child.

Communication Adjuncts

Visual communication systems, both print and electronic versions, have demonstrated efficacy in improving communication with children with ASD/DD.[58–61] Not only may such a system improve communication with the child; more importantly, it may be the only way the child can communicate with the clinicians. There are a numerous products, both free and commercial, which are readily available, such as Picture Exchange Communication System (Pyramid Educational Consultants Inc, Newark, DE), modified American Sign Language signs, PODD (Pragmatic Organization Dynamic Display) books and software (Dynavox Mayer-Johnson, Pittsburgh, PA), iPad (Apple Inc, Cupertino, CA) with iCommunicate (Grembe Apps, Marston Mills, MA), and Proloquo2go (AssistiveWare, Amsterdam, Netherlands). Alternatively, a system customized to a particular setting can easily be made with digital photographs and/or computerized clip art. A custom visual communication tool has the advantage of containing pictures specific to the site. The disadvantage of such a system, however, is that the child may not be familiar with it.

REFERENCES

1. Grupp-Phelan J, Harman JS, Kelleher KJ. Trends in mental health and chronic condition visits by children presenting for care at U.S. emergency departments. Public Health Rep 2007;122(1):55–61 PubMed PMID: 17236609; PubMed Central PMCID: PMC1802106.
2. Kessler RC, Demler O, Frank RG, et al. Prevalence and treatment of mental disorders, 1990 to 2003. N Engl J Med 2005;352(24):2515–23. http://dx.doi.org/10.1056/NEJMsa043266 PubMed PMID: 15958807; PubMed Central PMCID: PMC2847367.
3. Lewis M. Child psychiatric consultation in pediatrics. Pediatrics 1978;62(3): 359–64 PubMed PMID: 704211.
4. Sills MR, Bland SD. Summary statistics for pediatric psychiatric visits to US emergency departments, 1993-1999. Pediatrics 2002;110(4):e40 PubMed PMID: 12359813.
5. Wang PS, Demler O, Olfson M, et al. Changing profiles of service sectors used for mental health care in the United States. Am J Psychiatry 2006;163(7):1187–98. http://dx.doi.org/10.1176/appi.ajp.163.7.1187 PubMed PMID: 16816223; PubMed Central PMCID: PMC1941780.
6. Cooper S, Valleley RJ, Polaha J, et al. Running out of time: physician management of behavioral health concerns in rural pediatric primary care. Pediatrics 2006;118(1):e132–8. http://dx.doi.org/10.1542/peds.2005-2612 PubMed PMID: 16818528.
7. Heneghan A, Garner AS, Storfer-Isser A, et al. Pediatricians' role in providing mental health care for children and adolescents: do pediatricians and child and adolescent psychiatrists agree? J Dev Behav Pediatr 2008;29(4):262–9. http://dx.doi.org/10.1097/DBP.0b013e31817dbd97 PubMed PMID: 18698191.
8. Hoyle JD Jr, White LJ. Treatment of pediatric and adolescent mental health emergencies in the United States: current practices, models, barriers, and potential solutions. Prehosp Emerg Care 2003;7(1):66–73 PubMed PMID: 12540146.
9. Hoyle JD Jr, White LJ. Pediatric mental health emergencies: summary of a multidisciplinary panel. Prehosp Emerg Care 2003;7(1):60–5 PubMed PMID: 12540145.
10. Centers for Disease Control and Prevention. Leading causes of death 1999-2010. Atlanta (GA): Centers for Disease Control and Prevention; 2012.
11. Eaton DK, Kann L, Kinchen S, et al. Youth risk behavior surveillance—United States, 2011. MMWR Surveill Summ 2012;61(4):1–162 PubMed PMID: 22673000.
12. Ting SA, Sullivan AF, Boudreaux ED, et al. Trends in US emergency department visits for attempted suicide and self-inflicted injury, 1993-2008. Gen Hosp Psychiatry 2012;34(5):557–65. http://dx.doi.org/10.1016/j.genhosppsych.2012.03.020 PubMed PMID: 22554432; PubMed Central PMCID: PMC3428496.
13. Brown J, Cohen P, Johnson JG, et al. Childhood abuse and neglect: specificity of effects on adolescent and young adult depression and suicidality. J Am Acad Child Adolesc Psychiatry 1999;38(12):1490–6. http://dx.doi.org/10.1097/00004583-199912000-00009 PubMed PMID: 10596248.
14. Esposito-Smythers C, Spirito A. Adolescent substance use and suicidal behavior: a review with implications for treatment research. Alcohol Clin Exp Res 2004;28(Suppl 5):77S–88S PubMed PMID: 15166639.
15. Foley DL, Goldston DB, Costello EJ, et al. Proximal psychiatric risk factors for suicidality in youth: the Great Smoky Mountains Study. Arch Gen Psychiatry

2006;63(9):1017–24. http://dx.doi.org/10.1001/archpsyc.63.9.1017 PubMed PMID: 16953004.

16. Lewinsohn PM, Rohde P, Seeley JR. Psychosocial risk factors for future adolescent suicide attempts. J Consult Clin Psychol 1994;62(2):297–305 PubMed PMID: 8201067.

17. McDaniel JS, Purcell D, D'Augelli AR. The relationship between sexual orientation and risk for suicide: research findings and future directions for research and prevention. Suicide Life Threat Behav 2001;31(Suppl):84–105 PubMed PMID: 11326762.

18. McKeown RE, Garrison CZ, Cuffe SP, et al. Incidence and predictors of suicidal behaviors in a longitudinal sample of young adolescents. J Am Acad Child Adolesc Psychiatry 1998;37(6):612–9. http://dx.doi.org/10.1097/00004583-199806000-00011 PubMed PMID: 9628081.

19. Shaffer D, Craft L. Methods of adolescent suicide prevention. J Clin Psychiatry 1999;60(Suppl 2):70–4 [discussion 5–6, 113–6]. PubMed PMID: 10073391.

20. Shaffer D, Gould MS, Fisher P, et al. Psychiatric diagnosis in child and adolescent suicide. Arch Gen Psychiatry 1996;53(4):339–48 PubMed PMID: 8634012.

21. Smart RG, Walsh GW. Predictors of depression in street youth. Adolescence 1993;28(109):41–53 PubMed PMID: 8456615.

22. Brent DA, Emslie GJ, Clarke GN, et al. Predictors of spontaneous and systematically assessed suicidal adverse events in the treatment of SSRI-resistant depression in adolescents (TORDIA) study. Am J Psychiatry 2009;166(4):418–26. http://dx.doi.org/10.1176/appi.ajp.2008.08070976 PubMed PMID: 19223438; PubMed Central PMCID: PMC3593721.

23. Committee on Pathophysiology and Prevention of Adolescent and Adult Suicide, Board of Neuroscience and Behavioral Health, Institute of Medicine. Reducing suicide: a national imperative. Washington, DC: The National Academies Press; 2002.

24. Williams SB, O'Connor EA, Eder M, et al. Screening for child and adolescent depression in primary care settings: a systematic evidence review for the US Preventive Services Task Force. Pediatrics 2009;123(4):e716–35. http://dx.doi.org/10.1542/peds.2008-2415 PubMed PMID: 19336361.

25. Foy JM, Kelleher KJ, Laraque D. Enhancing pediatric mental health care: strategies for preparing a primary care practice. Pediatrics 2010;125(Suppl 3):S87–108. http://dx.doi.org/10.1542/peds.2010-0788E PubMed PMID: 20519566.

26. Wintersteen MB. Standardized screening for suicidal adolescents in primary care. Pediatrics 2010;125(5):938–44. http://dx.doi.org/10.1542/peds.2009-2458 PubMed PMID: 20385627.

27. National Center for Mental Health Checkups at Columbia University. TeenScreen: Columbia University. Available at: www.teenscreen.org. Accessed April 14, 2013.

28. Overholser JC. Predisposing factors in suicide attempts: life stressors. In: Spirito A, Overholser JC, editors. Evaluating and treating adolescent suicide attempters: from research to practice. New York: Academic Press; 2002. p. 42–54.

29. Swahn MH, Potter LB. Factors associated with the medical severity of suicide attempts in youths and young adults. Suicide Life Threat Behav 2001;32(Suppl 1):21–9 PubMed PMID: 11924691.

30. Brown GK, Henriques GR, Sosdjan D, et al. Suicide intent and accurate expectations of lethality: predictors of medical lethality of suicide attempts. J Consult Clin Psychol 2004;72(6):1170–4. http://dx.doi.org/10.1037/0022-006X.72.6.1170 PubMed PMID: 15612863.

31. Henneman PL, Mendoza R, Lewis RJ. Prospective evaluation of emergency department medical clearance. Ann Emerg Med 1994;24(4):672–7 PubMed PMID: 7619102.
32. Janiak BD, Atteberry S. Medical clearance of the psychiatric patient in the emergency department. J Emerg Med 2012;43(5):866–70. http://dx.doi.org/10.1016/j.jemermed.2009.10.026 PubMed PMID: 20117904.
33. Olshaker JS, Browne B, Jerrard DA, et al. Medical clearance and screening of psychiatric patients in the emergency department. Acad Emerg Med 1997;4(2): 124–8 PubMed PMID: 9043539.
34. Hetrick SE, McKenzie JE, Cox GR, et al. Newer generation antidepressants for depressive disorders in children and adolescents. Cochrane Database Syst Rev 2012;(11):CD004851. http://dx.doi.org/10.1002/14651858.CD004851.pub3. PubMed PMID: 23152227.
35. Spirito A, Plummer B, Gispert M, et al. Adolescent suicide attempts: outcomes at follow-up. Am J Orthopsychiatry 1992;62(3):464–8 PubMed PMID: 1497112.
36. Prinstein MJ, Nock MK, Simon V, et al. Longitudinal trajectories and predictors of adolescent suicidal ideation and attempts following inpatient hospitalization. J Consult Clin Psychol 2008;76(1):92–103. http://dx.doi.org/10.1037/0022-006X.76.1.92 PubMed PMID: 18229987.
37. Yen S, Weinstock LM, Andover MS, et al. Prospective predictors of adolescent suicidality: 6-month post-hospitalization follow-up. Psychol Med 2013; 43(5):983–93. http://dx.doi.org/10.1017/S0033291712001912 PubMed PMID: 22932393.
38. Cheung AH, Zuckerbrot RA, Jensen PS, et al. Guidelines for adolescent depression in primary care (GLAD-PC): II. Treatment and ongoing management. Pediatrics 2007;120(5):e1313–26. http://dx.doi.org/10.1542/peds.2006-1395 PubMed PMID: 17974724.
39. American Academy of Child and Adolescent Psychiatry. Practice parameter for the assessment and treatment of children and adolescents with suicidal behavior. American Academy of Child and Adolescent Psychiatry. J Am Acad Child Adolesc Psychiatry 2001;40(Suppl 7):24S–51S PubMed PMID: 11434483.
40. Sher L, LaBode V. Teaching health care professionals about suicide safety planning. Psychiatr Danub 2011;23(4):396–7 PubMed PMID: 22075742.
41. Simon OR, Swann AC, Powell KE, et al. Characteristics of impulsive suicide attempts and attempters. Suicide Life Threat Behav 2001;32(Suppl 1):49–59 PubMed PMID: 11924695.
42. Plutchik R, van Praag HM, Picard S, et al. Is there a relation between the seriousness of suicidal intent and the lethality of the suicide attempt? Psychiatry Res 1989;27(1):71–9 PubMed PMID: 2922447.
43. Vyrostek SB, Annest JL, Ryan GW. Surveillance for fatal and nonfatal injuries—United States, 2001. MMWR Surveill Summ 2004;53(7):1–57 PubMed PMID: 15343143.
44. Baxley F, Miller M. Parental misperceptions about children and firearms. Arch Pediatr Adolesc Med 2006;160(5):542–7. http://dx.doi.org/10.1001/archpedi.160.5.542 PubMed PMID: 16651499.
45. Brent DA, Perper JA, Allman CJ, et al. The presence and accessibility of firearms in the homes of adolescent suicides. A case-control study. JAMA 1991; 266(21):2989–95 PubMed PMID: 1820470.
46. McAneney CM, Shaw KN. Violence in the pediatric emergency department. Ann Emerg Med 1994;23(6):1248–51 PubMed PMID: 8198298.

47. Knott JC, Bennett D, Rawet J, et al. Epidemiology of unarmed threats in the emergency department. Emerg Med Australas 2005;17(4):351–8. http://dx.doi.org/10.1111/j.1742-6723.2005.00756.x PubMed PMID: 16091097.

48. Felthous AR. The clinician's duty to protect third parties. Psychiatr Clin North Am 1999;22(1):49–60 PubMed PMID: 10083944.

49. Busch AB, Shore MF. Seclusion and restraint: a review of recent literature. Harv Rev Psychiatry 2000;8(5):261–70 PubMed PMID: 11118235.

50. Centers for Medicare and Medicaid. Medicare and Medicaid programs; hospital conditions of participation: patients' rights. Fed Regist 2006;71(236): 71378–428.

51. Hilt RJ, Woodward TA. Agitation treatment for pediatric emergency patients. J Am Acad Child Adolesc Psychiatry 2008;47(2):132–8. http://dx.doi.org/10.1097/chi.0b013e31815d95fd PubMed PMID: 18216715.

52. Christian R, Saavedra L, Gaynes BN, et al. Future research needs for first- and second-generation antipsychotics for children and young adults. Rockville (MD): AHRQ; 2012.

53. Chan EW, Taylor DM, Knott JC, et al. Intravenous droperidol or olanzapine as an adjunct to midazolam for the acutely agitated patient: a multicenter, randomized, double-blind, placebo-controlled clinical trial. Ann Emerg Med 2013; 61(1):72–81. http://dx.doi.org/10.1016/j.annemergmed.2012.07.118 PubMed PMID: 22981685.

54. Huf G, Coutinho ES, Adams CE. Rapid tranquillisation in psychiatric emergency settings in Brazil: pragmatic randomised controlled trial of intramuscular haloperidol versus intramuscular haloperidol plus promethazine. BMJ 2007; 335(7625):869. http://dx.doi.org/10.1136/bmj.39339.448819.AE PubMed PMID: 17954515; PubMed Central PMCID: PMC2043463.

55. Knott JC, Taylor DM, Castle DJ. Randomized clinical trial comparing intravenous midazolam and droperidol for sedation of the acutely agitated patient in the emergency department. Ann Emerg Med 2006;47(1):61–7. http://dx.doi.org/10.1016/j.annemergmed.2005.07.003 PubMed PMID: 16387219.

56. Hsu WY, Huang SS, Lee BS, et al. Comparison of intramuscular olanzapine, orally disintegrating olanzapine tablets, oral risperidone solution, and intramuscular haloperidol in the management of acute agitation in an acute care psychiatric ward in Taiwan. J Clin Psychopharmacol 2010;30(3):230–4. http://dx.doi.org/10.1097/JCP.0b013e3181db8715 PubMed PMID: 20473056.

57. Centers for Disease Control and Prevention, Autism and Developmental Disabilities Monitoring Network Surveillance Year 2008. Prevalence of autism spectrum disorders—Autism and Developmental Disabilities Monitoring Network, 14 sites, United States, 2008. MMWR Surveill Summ 2012;61(3):1–19 PubMed PMID: 22456193.

58. Ganz JB, Davis JL, Lund EM, et al. Meta-analysis of PECS with individuals with ASD: investigation of targeted versus non-targeted outcomes, participant characteristics, and implementation phase. Res Dev Disabil 2012;33(2):406–18. http://dx.doi.org/10.1016/j.ridd.2011.09.023 PubMed PMID: 22119688.

59. Gordon K, Pasco G, McElduff F, et al. A communication-based intervention for nonverbal children with autism: what changes? Who benefits? J Consult Clin Psychol 2011;79(4):447–57. http://dx.doi.org/10.1037/a0024379 PubMed PMID: 21787048.

60. Howlin P, Gordon RK, Pasco G, et al. The effectiveness of Picture Exchange Communication System (PECS) training for teachers of children with autism: a pragmatic, group randomised controlled trial. J Child Psychol Psychiatry

2007;48(5):473–81.   http://dx.doi.org/10.1111/j.1469-7610.2006.01707.x
PubMed PMID: 17501728.

61. Yoder PJ, Lieberman RG. Brief report: randomized test of the efficacy of picture exchange communication system on highly generalized picture exchanges in children with ASD. J Autism Dev Disord 2010;40(5):629–32. http://dx.doi.org/10.1007/s10803-009-0897-y PubMed PMID: 19904596.

Updates in the General Approach to the Pediatric Poisoned Patient

Fermin Barrueto Jr, MD[a,b],*, Rajender Gattu, MD[c],
Maryann Mazer-Amirshahi, PharmD, MD[d,e]

KEYWORDS

• Toxicology • Poison • Overdose • Synthetic drugs • Marijuana • Opioids • Intralipid

KEY POINTS

• Poison prevention remains a challenge and necessity to prevent the most vulnerable population from becoming exposed to potentially lethal drugs and toxins.
• The evaluation of a child presumed to have been exposed to a toxic substance should include a precise history of the exposure, a physical examination, and knowledge of current ingestions and recreational practices.
• Cutting-edge treatments and new research guiding therapy continue to evolve.
• Poison centers and medical toxicologists can be consulted to assist with the diagnosis of medicinal/drug overdoses, for advice about the pitfalls inherent in stabilizing children who have been exposed to toxic compounds, and for treatment recommendations based on the latest research.

INTRODUCTION

Children constitute the population that is most vulnerable to unintentional and preventable poisonings. The National Poison Data System reported that children younger than 6 years of age accounted for 48.9% of the more than 2.3 million calls received by poison centers in the United States in 2011. The top 5 exposures were cosmetics/personal care items (14%), analgesics (9.9%), household cleaning supplies (9.2%), foreign bodies (6.9%), and topical preparations (6.6%).[1] These numbers show that poison prevention should remain a top priority in protecting children. As children

[a] Department of Emergency Medicine, University of Maryland School of Medicine, Baltimore, MD, USA; [b] Department of Emergency Medicine, Upper Chesapeake Health Systems, Bel Air, MD, USA; [c] Division of Pediatrics, University of Maryland School of Medicine, Baltimore, MD, USA; [d] Department of Emergency Medicine, George Washington University, Washington, DC, USA; [e] Department of Clinical Pharmacology, Children's National Medical Center, Washington, DC, USA
* Corresponding author. Department of Emergency Medicine – EM Administrative Office, Upper Chesapeake Medical Center, 500 Upper Chesapeake Drive, Bel Air, MD 21014.
E-mail address: fbarrueto1215@gmail.com

Pediatr Clin N Am 60 (2013) 1203–1220
http://dx.doi.org/10.1016/j.pcl.2013.06.002
0031-3955/13/$ – see front matter © 2013 Elsevier Inc. All rights reserved.

move past the age of 6 years and into adolescence, their types of exposure to poisons change. They have increased access to illicit drugs and alcohol, and their use of designer drugs and over-the-counter (OTC) preparations has proliferated, fueled by use of the Internet and social media.[1]

This article discusses the general approach to the poisoned pediatric patient, with an emphasis on new exposures and cutting-edge treatment modalities. Neonatal abstinence syndrome, which is increasingly seen, is also discussed. Gastrointestinal (GI) decontamination, single-pill/single-dose killers, designer drugs, energy drinks, prescription drug abuse, and OTC medications are also discussed.

GI DECONTAMINATION
Syrup of Ipecac

In 2003, the American Academy of Pediatrics (AAP) released a policy statement advising that syrup of ipecac should no longer be used in the home as a treatment of poisoning and that bottles of it being stored in medicine cabinets should be discarded.[2] This product is no longer manufactured in the United States and has been removed from emergency medical services (EMS), poison center, and hospital protocols.

Activated Charcoal

Administration of activated charcoal (AC) can be an effective intervention for reducing the bioavailability of ingested substances.[3] Charcoal works by adsorbing the toxin onto its surface, thus preventing enterohepatic and enteroenteric recirculation of ingested toxin. If AC is used, a charcoal/drug ratio of 10:1 is recommended (1–2 g per kg).[4] AC should not be used as a treatment in the symptomatic child but as a highly effective adjunct for GI decontamination.

The maximum benefit from AC is usually seen when it is administered within 60 minutes after ingestion.[5] The decision to use AC depends on the time since ingestion, the patient's clinical status, and the type of toxin that was ingested. A large single dose is effective in preventing drug absorption by mass action. Elimination is also enhanced by the administration of multiple doses of AC after ingestion of drugs that undergo enterohepatic recirculation (eg, digoxin, carbamazepine, and phenobarbital).[6,7] Multiple doses can also be used to counter overdoses that cause bezoars or concretions, such as aspirin and buproprion, as well as ingestion of slow-release/continuous-release preparations.[7] AC is unpalatable, messy, and poorly accepted by young children and their caregivers. Children often vomit after its administration, decreasing the likelihood that the recommended dose will be given.[8] Using charcoal with a flavored syrup may be beneficial to improve palatability. AC does not bind well with xenobiotics that are highly ionized (eg, metals, electrolytes, acids, and alkali; **Box 1**). In addition, AC is contraindicated in patients who have ingested corrosives or hydrocarbons, in those with bowel obstruction or perforation, and in patients with a depressed level of consciousness (because of the risk of pulmonary aspiration).

The AAP does not support the routine administration of AC in the home, because its efficacy and safety in that setting have not been shown.[2] The first action for a caregiver of a child who may have ingested a toxic substance should be to consult with the local poison control center.

Whole-bowel Irrigation

Whole-bowel irrigation (WBI) involves administration of large volumes of polyethylene glycol solution orally to decontaminate the GI tract without causing fluid or electrolyte

Box 1
Xenobiotics that do not adsorb to charcoal
Ethylene glycol
Alcohols such as ethanol and methanol
Acids such as hydrochloric acid
Alkalis such as bleach
Iron
Potassium
Lithium salts

shifts. The pediatric dose is 25 mL/kg/h, up to 500 mL/h in young children and up to 1 L/h in adolescents. Although indications and use have been decreasing, the theoretic objective of WBI is to propel the toxic substance through the GI tract before it is fully absorbed. The American College of Medical Toxicology position paper on WBI states that there are few indications for this approach and that few studies have shown efficacy.[9] It may be useful when a drug or toxicant does not have an antidote or treatment and the substance ingested is an enteric pill, sustained-release preparation, or agents poorly adsorbed by AC. Examples are lithium, iron, and lead. WBI can be used in body packers and body stuffers to accelerate the passage of drug-filled packets.[9] Adverse effects of WBI include vomiting; abdominal cramps; bloating; and, rarely, aspiration pneumonitis.

New Interventions: Enhanced Elimination

Active elimination techniques should be considered only when exposure to high concentrations of a toxin is a known hazard or a patient's recovery would otherwise be unlikely. Enhanced elimination techniques are indicated in patients who are hemodynamically unstable and have end-organ failure despite supportive measures. The available procedures are multidose AC, hemodialysis (HD), hemofiltration, hemoperfusion (HP), and extracorporeal devices.

Extracorporeal elimination (HD, HP, and hemofiltration) is usually reserved for specific toxins, depending on their pharmacokinetic properties. HD is considered for patients who have ingested drugs with small volume of distribution, poor plasma protein binding, low molecular weight, and weak lipid solubility. Examples are atenolol, ethylene glycol, methanol, and salicylates. HD is helpful when the patient has a coexisting acid-base or electrolyte imbalance (**Table 1**).

The molecular adsorbent recycling system (MARS) is an extracorporeal device with an albumin-impregnated membrane combined with a conventional HD technique. MARS has been used in adults for bioartificial liver support. In theory, it could be used in the treatment of acetaminophen toxicity and other severe poisonings with highly protein-bound drugs that are hepatotoxic.[10] This technique has not been studied in children.

HP, using a charcoal filter in an HD machine, can remove toxins with high molecular weight and small volume of distribution. The compounds amenable to HP include barbiturates, carbamazepine, chloral hydrate, dapsone, isoniazid, procainamide, organophosphates, and diphenhydramine.

Exchange transfusion (ET) is an alternative procedure that can be used for a small group of children who are not eligible for HD for technical reasons. This procedure

Table 1 Drugs that can undergo enhanced elimination	
Drug	**HD or HP**
Atenolol	HD
Carbamazepine	HP
Ethylene glycol	HD
Isopropanol	HD
Lithium	HD
Methanol	HD
Phenobarbital	HP
Phenytoin	HP
Salicylate	HD
Theophylline	HP > HD

can be life saving for those with severe jaundice or drug toxicities. Several case reports have shown the beneficial effect of ET with salicylate, theophylline, phenobarbital, chloramphenicol, lithium, and aniline toxicity. In isolated cases, ET has been effective for chloral hydrate, salicylate, quinine, and methemoglobinemia.[11–19] Extracorporeal membrane oxygenation (ECMO) has been used for hydrocarbon-induced lung injury,[20] bupropion,[21] amiodarone,[22] calcium channel blocker (CCB) overdose,[23] and a severe ibuprofen poisoning.[24]

Neonatal Abstinence Syndrome

A precise history of ingestion and evaluation for toxidromes help guide both diagnosis and management of the poisoned patient. One toxidrome, opioid withdrawal, is characterized by piloerection, diarrhea, vomiting, and diaphoresis. The patient must be physiologically dependent on opioids for withdrawal to occur. Until recently, opioid withdrawal was not seen often in the pediatric population. It now occurs in neonates whose mothers are opioid dependent or who took opioid replacement therapy (methadone) while they were pregnant. In addition, opioid withdrawal is being seen more frequently in the adolescent population as a result of the epidemic of prescription drug abuse.[1]

Opioid withdrawal syndrome in the neonate, also called neonatal abstinence syndrome (NAS), is induced by a variety of drugs. It is characterized by fussy behavior, decreased feeding, and seizures; unlike adult opioid withdrawal, the NAS carries a significant mortality.[25] The modified Finnegan NAS scoring tool is commonly used, and its accuracy has been verified in the literature. It assists with diagnosis, disposition, and treatment. Every neonatal unit should have a NAS protocol based on a scoring system to guide treatment.[25]

Prescription Drug Abuse

Over the past decade, efforts to improve the identification and treatment of causes of pain have translated into increased use of prescription opioid analgesics by adults and children.[26–29] This increase has been paralleled by even more dramatic increases in prescription opioid misuse, abuse, and related fatalities.[30–34] Adolescents are more likely than other age groups to experiment with the nonmedical use of prescription opioids.[29,35]

According to the 2010 National Survey on Drug Use and Health, prescription analgesics were the second most commonly abused substances by adolescents and young adults, surpassed only by marijuana.[34] One study found that 21% of high school seniors in an urban metropolitan area reported nonmedical use of a prescription opioid.[36] Up to 80% of high school students who were nonmedical users reported obtaining opioids from a previous medical prescription.[35] These trends generate concern in light of the increasing number of narcotics and controlled substance prescriptions that are written for adolescents and young adults, which nearly doubled between 1994 and 2007.[37]

Prescription medications, especially opioids, may be easier for adolescents to obtain than illicit drugs. Often, opioid analgesics are obtained from prior medical prescriptions, friends, and relatives.[38,39] Opioids and other prescription medications can be misused or abused by the oral route; however, studies have shown that a significant percentage of adolescents use alternative routes of administration, such as injection or insufflation.[40,41] Increasing prescription rates and the easy accessibility of opioid analgesics have led to a significant increase in the frequency and severity of overdoses, concomitant substance abuse, trauma, as well as long-term addiction in adolescents and young adults.[42–44] Even more disturbing is the increase in opioid-related fatalities in adolescents, which more than doubled between 1980 and 2008.[32]

A variety of methods have been proposed to mitigate prescription drug abuse in adolescents and adults. The US Food and Drug Administration (FDA) has established Risk Mitigation and Evaluation Strategies (REMS) for long-acting opioids, which require patient medication guides and expanded health care provider education.[37] Some states have instituted prescription drug–monitoring programs (PDMPs) that collect statewide data about medication-prescribing practices and pharmacy-filing patterns. Preliminary data suggest that these programs might be having a positive impact on opioid prescribing and drug diversion. However, the true impact and optimal organization of these programs has yet to be elucidated.[45,46] Some states, such as Washington, have developed opioid-prescribing guidelines in an effort to promote safe and appropriate use of these medications.[47] In addition, several specialties have developed clinical practice guidelines. For example, the American College of Emergency Physicians issued a clinical policy statement regarding the prescribing of opioids in adult emergency department patients in 2012.[48] On a more local level, many individual practices and institutions have implemented opioid-prescribing guidelines. Industry efforts have focused on developing abuse-deterrent formulations, especially for agents with high abuse potential, such as sustained-release oxycodone.[49]

Individual medical care providers can mitigate prescription drug abuse through patient and family counseling and by implementing good prescribing practices. If an opioid is indicated, only the necessary duration of therapy should be prescribed. This restriction decreases the likelihood that unused medication might be used inappropriately. Health care providers should be encouraged to discuss prescription drug abuse with children and adolescents at an early age, which can prevent later experimentation and abuse. Parents should be instructed on how to administer prescribed drugs and how to properly store and dispose of remaining medication. In addition, parents should be counseled regarding the signs of prescription drug abuse and where to seek help.

SINGLE-PILL/SINGLE-DOSE KILLERS

The substances that are most toxic (potentially lethal even in 1 dose) to small children include hypoglycemics, certain cardiovascular drugs, opioids, and methylsalicylates (**Box 2**).

Box 2	
Drugs and other agents that are poisonous to children in a single or small dose	
Pharmacologic agents	*Nonpharmacologic agents*
• Antimalarials	• Alcohols
Chloroquine	Ethanol
Quinidine	Ethylene glycol (antifreeze)
Quinine	Methanol (windshield wiper fluid)
• Cardiovascular agents	• Caustic agents
β-Blockers	Acids (antirust compounds, toilet cleaners)
CCBs	Alkalis (drain cleaners, perm relaxers)
Clonidine	Cleaning agents
• Opioids	• Hydrocarbons
Methadone	Kerosene
Oxycodone	Lamp oil
Diphenoxylate/atropine	Mineral seal oil (furniture polish)
• Oral hypoglycemic agents	• Industrial chemicals
Sulfonylureas	Methylene chloride
• Topical agents	Selenious acid (gun bluing)
Benzocaine	Zinc chloride (soldering fluid)
Lindane	• Nail products
Methyl salicylate (oil of wintergreen)	Acetonitrite
• Other agents	Methacrylic acid (artificial nail primer)
Isoniazid	Nitromethane (artificial nail remover)
Theophylline	• Pesticides
	Organophosphates
	Paraquat

Sulfonylurea

The management of an asymptomatic, euglycemic child who has been exposed to a sulfonylurea is difficult because of the risk of late-onset hypoglycemia. Ingestion of as little as 2 mg of glimepiride can cause profound hypoglycemia that can lead to permanent neurologic disability or death.[50,51] A normal blood sugar concentration during the first few hours after ingestion does not predict the late onset of hypoglycemia. For this reason, in-hospital observation is required for at least 24 hours for all children who have ingested a sulfonylurea, even if they are asymptomatic. Symptomatic hypoglycemia induced by sulfonylurea toxicity should be treated with both intravenous (IV) dextrose and octreotide (pediatric dosing: 4 or 5 μg/kg/d, divided every 6 hours).[52]

Octreotide is a somatostatin analogue that inhibits insulin release from pancreatic beta islet cells. Its administration decreases the number of hypoglycemic events and increases blood glucose concentration for the treatment of sulfonylurea-induced hypoglycemia.[52] Octreotide is considered safe antidotal therapy for xenobiotic-induced endogenous secretion of insulin (as induced by sulfonylureas and quinine).

CCBs and β-Blockers

Toxicity from CCBs includes bradycardia, hypotension, cardiac conduction delay, and hyperglycemia. Despite hypotension, CCB-poisoned patients might maintain normal mental status until cerebral perfusion is critically limited, perhaps because of CCBs' neuroprotective effect. The types of CCBs are listed in **Table 2**, and CCBs' clinical effects are compared with those of β-blockers in **Table 3**. Diltiazem and verapamil cause bradycardia initially, whereas dihydropyridines initially cause vasodilation and a reflex tachycardia. Dihydropyridines have specificity for the L-type calcium channels in the vasculature and less effect on the electrical conducting system of the heart.

Specific treatment of CCB and β-blocker toxicity is designed primarily to address bradycardia and hypotension. Treatment has traditionally included IV fluids, atropine, glucagon, and calcium. A high-dose continuous infusion of calcium was used in one severe nifedipine overdose.[53] Norepinephrine is the initial vasopressor of choice, because of its positive inotropy, chronotropy, and vasoconstrictive effects. Recent case reports of CCB overdose have shown efficacy of administration of high-dose insulin infusion (1 unit/kg/h of regular insulin) and maintaining of euglycemia through dextrose infusion.[54] Although the mechanism is not clear, this high-dose insulin/ euglycemia (HIE) therapy has shown improvement in inotropy and peripheral vascular resistance, particularly in CCB toxicity.[54] As a result, HIE improves mean arterial pressure and pH and decreases the need for vasopressors. Bradycardia and heart block might not respond to HIE therapy.[54]

IV lipid emulsion (ILE) is being studied as therapy for hemodynamically unstable patients poisoned with several lipophilic medications. Its mechanism of action is not completely understood, but the application came from its impressive effects on patients poisoned by local anesthetics (www.lipidrescue.org). The dosing is 1.5 mL/kg of 20% lipid emulsion, delivered over 1 minute; the bolus can be repeated in 5 minutes, with a maximum dose of 3 mL/kg. ILE has been used on patients with severe exposures to verapamil,[55] β-blockers,[56] tricyclic antidepressants,[57] and bupivacaine.[58] HIE and IV lipid emulsion therapies are both developing treatment adjuncts for severe poisoning that need to be considered (**Table 4**).

Opioids

Multiple forms of opioids are prescribed at present: natural (eg, morphine, codeine), semisynthetic (oxycodone, hydrocodone), and synthetic (methadone, meperidine). Methadone is the most toxic of the opioids for children younger than 6 years of age.[1,59] Ingestion of a single 5-mg tablet of methadone can be very toxic and can lead to death in this age group.[59] Transdermal fentanyl is prone to misuse by adolescents and could be fatal.[60] Death from an overdose of opioids usually results from

Table 2 Types of CCBs	
Direct Vasodilation and Secondary Reflex Tachycardia	**Direct Negative Chronotropy and Inotropy**
Dihydropyridines	Phenylalkylamine
Nicardipine	Verapamil
Nifedipine	Benzothiazepine
Isradipine	Diltiazem
Amlodipine	
Felodipine	
Nimodipine	

Table 3
Physiologic effects of CCBs and β-blockers

	Dihydropyridines	Verapamil, Diltiazem	β-Blockers
Pulse	Reflex tachycardia	Bradycardia	Bradycardia
Blood pressure	Hypotension	Hypotension	Hypotension
Potassium	No change	No change	Hyperkalemia
Glucose	Hyperglycemia	Hyperglycemia	Hypoglycemia
Lungs	No examination findings	No examination findings	Bronchoconstriction
Neurologic	Alert	Alert	Sedating

respiratory failure. Most opioid exposures in children younger than 6 years of age occur with analgesic combinations[1]; therefore, toxicity from acetaminophen or aspirin must be considered when evaluating children who have been poisoned with one of these compounds.

Naloxone is antidotal therapy and a specific opioid antagonist that should be given to children who show respiratory depression. If an extended-release preparation such as oxycodone or morphine or a long-acting opioid such as methadone was ingested then a naloxone infusion and prolonged observation or admission should be considered. A good general rule is that when more than 1 dose of naloxone is administered to prevent apnea, the child is a likely candidate for continuous infusion of naloxone.[59] The standard dose of naloxone for acute opioid toxicity is 0.1 mg/kg, administered intravenously, for newborns (including premature infants) and children up to 5 years of age or 20 kg of weight. For patients weighing more than 20 kg, a minimum of 2 mg should be used. Naloxone can also be given intramuscularly or through a nebulizer.[61]

Methylsalicylate (Oil of Wintergreen)

Oil of wintergreen is sold as a component of herbal products, aroma therapy, and topical agents for management of musculoskeletal pain. Five milliliters of the oil contains 7 g of salicylate. Ingestion of as little as 4 mL can be fatal for an infant (<10 kg).[62]

Table 4
Pediatric dosing of new or rarely used antidotes and treatments

Antidote	Toxin Treated	Dose	Monitor
Octreotide	Sulfonylurea, quinine, hyperinsulinemic states	4–5 µg/kg/d divided every 6 h subcutaneously (maximum 50 µg every 6 h)	Glucose
Hyperinsulinemia/ euglycemia	Evidence for calcium channel and β-blockers	Goal: 1 unit of regular insulin/kg/h infusion	Glucose
20% Lipid emulsion	Any hemodynamic unstable poisoning (effective with lipophilic drugs)	1.5 mL/kg bolus; can repeat in 5 min; maximum 3 mL/kg total	Hemodynamic response
Physostigmine	Anticholinergic symptoms, especially agitation and hallucinations	0.02 mg/kg slow IV over 1–2 min; can repeat if symptoms are not resolving	Watch for cholinergic crisis, monitor pulse, atropine at bedside

All salicylate intoxications have similar manifestations; their management is similar as well. The plasma salicylate concentration has no absolute correlation with the patient's symptoms. When salicylate toxicity is suspected, the plasma salicylate concentration should be measured but the results should be interpreted in conjunction with the clinical findings. A concentration greater than 100 mg/dL after an acute intoxication is an indication for HD. The goals of treatment are to provide supportive care, correct fluid and electrolyte imbalances, and enhance excretion. The primary methods of enhancing elimination of salicylates are urinary alkalinization and HD. The goal of urinary alkalinization is to achieve a urine pH greater than 7.5 while maintaining a serum pH of no more than 7.55, which can be done by providing 1.5 to 2 times maintenance fluids containing 150 mEq of sodium bicarbonate per 1 L 5% dextrose water solution.[63]

Indications for HD include persistent central nervous system dysfunction (seizures, coma), pulmonary edema, renal insufficiency, intractable metabolic acidosis, clinical deterioration despite aggressive therapy, and a plasma salicylate level greater than 100 mg/dL. A case report suggested that a peri-intubation death was caused by transient respiratory acidosis and subsequent influx of salicylate into the brain of a man who had attempted suicide.[64]

DESIGNER DRUGS
Synthetic Marijuana

Synthetic cannabinoids were developed by pharmaceutical companies in the 1960s in an effort to study the cannabinoid system as a potential therapeutic target.[65,66] Dr John W. Huffman and his team synthesized many of these compounds to study their antiemetic and appetite stimulation properties (Dr Huffman's initials are used in the names of many of these compounds [listed later]). In the early 2000s, synthetic cannabinoids began to emerge as drugs of abuse in Europe and eventually the United States.[67–69] These agents are marketed as incense or legal alternatives to traditional marijuana. Because of the increasing rates of abuse, the US Drug Enforcement Agency made 5 commonly used synthetic cannabinoids (JWH-018, JWH-073, JWH-200, CP-47,497, and cannabicyclohexanol) schedule I controlled substances in 2011.[58] The content of individual products such as spice and K2 can be highly variable.[69] Synthetic cannabinoids are typically combined with a herbal mixture and smoked; they can also be ingested.[70–72]

These compounds bind with high affinity to the CB1 and CB2 receptors, but they also affect other receptors, including the serotonin and NDMA systems.[73,74] Substances present in the herbal mixture may have additional pharmacologic effects.[68] The clinical presentation of patients with synthetic cannabinoid intoxication can include agitation, psychosis, dystonia, tachycardia, diaphoresis, GI disturbances, seizures, and coma. Secondary trauma and rhabdomyolysis can also occur.[70,71,75–79] Prolonged psychiatric manifestations and withdrawal symptoms have been reported with prolonged use.[80–82] There is no specific antidote for synthetic cannabinoid intoxication and care is largely supportive. Benzodiazepines are the mainstay of therapy for agitation and seizures, in addition to aggressive supportive care.[70] Potential diagnostic tests include an electrocardiogram, glucose and electrolyte determination, serum creatinine, creatinine phosphokinase, liver function tests, and evaluation for coingestants, as indicated. Specific assays can detect selected synthetic cannabinoids; however, results are often not available in a timely manner and generally do not change management.[70,79] A urine toxicology screen for marijuana is generally negative in patients who have used synthetic cannabinoid. Patients should be kept in a safe environment and observed until symptoms resolve, which could be as long as 24 hours. Psychosis has been irreversible in some cases.[70,77]

Bath Salts (Synthetic Cathinones)

Synthetic cathinones recently emerged as drugs of abuse; however, cathinone derivatives have been used for centuries.[83,84] In the Middle East and Africa, the leaves of the khat plant (Catha edulis) are commonly chewed for their stimulant effects.[85] In the twentieth century, cathinone derivatives were synthesized, but it was not until several decades later that they gained popularity as drugs of abuse. The synthetic cathinones that are most commonly used as drugs of abuse are mephedrone, methylone, and 3,4-methylenedioxypyrovalerone (MDPV). Many other analogues exist and products can have significant variations.[70,83,85] Synthetic cathinones are commonly sold as bath salts or plant food under product names such as Ivory Wave, Vanilla Sky, and Meow Meow,[70,83] and are marketed as so-called legal highs. Concerns about increased rates of abuse prompted the US Drug Enforcement Agency to make 3 synthetic cathinones schedule I controlled substances.

Cathinones are structurally related to amphetamines. As such, they increase the concentrations of multiple neurotransmitters, including dopamine, norepinephrine, and serotonin.[83,86,87] Cathinones are available as a powder but can also be made into tablets or capsules. Their routes of administration include oral, insufflation, and injection.[83,88] Effects reported by synthetic cathinone users include euphoria and increased awareness, alertness, openness, and sexual libido.[70,83,85] In contrast, a variety of adverse effects have been reported, including agitation, psychosis, paranoia, tremors, insomnia, seizures, and mood disturbances.[83,84,88–90] Other physical signs and symptoms include hyperthermia, tachycardia, dehydration, GI disturbances, rhabdomyolysis, and myocardial infarction. Infectious complications can occur as a result of parenteral abuse.[91] Secondary trauma may occur as a result of altered mental status.

Routine urine drug screens do not detect synthetic cathinones; however, an amphetamine screen could be falsely positive. Tests for common cathinone derivatives are available, but their results generally do not influence clinical management and are often not available in a timely manner.[92] Diagnostic tests that are potentially useful include an electrocardiogram, glucose and electrolyte determination, serum creatinine, creatinine phosphokinase, liver function tests, and evaluation for coingestants as indicated.

There is no specific antidote for synthetic cathinones, so care is largely supportive. The patient should be kept safe. The treatment of agitation, seizures, and sympathetic symptoms could require the liberal use of benzodiazepines.[93] Vasodilators, such as phentolamine or hydralazine, should be used for persistent hypertension (beta-adrenergic blockers should be avoided). Cooling measures should be instituted for patients with significant hyperthermia. Fluid resuscitation is indicated for those with dehydration or evidence of rhabdomyolysis.[83] The effects of synthetic cathinones generally last for several hours, depending on the agent, although symptoms have been reported to last for days.[70] Patients should be monitored until they become asymptomatic, and those with prolonged symptoms or medical complications should be admitted.

Energy Drinks

Energy drinks (eg, Red Bull, Monster, Rockstar) contain caffeine and other energy-promoting substances.[94,95] First marketed in the late 1990s, these beverages have gained widespread popularity. Energy shots contain comparable amounts of caffeine and stimulant ingredients, but in a more concentrated volume.[94] These products are marketed aggressively to adolescents and young adults; nearly a third of teenagers report regular consumption.[95] The primary ingredient in energy drinks is caffeine, ranging from 80 to 140 mg per 237-mL (8-ounce) serving, approximately 2 to 3 times that of an equivalent serving of soda.[96,97] Energy shots and large bottles of energy drinks can contain even greater amounts of caffeine (**Table 5**).[98] In addition to caffeine, these beverages contain ingredients with caffeinelike effects, including guarana.[99]

Consumption of excessive quantities of these beverages can lead to central nervous system excitation, seizures, tachycardia, and ventricular dysrhythmias.[94] Beta-adrenergic stimulation can also lead to hypokalemia and hyperglycemia. The few deaths that have been associated with caffeine and energy drink consumption were attributed to cardiac dysrhythmias.[100–102] A more recent and also potentially dangerous trend is mixing energy drinks with ethanol,[95] as in products such as Four Loco. In combinations of ethanol and caffeine, the caffeine might decrease the sedative effects of alcohol, leading to impaired judgment and risk-taking behaviors, such as driving while intoxicated.[97]

Diagnosis is based largely on history and clinical presentation. An electrocardiogram and electrolyte and glucose determinations are indicated. Caffeine levels are of limited usefulness.

There is no specific antidote for toxicity resulting from consumption of energy drinks. Benzodiazepines are first-line therapy for agitation and seizures. Dysrhythmias should be treated with beta-adrenergic blockers or lidocaine and by correcting hypokalemia. Concomitant ethanol intoxication and any subsequent complications should also be addressed. Patients should be monitored until symptoms resolve, and those with seizures, dysrhythmias, or cardiovascular compromise should be admitted.

Internet Phenomena, OTC Products, and Topical Patches

Most children younger than 18 years of age have limited access to illicit drugs such as heroin, cocaine, and methamphetamine. However, because of the proliferation of

| Table 5 | | |
| Caffeine concentrations in energy drinks | | |
Product	Serving Size (mL)	Caffeine Content (mg)
Cola	355	46.5
Mountain Dew	355	54.4
Coffee	148	85–200
Espresso	60	100
Black tea	148	50
Amp	248	69.6
Four Loco	695	135
Five-Hour Energy	59	120
Java Monster	444	160
Jolt Energy Drink	695	280
Monster Energy Drink	473	160
Red Bull	251	80
Rockstar	473	160
Spider	473	240

designer drugs and ubiquitous access to the Internet, options for access are virtually endless for the adolescent who wants to experiment with OTC preparations and designer drugs.

With access to Internet sites such as www.erowid.org, anyone can learn about the effects of psychoactive plants and chemicals. For example, anticholinergics such as dimenhydrinate and scopolamine are used to cause hallucinations (although the urinary retention that they cause might act as a deterrent).[103] Anticholinergic hallucinations produce spatial distortions (Lilliputian hallucinations) such as the dysmorphic exaggerations described in *Gulliver's Travels*. Asking the patient to perform a simple task such as drawing a clock (**Fig. 1**) can reveal the distortion induced by psychotropic compounds. **Fig. 1** also shows the effect of the antidote, physostigmine, being administered to an anticholinergic patient.

Dextromethorphan is classified as an opioid but it chemically resembles arylhexamines (eg, phencyclidine [PCP]). This drug can be purchased over the Internet and is a readily available OTC medication. At high doses, it can cause PCP-like effects (agitation and psychosis).[104] The FDA removed OTC cough remedies for children less than the age of 6 years because of the incidence of unintentional overdoses, adverse drug reactions in this age group, and the questionable efficacy of the medications. The main tenets when treating a patient suspected of dextromethorphan overdose is monitoring for serotonin syndrome and hyperthermia, controlling agitation with benzodiazepines, searching for occult trauma, and providing supportive care.[105]

Patches are another vehicle of drug use/abuse that is not unique to the pediatric population but is within the realm of poison prevention. Topically applied medication patches deliver a drug over a period of 24 to 72 hours. They use a simple diffusion gradient and matrix to facilitate diffusion through the skin.[60] A large concentration of drug must be stored within the patch so that it can cross through the matrix and skin to reach the blood stream. A fentanyl patch labeled as delivering 100 μg/h contains 10 mg of the drug. Even when the patch is scheduled to be removed, several lethal doses remain in it.[36] The contents can be eaten, or the gel can be extracted and injected intravenously or intramuscularly, smoked, or even insufflated. Patches, especially those containing the synthetic opioid fentanyl, have been implicated in lethal exposures.[106] Family members should be educated about the proper disposal of these patches and their abuse potential. Assessment is designed to address the symptoms of narcotic overdose and treatment is likewise geared to ameliorating life-threatening symptoms.

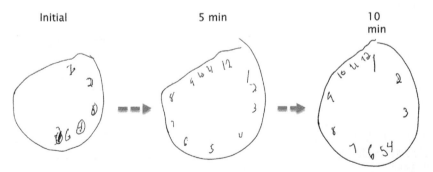

Initial   5 min   10 min

Fig. 1. A 15-year-ld boy who had overdosed on dimenhydrinate was asked to draw a clock. Physostigmine, 2 mg IV, was administered, and he made these drawings after 5 and 10 minutes of treatment.

SUMMARY

Poison prevention remains a challenge and a necessity to prevent the most vulnerable population from becoming exposed to potentially lethal drugs and toxins. The evaluation of a child presumed to have been exposed to a toxic substance should include a precise history of the exposure, a physical examination, and knowledge of current ingestions and recreational practices. Cutting-edge treatments and new research guiding therapy continue to evolve. Poison centers and medical toxicologists can be consulted to assist with the diagnosis of medicinal/drug overdoses, for advice about the pitfalls inherent in stabilizing children who have been exposed to toxic compounds, and for treatment recommendations based on the latest research.

REFERENCES

1. Bronstein AC, Spyker DA, Cantilena LR Jr, et al. 2011 Annual report of the American Association of Poison Control Centers' National Poison Data System (NPDS): 29th Annual Report. Clin Toxicol (Phila) 2012;50(10):911–1164.
2. American Academy of Pediatrics. Policy statement: poison treatment in the home. Pediatrics 2003;112:1182–5.
3. McGuigan MA. Activated charcoal in the home. Clin Pediatr Emerg Med 2000;1: 191–4.
4. Levy G, Tsuchiya T. Effect of activated charcoal on aspirin absorption in man. Part 1. Clin Pharmacol Ther 1972;13:317–22.
5. Chyka PA, Seger D, Krenzelok EP, et al. Position paper: single-dose activated charcoal. Clin Toxicol (Phila) 2005;43(2):61–87.
6. Roberts DM, Southcott E, Potter JM, et al. Pharmacokinetics of digoxin cross-reacting substances in patients with acute yellow Oleander (*Thevetia peruviana*) poisoning, including the effect of activated charcoal. Ther Drug Monit 2006; 28(6):784–92.
7. Christophersen AJ, Hoegberg LC. Techniques used to prevent gastrointestinal absorption. In: Flomenbaum NE, Goldfrank LR, Hoffman RS, et al, editors. Goldfrank's toxicologic emergencies. 8th edition. New York: McGraw-Hill; 2006. p. 115–6.
8. Dilger I, Brockstedt M, Oberdisse U, et al. Activated charcoal is needed rarely in children but can be administered safely by the lay public [abstract]. J Toxicol Clin Toxicol 1999;37:402–3.
9. Position paper: whole bowel irrigation. J Toxicol Clin Toxicol 2004;42(6):843–54.
10. Strange J, Mitzner SR, Risler T, et al. Molecular adsorbent recycling system (MARS): clinical results of a new membrane-based blood purification system for bioartificial liver support. Artif Organs 1999;23:319–30.
11. Osborn HH, Henry G, Wax P, et al. Theophylline toxicity in a premature neonate-elimination kinetics of exchange transfusion. J Toxicol Clin Toxicol 1993;31: 639–44.
12. Sancak R, Kucukoduk S, Tasdemir HA, et al. Exchange transfusion treatment in a newborn with phenobarbital intoxication. Pediatr Emerg Care 1999;15:268–70.
13. Stevens DC, Kleiman MB, Lietman PS, et al. Exchange transfusion in acute chloramphenicol toxicity. J Pediatr 1981;99:651–3.
14. Jenniskens-Bruins JJ, Gerards LJ. Lithium poisoning in a newborn infant. Tijdschr Kindergeneeskd 1992;60:76–8 [in Dutch].
15. Mier RJ. Treatment of aniline poisoning with exchange transfusion. J Toxicol Clin Toxicol 1988;26:357–64.
16. Mowry JB. Effect of exchange transfusion in chloral hydrate overdose. Vet Hum Toxicol 1983;25:15–21.

17. Leiken SL, Emmanouilides GC. The use of exchange transfusion in salicylate intoxication. J Pediatr 1960;57:715–20.
18. Burrows AW, Hambleton G, Hardman MJ, et al. Quinine intoxication in a child treated by exchange transfusion. Arch Dis Child 1972;47:304–5.
19. Berlin G, Brodin B, Hilden JO, et al. Acute dapsone intoxication: a case treatment with continuous infusion of methylene blue, forced diuresis and plasma exchange. J Toxicol Clin Toxicol 1984–1985;22:537–48.
20. Langham MR Jr, Kays DW, Beierle EA, et al. Expanded application of extracorporeal membrane oxygenation in a pediatric surgery practice. Ann Surg 2003; 237(6):766–72.
21. Shenoi AN, Gertz SJ, Mikkilineni S, et al. Refractory hypotension from massive bupropion overdose successfully treated with extracorporeal membrane oxygenation. Pediatr Emerg Care 2011;27(1):43–5.
22. Haas NA, Wegendt C, Schäffler R, et al. ECMO for cardiac rescue in a neonate with accidental amiodarone overdose. Clin Res Cardiol 2008;97(12):878–81.
23. Kolcz J, Pietrzyk J, Januszewska K, et al. Extracorporeal life support in severe propranolol and verapamil intoxication. J Intensive Care Med 2007;22(6):381–5.
24. Marciniak KE, Thomas IH, Brogan TV, et al. Massive ibuprofen overdose requiring extracorporeal membrane oxygenation for cardiovascular support. Pediatr Crit Care Med 2007;8(2):180–2.
25. Hudak ML, Tan RC, Committee on Drugs, Committee on Fetus and Newborn, American Academy of Pediatrics. Neonatal drug withdrawal. Pediatrics 2012; 129(2):e540–60.
26. Philips DM. Joint Commission on Accreditation of Healthcare Organizations: JCAHO pain management standards are unveiled. JAMA 2000;284:428–9.
27. Fein JA, Zepmsky WT, Craver JP, et al. Relief of pain and anxiety in pediatric patients in emergency medical systems. Pediatrics 2012;130(5):e1391–405.
28. Pletcher MJ, Kertesz SG, Kohn MA, et al. Trends in opioid prescribing by race/ethnicity for patients seeking care in US emergency departments. JAMA 2008; 299(1):70–8.
29. Fortuna RJ, Robbins BW, Caiola E, et al. Prescribing of controlled medications to adolescents and young adults in the United States. Pediatrics 2010;126(6): 1108–16.
30. Manchikanti L, Helm S, Fellows B, et al. Opioid epidemic in the United States. Pain Physician 2012;15(Suppl 3):ES9–38.
31. Manchikanti L, Singh A. Therapeutic opioids: a ten-year perspective on the complexities and complications of the escalating use, abuse, and nonmedical use of opioids. Pain Physician 2008;11(Suppl 2):S63–88.
32. Centers for Disease Control and Prevention 2011. Drug poisoning deaths in the United States, 1980–2008. Available at: www.cdc.gov/nchs/data/databriefs/db81.pdf. Accessed April 23, 2013.
33. Johnston LD, O'Malley PM, Bachman JF, et al. Monitoring the future. National Survey Results on Drug Use, 1975-2008. In: Secondary School Students, vol. I. Bethesda (MD): National Institute on Drug Abuse; 2009. NIH Publication 09–742.
34. Substance Abuse and Mental Health Services Administration. Results from the 2010 National Survey on Drug Use and Health: summary of national findings. Rockville (MD): Substance Abuse and Mental Health Services Administration; 2010. NSDUH Series H-4, HHS Publication No. (SMA) 11–4658.
35. Esteban-McCabe S, West BT, Teter CJ, et al. Medical and nonmedical use of prescription opioids among high school seniors in the United States. Arch Pediatr Adolesc Med 2012;166(9):797–802.

36. Meier EA, Troost JP, Anthony JC. Extramedical use of prescription pain relievers by youth aged 12 to 21 years in the United States. Arch Pediatr Adolesc Med 2012;166(9):803–7.
37. Department of Health and Human Services, Food and Drug Administration. Draft blueprint for prescriber education for long-acting/extended-release opioid class-wide risk evaluation and mitigation strategy. Fed Reg 2011;76: 68766–7.
38. Garnier LM, Arria AM, Caldeira KM, et al. Sharing and selling of prescription medications in a college student sample. J Clin Psychiatry 2010;71(3):262–9.
39. Results from the 2011 National Survey on Drug Use and Health: Summary of National Findings. The DAWN Report 2011. Available at: www.samhsa.gov/data/NSDUH/2k11Results/NSDUHresults2011.htm. Accessed April 23, 2013.
40. Osgood ED, Eaton TA, Trudeau JJ, et al. A brief survey to characterize oxycodone abuse patterns in adolescents enrolled in two substance abuse recovery high schools. Am J Drug Alcohol Abuse 2012;38(2):166–70.
41. Wightman R, Perrone J, Portelli I, et al. Likeability and abuse liability of commonly prescribed opioids. J Med Toxicol 2012;8(4):335–40.
42. Esteban-McCabe S, Cranford JA, West BT. Trends in prescription drug abuse and dependence, co-occurrence with other substance use disorders, and treatment utilization: results from two national surveys. Addict Behav 2008;33(10):1297–305.
43. Sung HE, Richter L, Vaughan R, et al. Nonmedical use of prescription opioids among teenagers in the United States: trends and correlates. J Adolesc Health 2005;37(1):44–51.
44. Tormoehlen LM, Mowry JB, Bodle JD, et al. Increased adolescent opioid use and complications reported to a poison control center follow the 2000 JCAHO pain initiative. Clin Toxicol 2011;49:492–8.
45. Sehgal N, Manchikanti L, Smith HS. Prescription opioid abuse in chronic pain: a review of opioid abuse predictors and strategies to curb opioid abuse. Pain Physician 2012;15(Suppl 3):ES67–92.
46. Gugelmann HM, Perrone J. Can prescription drug monitoring programs help limit opioid abuse? JAMA 2011;306(20):2258–9.
47. Neven DE, Sabel JC, Howell DN, et al. The development of the Washington State emergency department opioid prescribing guidelines. J Med Toxicol 2012;8(4):353–9.
48. Cantrill SV, Brown MD, Carlisle RJ, et al. Clinical policy: critical issues in the prescribing of opioids for adult patients in the emergency department. Ann Emerg Med 2012;60:499–525.
49. Schaeffer T. Abuse-deterrent formulations, an evolving technology against the abuse and misuse of opioid analgesics. J Med Toxicol 2012;8(4):400–7.
50. Quadrani DA, Spiller HA, Widder P. Five year retrospective evaluation of sulfonylurea ingestion in children. J Toxicol Clin Toxicol 1996;34:267–70.
51. Harrigan RA, Nathan MS, Beattie P. Oral agents for the treatment of type 2 diabetes mellitus: pharmacology, toxicity, and treatment. Ann Emerg Med 2001;38: 68–78.
52. Dougherty PP, Lee SC, Lung D, et al. Evaluation of the use and safety of octreotide as antidotal therapy for sulfonylurea overdose in children. Pediatr Emerg Care 2013;29(3):292–5.
53. Lam YM, Tse HF, Lau CP. Continuous calcium chloride infusion for massive nifedipine overdose. Chest 2001;119:1280–2.
54. Levine MD, Boyer E. Hyperinsulinemia-euglycemia: a useful tool in treating calcium channel blocker poisoning. Crit Care 2006;10(4):149.

55. French D, Armenian P, Ruan W, et al. Serum verapamil concentrations before and after Intralipid therapy during treatment of an overdose. Clin Toxicol 2011;49(4):340–4.
56. Jovic-Stosic J, Gligic B, Putic V, et al. Severe propranolol and ethanol overdose with wide complex tachycardia treated with intravenous lipid emulsion: a case report. Clin Toxicol 2011;49(5):429–30.
57. Nair A, Paul F, Protopapas M. Management of near fatal mixed tricyclic antide-pressant and selective serotonin reuptake inhibitor overdose with Intralipid 20% emulsion. Anaesth Intensive Care 2013;41(2):264–5.
58. Patil K. Use of Intralipid for local anesthetic toxicity in neonates. Paediatr Anaesth 2011;21(12):1268–9.
59. Sachdeva DK, Stadnyk JM. Are one or two dangerous? Opioid exposure in tod-dlers. J Emerg Med 2005;29(1):77–84.
60. Barrueto F Jr, Howland MA, Hoffman RS, et al. The fentanyl tea bag. Vet Hum Toxicol 2004;46(1):30–1.
61. American Academy of Pediatrics Committee on Drugs. Emergency drug doses for infants and children. Pediatrics 1988;81:462–5.
62. Botma M, Colquhoun-Flannery W, Leighton S. Laryngeal oedema caused by accidental ingestion of Oil of Wintergreen. Int J Pediatr Otorhinolaryngol 2001; 58(3):229–32.
63. Davis JE. Are one or two dangerous? Methyl salicylate exposure in toddlers. J Emerg Med 2007;32(1):63–9.
64. Greenberg MI, Hendrickson RG, Hofman M. Deleterious effects of endotracheal intubation in salicylate poisoning. Ann Emerg Med 2003;41(4):583–4.
65. Huffman JW. CB2 receptor ligands. Mini Rev Med Chem 2005;5:641–9.
66. Pavlopoulos S, Thakur GA, Nikas SP, et al. Cannabinoid receptors as therapeu-tic targets. Curr Pharm Des 2006;12:1751–69.
67. Di Marzo V, Bifuco M, De Petrocellis L. The endocannabinoid system and its therapeutic exploration. Nat Rev Drug Discov 2004;3:771–84.
68. European Monitoring Center for Drugs and Drug Addiction (EMCDDA) 2009. Thematic papers: understanding the spice phenomenon. Available at: www.emcdda.europa.eu/html.cmf/index90917EN.html. Accessed February 28, 2013.
69. US Department of Justice Drug Enforcement Administration. Scheduling update. Micr Bull 2011;44:1–4.
70. Rosenbaum CD, Carreiro SP, Babu KM. Here today, gone tomorrow...and back again? A review of herbal marijuana alternatives (K2, Spice), synthetic cathi-nones (bath salts), kratom, Salvia divinorum, methoxetamine, and piperazines. J Med Toxicol 2012;8:15–32.
71. Schneir AB, Cullen J, Ly BT. "Spice" girls: synthetic cannabinoid intoxication. J Emerg Med 2011;40:296–9.
72. Bonkowsky JL, Sarco D, Pomeroy SL. Ataxia and shaking in a 2-year-old girl: acute marijuana intoxication presenting as seizure. Pediatr Emerg Care 2005; 21(8):527–8.
73. Pertwee RG, Howlett AC, Abood ME, et al. International union of basic and clin-ical pharmacology. Cannabinoid receptors and their ligands. Beyond CB1 and CB2. Pharmacol Rev 2010;62:588–631.
74. Cohen J, Morrison S, Greenberg J, et al. Clinical presentation of intoxication due to synthetic cannabinoids. Pediatrics 2012;4:e1064–7.
75. Lapoint J, James LP, Moran CL, et al. Severe toxicity following synthetic canna-binoid ingestion. Clin Toxicol 2011;49:760–4.

76. Simmons JR, Skinner CG, Williams J, et al. Intoxication from smoking "spice". Ann Emerg Med 2011;57:187–8.
77. Simmons J, Cookman L, Kang C, et al. Three cases of "spice" exposure. Clin Toxicol 2011;49:431–3.
78. Schneir AB, Baumbacher T. Convulsions associated with the use of a synthetic cannabinoid product. J Med Toxicol 2012;8:62–4.
79. Harris CR, Brown A. Synthetic cannabinoid intoxication: a case series and review. J Emerg Med 2013;44:360–6.
80. Benford DM, Caplan JP. Psychiatric sequelae of spice, K2, and synthetic cannabinoid receptor agonists. Psychosomatics 2011;52:295.
81. Zimmermann US, Winkelmann PR, Pilhatsch M, et al. Withdrawal phenomena and dependence syndrome after the consumption of "spice gold". Dtsch Arztebl Int 2009;27:464–7.
82. US Department of Justice. Drug alert watch: increasing use of abuse of bath salts. Available at: www.justice.gov/ndic/pubs43/43474/sw0007p.pdf. Accessed March 7, 2013.
83. Prosser JM, Nelson LS. The toxicology of bath salts: a review of synthetic cathinones. J Med Toxicol 2012;8:33–42.
84. Al-Hebshi NN, Skaug N. Khat (*Catha edulis*)-an updated review. Addict Biol 2005;10:299–307.
85. Winstock A, Mitcheson L, Marsden J. Mephedrone: use, subjective effects and health risk. Addiction 2011;106:1991–6.
86. US Department of Justice Drug Enforcement Administration. Notice of intent-scheduled of controlled substances: temporary placement of three synthetic cathinones into schedule. Micr Bull 2011;44:57–65.
87. Gibbons S, Zloh M. Analysis of the "legal high" mephedrone. Bioorg Med Chem Lett 2010;20(14):4135–9.
88. US Department of Justice DEA. Request for information on synthetic cathinones. Micr Bull 2011. Contract No 4.
89. Centers for Disease Control and Prevention. Emergency department visits after use of a drug sold as "bath salts"-Michigan. MMWR Morb Mortal Wkly Rep 2011;60:624–7.
90. Fass JA, Fass AD, Garcia AS. Synthetic cathinone (bath salts): legal status and patterns of abuse. Ann Pharmacother 2012;46:436–41.
91. Russo R, Marks N, Morris K, et al. Life-threatening necrotizing fasciitis due to "bath salts". Orthopedics 2012;16:e124–7.
92. Torrence H, Cooper G. The detection of mephedrone (4-methylmethcathinone) in 4 fatalities in Scotland. Forensic Sci Int 2010;202:e62–3.
93. Olives TD, Orozco BS, Stellpflug SJ. Bath salt: the ivory wave of trouble. West J Emerg Med 2012;13:58–62.
94. Wolk BJ, Ganetsky M, Babu KM. Toxicity of energy drinks. Curr Opin Pediatr 2012;24:243–51.
95. O'Brien MC, McCoy TP, Rhodes SD, et al. Caffeinated cocktails: energy drink consumption, high-risk drinking, and alcohol-related consequences among college students. Acad Emerg Med 2008;15:453–60.
96. Seifert SM, Schaechter JL, Hershorin ER, et al. Health effects of energy drinks on children, adolescents, and young adults. Pediatrics 2011;127:511–28.
97. Howland J, Rohsenow DJ. Risk of energy drinks mixed with alcohol. JAMA 2013;309:245–6.
98. Reissig CJ, Strain EC, Griffiths RR. Caffeinated energy drinks: a growing problem. Drug Alcohol Depend 2009;99:1–10.

99. Babu KM, Church RJ, Lewander W. Energy drinks: the new eye-opener for adolescents. Clin Pediatr Emerg Med 2008;9:35–42.
100. Holgren P, Norden-Pettersson L, Ahlner J. Caffeine fatalities: four case reports. Forensic Sci Int 2004;139:71–3.
101. Berger AJ, Alford K. Cardiac arrest in a young man following excess consumption of caffeinated "energy drinks". Med J Aust 2009;190:41–3.
102. Sepkowitz KA. Energy drinks and caffeine-related adverse effects. JAMA 2013; 309:243–4.
103. Rowe C, Verjee Z, Koren G. Adolescent dimenhydrinate abuse: resurgence of an old problem. J Adolesc Health 1997;21(1):47–9.
104. Romanelli F, Smith KM. Dextromethorphan abuse: clinical effects and management. J Am Pharm Assoc (2003) 2009;49(2):e20–5.
105. Ganetsky M, Babu KM, Boyer EW. Serotonin syndrome in dextromethorphan ingestion responsive to propofol therapy. Pediatr Emerg Care 2007;23(11): 829–31.
106. Jumbelic MI. Deaths with transdermal fentanyl patches. Am J Forensic Med Pathol 2010;31(1):18–21.

Updates in Pediatric Gastrointestinal Foreign Bodies

Christian C. Wright, MD*, Forrest T. Closson, MD

KEYWORDS

- Foreign body • Ingestion • Coin • Magnet • Battery • Caustic • Children

KEY POINTS

- Foreign body ingestions are common in children, especially children younger than 5 years.
- Foreign bodies should be evaluated by radiograph so that high-risk foreign bodies are not misdiagnosed.
- Coins are the most commonly retained foreign body in children and may be managed conservatively in otherwise healthy, asymptomatic patients.
- Button batteries, high-powered magnets, sharp objects, and caustic liquids carry the risk of serious clinical complications and should be evaluated and managed urgently.

INTRODUCTION

The first recorded swallowed foreign object occurred in 1692, when the Crown Prince of Brandenburg, Frederick the Great, at the age of 4 years old, swallowed a shoe buckle.[1] Since then, reports of children placing objects into their mouths have continued. Children are naturally curious about the world they live in as well as the many openings of their bodies. When those 2 curiosities collide, foreign bodies often become lodged in a variety of body orifices. Pediatric foreign body ingestion is a common occurrence. Data from the American Association of Poison Control Centers' National Poison Data System (NPDS) show that more than 110,000 ingested foreign bodies were reported in the United States in 2011; of these, more than 85% occurred within the pediatric population.[2] However, exact numbers are difficult to determine because many cases are either unrecognized or are managed at home without the involvement of health care professionals.[3,4] It is estimated that up to 40% of foreign body ingestions in children are not witnessed, and the child may be asymptomatic in many cases. Consequently, the true incidence of pediatric foreign body ingestions is likely to be higher than what is reported by the available data.[5]

Disclosures: None.
Division of Emergency Medicine, Department of Pediatrics, University of Maryland School of Medicine, University of Maryland Children's Hospital, 22 South Greene Street, Baltimore, MD 21201, USA
* Corresponding author.
E-mail address: cwright@peds.umaryland.edu

Pediatr Clin N Am 60 (2013) 1221–1239
http://dx.doi.org/10.1016/j.pcl.2013.06.007   **pediatric.theclinics.com**
0031-3955/13/$ – see front matter © 2013 Elsevier Inc. All rights reserved.

AGE-APPROPRIATE BEHAVIORS

Most foreign body ingestions in children are unintentional. Approximately 98% of swallowed foreign objects are swallowed accidentally.[6] According to NPDS data, the peak age for foreign body ingestion is in the preschool years, and more than 73% of the foreign bodies ingested in 2011 occurred in children younger than 5 years.[2] Other studies performed outside the United States have also confirmed the peak incidence of foreign body ingestion is in children between the ages of 6 months and 6 years, with an equal incidence among boys and girls.[7–12] At this age, children are naturally inquisitive about their environment. As they explore and investigate the world, they often use their hands as well as their mouths. Often, children put the objects that they are investigating into their mouths and the object is swallowed. A young child may be fed the object by an older child or even by a caregiver as a form of child abuse.[6,8,13]

Older children and adolescents are not immune to swallowing foreign objects. They may do so as a result of poor eating habits, such as eating too quickly or chewing food inadequately; risky behaviors, such as using magnets to mimic tongue or lip piercings;[14] transporting objects in their mouths; or as a result of impaired judgment from substance abuse.[6,10,11,15,16] Other groups at risk for foreign object ingestion include children with underlying psychiatric conditions, mental retardation, developmental delay, or autism spectrum disorders, as well as children seeking secondary gain, such as prisoners hoping to gain access to a medical facility and leave a correctional institute.[17,18]

CAUSE

Common objects swallowed in children include coins, magnets, batteries, small toys, pieces of plastic, jewelry, buttons, bones, or pieces of food (**Box 1**).[6,12,19–22] Coins are the most common foreign object that is retained in the esophagus, comprising up to 80% of impacted foreign bodies.[19] In cultures in which fish is a large part of the diet, fish bones are a frequent cause of foreign body ingestion.[12] Although most children who swallow a foreign body are otherwise healthy, some have underlying conditions that may predispose them to having retained swallowed objects. Some of these conditions include impaired swallowing reflex, strictures, rings, dysmotility, achalasia, esophagitis (including eosinophilic esophagitis), a tight Nissen fundoplication operative procedure, or congenital defects of the esophagus requiring surgical repair, including esophageal atresia and trachea-esophageal fistula.[6,23,24] In addition, young children may be particularly vulnerable to retained foreign bodies because of the small diameter of their esophagus compared with older children, adolescents, and adults.[7]

CLINICAL MANIFESTATIONS

In most ingested foreign bodies, the patient is asymptomatic. One retrospective review found that 50% of children with confirmed foreign body ingestions were asymptomatic.[22] When symptoms are present, they are often nonspecific and are based on the foreign body type, location of the obstruction, size of the object, and duration of the impaction. Common signs and symptoms include dysphagia, vomiting, drooling, gagging, coughing, respiratory distress, and food refusal. Other symptoms include fussiness or irritability, blood-tinged sputum, foreign body sensation, or pain of the throat, neck, chest, or abdomen. If the foreign body has been present for an extended period, additional symptoms may include fever, failure to thrive, or recurrent aspiration pneumonia (**Box 2**).[5,6,9,12,19,25–27]

Box 1
Commonly ingested foreign bodies

- Batteries
- Coins
- Magnets
- Toys
- Balls
- Pieces of plastic
- Pins (safety and straight)
- Balloons
- Pen caps
- Buttons
- Pieces of jewelry
- Nails/screws
- Bones (fish and chicken)
- Food bolus
- Dentures
- Drugs

In most children with foreign body ingestion, the physical examination is unremarkable. As with all potential emergencies, airway and breathing should be initially assessed. Abnormal examination findings may include neck swelling or crepitus, suggesting possible esophageal perforation; inspiratory stridor or expiratory wheezing, suggesting possible obstruction; or abdominal tenderness, rebound tenderness, or rigidity, which may indicate possible intestinal or colonic perforation with subsequent peritonitis. In addition, inspection of the nose, ears, or anus may reveal additional foreign objects.[10]

DIAGNOSTIC EVALUATION

Because most children with an esophageal foreign body are initially asymptomatic, a chest radiograph with both frontal and lateral views should be obtained in all cases of suspected foreign object ingestion. In addition, radiographs of the soft tissues of the neck and abdomen should be considered to provide a complete view from the mouth to the anus. Limiting the evaluation to a chest radiograph alone may result in the failure to detect multiple foreign bodies, objects higher than the thoracic inlet, or objects past the pylorus.[12]

Foreign bodies in the gastrointestinal (GI) tract are typically located on radiographic evaluation in 3 areas: the upper esophageal sphincter, the midesophagus, and the lower esophageal sphincter.[5,6,9,12,20,24] The upper esophageal sphincter is the site of the transition from skeletal muscle into the smooth muscle of the esophagus. On chest radiograph, it is located at the thoracic inlet and can be identified as the area between the clavicles. It is the most common area where foreign bodies become impacted in the esophagus; up to 75% of impacted esophageal foreign bodies are found in this area. The midesophagus is where the aortic arch crosses over the

---

Box 2
Symptoms of ingested foreign bodies

Acute ingestion

- Gagging
- Drooling
- Coughing
- Vomiting
- Blood in saliva or vomit
- Food refusal
- Foreign body sensation
- Pain (neck, throat, chest, or abdomen)
- Respiratory distress
- Stridor
- Wheezing
- Fussiness or irritability

Chronic ingestion

- Fever
- Food refusal
- Weight loss
- Failure to thrive
- Vomiting
- Blood in saliva or vomit
- Blood in stool
- Chronic cough
- Persistent pain (neck, throat, chest, or abdomen)
- Recurrent pneumonia
- Respiratory distress
- Fussiness

---

esophagus and is the site of impaction for 10% to 20% of esophageal foreign bodies. The lower esophageal sphincter is located at the junction between the distal esophagus and the stomach and is the location for up to 20% of impacted esophageal foreign bodies.[6,11,12,28] Other common sites for retained foreign objects include the pylorus, the duodenum, the ileocecal valve, and the rectum. Foreign bodies may present with different symptoms depending on their location in the esophagus. Objects retained at the upper esophageal sphincter typically present with drooling, vomiting, and dysphagia, whereas objects retained at the lower esophageal sphincter present more often with pain.[24]

Approximately two-thirds of ingested foreign objects in children are radiopaque, likely because of the high prevalence of ingested coins.[22,27] Common radiolucent ingestions include food bolus, plastics, or aluminum. In addition, sharp, thin objects, such as pins or needles, may not be easily visualized by radiograph. In cases in which plain films are nondiagnostic but foreign body ingestion remains a concern, computed tomography (CT) can assist in the diagnosis. Although ultrasonography is useful for identifying retained foreign bodies in soft tissue[29,30] or in the vagina, this modality is less useful for detecting foreign bodies in the GI tract, because the object may be obscured by bowel gas. Gastric foreign bodies may be identified by ultrasonography if anechoic fluid is present in the stomach, which allows an acoustic shadow to be seen.[31,32] Studies with oral contrast generally should not be performed because of risk of aspiration; in addition, the presence of contrast makes examination of the esophagus more difficult during endoscopy.[10] There is little to no need for laboratory evaluation in cases of ingested foreign bodies, unless significant complications are suspected or present.

Special Radiographic Considerations

Coin-shaped foreign bodies present important diagnostic challenges. Because coins are the most commonly ingested foreign object, it is common to interpret any round radiopaque foreign object as a coin. However, misidentifying a button battery as a coin can have serious clinical consequences.[33] Twenty-millimeter batteries are similar in size to pennies (19 mm) and nickels (21 mm). Button batteries are bilaminar and appear to have a double ring or halo on radiographs (**Fig. 1**). They also have a visible step-off on lateral view where the cathode and anode separate, although this finding can be absent in very thin batteries and can be mimicked by multiple coins of different sizes stacked up each other.[34] In contrast, coins in the United States do not have a double-ring appearance on radiograph.

The location of a coin should be confirmed with frontal and lateral radiographs of the chest. Traditional teaching holds that a coin located in the esophagus presents in the coronal plane on chest radiograph (ie, en face on a frontal view) and that a coin located in the trachea presents in the sagittal plane (ie, en face on a lateral view). However, there are numerous reports of esophageal coins presenting in the sagittal plane.[35,36] The investigators of a recent case series of 8 esophageal coins presenting in the sagittal plane argue that because aspiration of coins into the trachea is rare and lodging in the esophagus is more common, a coin oriented in the sagittal plane on chest radiograph is still more likely to be located in the esophagus.[37] Consequently, lateral views of the chest are essential to correctly identify the location of the coin. Lateral views may also reveal the presence of additional objects, such as coins stacked together (**Fig. 2**).

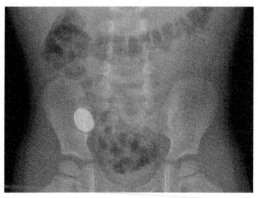

Fig. 1. Button battery. Button batteries may be distinguished from coins by the presence of a halo or double ring. (*Courtesy of* George W. Gross, MD, Baltimore, MD.)

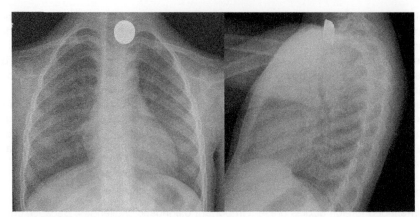

Fig. 2. Stack of coins at upper esophageal sphincter. The presence of multiple coins is revealed on lateral view. (*Courtesy of* George W. Gross, MD, Baltimore, MD.)

Another foreign object ingestion with significant radiographic findings is that of magnets. Classic findings include 2 or more metallic objects located adjacent to each other, sometimes with a small gap between them. Other findings may include distended loops of bowel or air fluid levels, which can represent obstruction, and free air, which can represent perforation. It has been suggested that the use of a compass may help to diagnose potential magnet ingestions when the object is located in the stomach and the type of object is unknown.[17]

Other evaluation may include the use of metal detectors. A systematic review of the use of metal detectors in locating coins concludes that they are accurate and cost-effective.[38] In addition, metal detectors have the benefits of being radiation free and requiring little to no training to use effectively.[39,40] A metal detector can also be helpful in the evaluation of radiolucent ingested foreign objects, such as aluminum soda can flip tops, and they may be helpful in the serial evaluation of known coin ingestions in which the coin has been previously determined to have passed into the stomach. However, metal detectors have several limitations: they may not reliably exclude other metallic objects, such as button batteries or needles,[41] and they are less accurate when children are obese or if they have metal implants, such as thoracotomy wires or clips. An algorithm for the detection of coins by metal detector has been developed by Lee and colleagues.[38] When a metal detector is used, a scan should be performed of the anterior neck, chest, and abdomen as well as posteriorly to the sacrum. Patients with a negative scan or a coin below the xiphisternum may be observed at home. The locations of coins in the neck or chest should be confirmed by chest radiograph.

MANAGEMENT

Once a foreign body ingestion is diagnosed, it must be decided whether or not intervention is necessary and what degree of urgency is indicated. Management decisions are influenced by several factors, including the patient's age and clinical condition, the size and shape of the foreign object, the type of object ingested, the anatomic location where the object has become embedded, and the removal techniques readily available. Most swallowed objects pass through the GI tract without intervention. Reported numbers vary from study to study; however, between 50% and 90% of foreign objects pass spontaneously, 10% to 20% require removal, and less than 1% require surgical intervention.[6,17,18,24,42]

Indications for urgent intervention are summarized in **Box 3**. If a patient has a blunt object such as a coin lodged in the esophagus and remains asymptomatic, the patient may be observed for 12 to 24 hours, because spontaneous passage to the stomach is common. Many objects can be observed if they have passed to the stomach, as they will likely transverse the remainder of the GI tract without difficulty. However, some objects in the stomach should still be removed urgently. These objects include sharp objects, long objects, high-powered magnets, or disk batteries if they cause GI symptoms or if they remain in the stomach for 4 days or more.

When watchful waiting is indicated, the stool can be inspected for passage of these objects, with follow-up radiographs every 2 weeks if it has not passed.[9,43] The time it takes an object to transverse the GI tract varies from person to person, but most ingested foreign bodies pass within 4 to 6 days, although some objects may take up to 4 weeks to pass.[10] Transit time may increase as children get older.[44] Children with a history of pyloromyotomy may have prolonged retention of gastric foreign bodies such as coins and marbles.[45,46] Children with Down syndrome are also at risk of duodenal anomalies that can cause coins to become impacted.[47]

Removal Techniques

Foreign bodies may be removed by several techniques. Flexible endoscopy is used most often because it offers many advantages: the foreign body can be directly visualized and manipulated, and the GI tract can be examined for underlying disease or for complications of the ingestion. A protector hood is placed over the tip of the endoscope to protect the esophagus if the object is sharp. Rigid endoscopy uses a nonflexible device and is useful for sharp objects in the proximal esophagus.

Magill forceps are useful for objects in the oropharynx or upper esophagus. Often, the foreign body may be visualized directly with the use of a laryngoscope and removed with the forceps. This approach has been used successfully with coins in the esophagus.[48]

Bougienage refers to the practice of using a dilator to push objects into the stomach. It has been used successfully to push coins into the stomach,[49,50] although it has the disadvantage that the esophagus cannot be visualized. This technique should be used only if the object is likely to pass through the stomach and through the remainder of the GI tract without complications and when there is a low risk of injury to the esophagus.

In the Foley catheter technique, an uninflated Foley catheter is passed beyond the object, the balloon is filled with radiopaque contrast, and the catheter is slowly drawn

---

Box 3
Indications for urgent intervention

- Signs of airway compromise
- Evidence of esophageal obstruction, such as an inability to manage secretions
- Disk battery in the esophagus
- Sharp or long (>5 cm) objects in the esophagus or stomach
- High-powered magnets
- Signs and symptoms of inflammation or intestinal obstruction, such as fever, abdominal pain, or vomiting
- A foreign body has been impacted in the esophagus for more than 24 hours or for an unknown period

back under fluoroscopy until the object is in the patient's mouth.[51] This technique carries many risks, including aspiration of the foreign body and esophageal perforation, and it does not allow the esophagus to be visualized.

In the penny pincher technique, a grasping endoscopic forceps is inserted though a soft rubber catheter and is then inserted like an orogastric tube under fluoroscopy. After the forceps reaches the object, the prongs of the forceps are deployed and the object is grasped and removed. This technique does not require sedation or placement of an advanced airway.[52]

SPECIFIC TYPES OF FOREIGN BODIES
Coins

Coins are frequently ingested by children and are the most common foreign object to be retained in the esophagus. The most commonly swallowed coins are pennies, followed by quarters, nickels, and dimes.[1] Symptoms of coin ingestion vary depending on where the coin is located. Children with a coin in the proximal esophagus may present with symptoms of airway obstruction, such as cough, stridor, and respiratory distress. Children with a coin in the middle or distal esophagus may present with chest pain, drooling, and dysphagia.[9]

Management of coin ingestion depends on the location of the coin and if the patient is symptomatic. If the coin is located in the stomach, it can be managed expectantly, because it will most likely pass on its own. Parents may inspect the stool for passage of the coin. Repeat abdominal films can be performed at 2 to 3 weeks and again at 4 to 6 weeks if passage has not occurred.[9]

Patients with retained esophageal coins are at risk of numerous complications, including esophageal strictures, perforation, aortoesophageal or tracheoesophageal fistulas, and respiratory distress, which may progress to death.[9] However, many esophageal coins pass spontaneously to the stomach. One retrospective study showed different rates of spontaneous passage from the esophagus to the stomach: 14% of coins in the proximal third of the esophagus, 43% of coins in the middle third, and 67% in the distal third. Seventy-five percent of coins that passed did so within 6 to 10 hours, and the rest passed within 19 hours.[53] Consequently, an asymptomatic child with an esophageal coin and no underlying abnormalities of the esophagus or trachea can be observed for 8 to 16 hours, with a repeat radiograph in 12 to 24 hours.[9]

Symptomatic patients should have the coin removed promptly. Endoscopy has been used successfully for many years, but other options have become available that can be performed more quickly, less expensively, and often without need for sedation. Bougienage has been used successfully to push esophageal coins into the stomach; it can be performed by providers in the emergency department and usually does not require sedation.[49,50] However, this technique should not be used if multiple coins have been ingested, if there is a previous history of foreign body ingestion, or if there is a history of previous esophageal disease or injury, because there is a risk of serious complications, such as esophageal perforation or tracheoesophageal fistula.[54] It has been proposed that in selected cases, water or bread can be given to the child to help push the coin into the stomach.[43]

Magill forceps may also be used to remove coins in the proximal esophagus under direct laryngoscopy.[48] In the penny pincher technique, the coin is grasped directly using a grasping endoscopic forceps, which has been covered with a soft rubber catheter. This procedure is performed under fluoroscopy, which allows the coin to be extracted quickly without needing sedation.[52] Glucagon is not recommended for use in coin ingestions[55] because of risk of vomiting, which could lead to aspiration, esophageal perforation, and death.[56]

Sharp Objects

Children may ingest a wide variety of sharp objects, including chicken and fish bones, pins, razor blades, needles, straightened paper clips, nails, and toothpicks. There is a higher risk of complications after ingestions with sharp objects than with other foreign bodies, including risk of perforation anywhere along the GI tract. Sharp objects in the esophagus can result in esophageal perforation and formation of an aortoesophageal fistula.[57] Perforation is more likely to occur at angulated areas, such as the C loop of the duodenum and ileocecal valve.[58] Retropharyngeal abscess and mediastinitis may also occur.[59]

Radiographs should be obtained to localize and characterize the foreign body. However, many sharp objects are not visible on a radiograph, so endoscopy should still be performed if the radiograph is negative. Sharp objects in the esophagus should be removed immediately. Objects in the oropharynx can often be removed under direct laryngoscopy. Most sharp objects in the stomach or duodenum pass through the GI tract uneventfully; because these objects still carry a high risk of complications, they should be removed endoscopically if possible. During removal, a protector hood on the end of the endoscope or an overtube can be used to minimize tissue injury; retrieval forceps, or a polypectomy snare or retrieval net can also be used. The sharp object should be removed so that the sharp end trails behind during extraction. If the object has passed beyond the duodenum, it should be followed with serial radiographs. If the object does not move downward for 3 days, consider surgical intervention. In addition, watch for signs and symptoms of GI obstruction or bleeding such as abdominal pain, vomiting, fever, hematemesis, or melena.[60]

Long Objects

Long objects such as toothbrushes and spoons are typically ingested by adolescents and adults; these ingestions are usually intentional. They can become impacted in the esophagus, the pylorus, the duodenal C loop, and the ileocecal valve. They have a high risk of complications, such as pressure necrosis, obstruction, and perforation.[6] In an adult-sized patient, objects longer than 6 cm are unlikely to pass through the duodenum successfully and should be removed.[60] In addition, ovoid objects greater than 5 cm by 2 cm are unlikely to pass through the pylorus.[6] In younger children, objects larger than 1 cm by 3 cm should be removed endoscopically, although size criteria for objects that pass though the pylorus do not exist.[58]

Food Bolus

Food impactions in the esophagus are more common in adults but can also occur in children. In the largest retrospective study to date of esophageal food impactions in children,[61] the mean age was 9.9 years and 62% were males. The most commonly impacted food was meat. Food impactions typically present with dysphagia that starts with eating. Children with food impaction have an increased incidence of esophageal pathology. In 1 study,[62] 39% of children with food impaction were diagnosed with eosinophilic esophagitis. Esophageal strictures, esophagitis secondary to gastroesophageal reflux, and motility disorders can also make food impactions more likely.[61,63]

A child with a food impaction who is unable to handle their secretions should undergo immediate endoscopic disimpaction. If they are able to handle their secretions, endoscopic disimpaction should be performed within 12 hours.[6] Many food impactions resolve spontaneously; in 1 study this occurred in 25% of patients.[61]

Oral contrast should not be given when evaluating a food impaction, because there is a risk that the contrast will pool above the impaction and subsequently will be aspirated.[6] Proteolytic enzymes such as papain are not recommended,[64] because they carry the risk of aspiration pneumonitis[65] and esophageal perforation, leading to death.[66] As with coin impaction, glucagon administration is not recommended.[56]

Removal by endoscopy with a protected airway is recommended, because of the risk of aspiration. A food bolus should not be blindly pushed into the stomach as with bougienage. The food bolus may be removed piecemeal, with the remainder pushed into the stomach. Because of the high rate of esophageal disease in these children, the esophagus should be examined and biopsies of the distal and middle esophagus should be performed.[6]

Caustic Liquids

In children, caustic ingestions are typically accidental and involve small volumes of ingested material. In contrast, caustic ingestions in adolescents and adults are usually intentional and may involve larger volumes. Caustic ingestions occur most frequently in children younger than 6 years; most cases are in children between 12 and 48 months of age.[67] Alkali ingestions are more common than acidic ingestions, and household bleach is a common cause of ingestions.[68]

Alkalis and acids have different mechanisms of injury to tissues. Alkalis cause liquefaction necrosis of the mucosa, which can lead to deep penetration and perforation. The degree of tissue damage is related to the alkalinity of the product: alkalis of pH 9 to 11 rarely cause significant injury, but alkalis of pH 11 or higher can cause severe burns.[67] Products that are sold as granules or crystals are even more dangerous because they adhere to areas where the esophagus is most narrow.[68] Unlike acids, alkalis usually have an innocuous taste and as a result are often ingested in larger quantities. Alkalis include detergents, drain cleaners, oven cleaners, and lyes.

In African American populations, hair relaxers are a common alkali ingestion. These patients typically present with drooling and burns to the lips and oropharynx. However, hair relaxer ingestion has not been associated with significant esophageal or gastric injury. The investigators of the largest retrospective study of hair relaxer ingestion to date[69] recommend that these patients should be managed with overnight observation and giving oral feeds. Endoscopy should be performed if symptoms persist.

Acid ingestion results in coagulation necrosis, which can limit the damage done to the esophagus. However, acids quickly move to the stomach, resulting in a higher incidence of gastric injury than with alkalis.[67] Acids have an unpleasant taste and are typically not ingested in large quantities. However, they also have an increased incidence of upper airway injury because the child may gag, choke, or attempt to spit out the acid. Common acids may be found in toilet bowl cleaners, drain cleaners, or pool cleaners.

Ingestions of household bleach manufactured in the United States are usually associated with a benign clinical course with no long-term or short-term sequelae. This situation is because household bleach typically has a concentration between 5% and 10% and pH between 11 and 12, both of which are lower than the threshold for injury to the esophagus. As a result, household bleach typically causes irritation of the pharynx and esophagus rather than burns. These cases usually do not require endoscopy or other interventions unless significant symptoms are present.[70]

Common presenting symptoms after a caustic ingestion include dysphagia, drooling, vomiting, refusing to take anything by mouth, abdominal pain, and substernal chest pain. Signs include lip swelling, tongue erythema, and oral ulcerations or leukoplakia.[68] However, the presence or absence of symptoms or oral lesions does not correlate with the degree of injury to the esophagus.[67] In the week after the initial injury, continued destruction of the esophageal wall continues, which causes an increased risk of perforation. Esophageal strictures develop after between 3 and 8 weeks of an ingestion.[67]

Management of caustic ingestions depends on the history of ingestion and the patient's symptoms. If there is a questionable history of ingestion and the patient is asymptomatic and has no oral burns, the patient may be observed and offered oral fluids. If dysphagia develops, an upper GI series should be performed to identify an esophageal stricture. As noted earlier, household bleach ingestions may be managed conservatively, unless the patient has significant symptoms or burns of the oropharynx. If there is a definite history of ingestion, the patient is symptomatic, or the patient has oral burns, endoscopy should be performed within 24 hours. If the ingestion was intentional, endoscopy should be performed even if the patient is asymptomatic. The caustic material is likely to have been swallowed quickly, and thus, the absence of oral burns does not correlate with esophageal or gastric injury.[67]

Administration of ipecac or diluting or neutralizing agents is contraindicated because vomiting exposes the esophagus to the caustic ingestion a second time, leading to increased injury. Nasogastric tubes should not be placed blindly because of the risk of esophageal perforation.[67] Corticosteroids are not recommended, because they have not been shown to prevent stricture formation and may lead to worse outcomes.[71,72]

Management then proceeds according to the findings on endoscopy. If there is a grade 1 esophageal burn (mucosal erythema), the patient may be fed by mouth and discharged home. An upper GI series should be performed within 3 to 6 weeks or if the patient develops dysphagia. Patients with higher-grade lesions require intravenous nutrition and may require esophageal dilation or stenting.[67]

Batteries

There are up to 15 button battery ingestions per million people in the United States each year. Although the frequency of ingestions is stable, there is an increase in clinically significant outcomes. According to data from the NPDS, the percentage of button battery ingestions with major or fatal outcomes had a 6.7-fold increase from 1985 to 2009. In addition, there has been an increase in ingestions of 20-mm-diameter to 25-mm-diameter cells and lithium button batteries (virtually all large-diameter button cells on the market are lithium cells). This increase in severe outcomes is believed to be caused by the increasing popularity of lithium button batteries.[73] These batteries can be found in a wide variety of products, including remote controls, musical greeting cards, watches, calculators, and other electronics. Children younger than 6 years who ingested a battery most often obtain the battery directly from the product containing it, such as in remote controls; these children may also ingest batteries that are loose or in their packaging.[74]

There are several mechanisms for injury by ingesting a battery.[73]

1. Electrical discharge: electric current flows from the negative pole of the battery through surrounding tissue, causing local hydrolysis of tissues, production of hydroxide at the negative pole, and corrosive tissue injury.
2. Leakage of battery contents: the crimp or seal of the battery may be compromised through the action of stomach acid, leading to leakage of alkaline hydroxides.
3. Pressure necrosis: the battery presses on GI mucosa, causing tissue injury over time.

Although there is a possibility that heavy metals can be released from a battery, heavy metal poisoning after battery ingestion is rare. Button cells containing mercuric oxide have been off the market since 1996, and no ingestions of this type of battery have been reported to the National Battery Ingestion Hotline since 2004.[73] It is not necessary to obtain mercury levels in blood or urine after a battery ingestion has occurred.[75] There is a case report of a 5-year-old boy who swallowed a lithium, button battery and subsequently had a peak serum lithium level of 0.7 mEq/L.[76]

Cylindrical batteries are ingested less frequently than button batteries. They carry a lower risk of caustic injury or major outcomes, and most pass through the GI tract uneventfully. Cylindrical batteries that lodge in the esophagus or that remain in the stomach for more than 48 hours should be removed endoscopically.[60]

Button batteries are at high risk for serious complications and may be difficult to distinguish from coins on radiographs. Lithium batteries pose particular challenges. Twenty-millimeter lithium cells have a higher voltage and capacitance than other button cells and generate more current, leading to more hydroxide production and increased tissue injury. As a result, lithium cells are more likely to be associated with significant clinical outcomes than other types of batteries.[73] Even dead cells can still produce an electrical current.

The National Battery Ingestion Hotline has developed a guideline for the management of ingested button batteries, which is available on their Web site.[75] The hotline is available at 202-625-3333 for help with battery ingestions. The battery can be identified by the imprint code on a matching battery, the product, or its packaging. Anteroposterior and lateral radiographs of the neck, chest, and abdomen should be obtained immediately in children 12 years of age or younger or if the battery diameter is greater than 12 mm or unknown. Esophageal burns can occur as quickly as 2 hours, so immediate radiographs are necessary even if the patient is asymptomatic. An immediate radiograph is not necessary if the patient is older than 12 years, the battery has been reliably identified as being 12 mm or smaller, the patient is asymptomatic, only 1 battery was ingested, there was no coingestion of a magnet, and there is no previous history of esophageal disease, if the caregiver is reliable and is able to promptly seek evaluation and treatment in case the patient becomes symptomatic.

Button batteries in the esophagus should be removed immediately. Endoscopic removal is recommended because it allows tissue injury to be visualized. Other techniques such as removal with a Foley catheter or with a magnet attached to an orogastric tube are not recommended, because they do not allow evaluation of the esophageal mucosa. In addition, these techniques carry the risk of the battery becoming lodged in the esophagus and esophageal perforation.

If the button battery has already passed beyond the esophagus and the patient is asymptomatic, the patient can be observed at home. Stools can be checked to verify that the battery has passed; repeat radiographs can be obtained in 10 to 14 days if the battery has not yet passed. The battery should be removed from the stomach or beyond if a magnet was also ingested, the patient develops GI symptoms, or if a child younger than 6 years ingests a battery 15 mm or larger and it remains in the stomach for 4 days or more.[75] Necrosis of gastric mucosa may be seen within 4 hours of battery ingestion[77]; consequently, batteries in the stomach should still be monitored carefully.

After removal of a button battery, the child should be observed for complications. These complications include tracheoesophageal fistulas, other perforations of the esophagus, esophageal strictures or stenosis, vocal cord paralysis caused by paralysis of the recurrent laryngeal nerve, mediastinitis, respiratory or cardiac arrest, pneumothorax, pneumoperitoneum, tracheal stenosis or tracheomalacia, aspiration pneumonia, empyema, lung abscess, and spondylodiscitis.[73] The most common cause of death after button battery ingestion is aortoesophageal fistula, which may occur up to 27 days after removal.[75] Most fatal cases occur after the battery has been removed, so close observation is warranted. In a retrospective study of 10 fatal cases of hemorrhage after battery ingestion,[78] 70% had mild bleeding before the onset of bleeding leading to exsanguinations. These sentinel bleeds may provide early warning of serious complications in a patient with a history of battery ingestion. Esophageal strictures may present weeks to months after an ingestion. Risk factors for worse clinical outcomes are found in **Box 4**.[74]

Magnets

The first report of bowel perforation caused by the ingestion of multiple magnets was made in 1995.[79] Since that time, magnet ingestion has been increasingly recognized as a serious cause of morbidity and mortality in children. This finding is especially true because small, high-powered magnets are found in many products. These high-powered magnets, also known as rare earth magnets, are typically made of iron, boron, and neodymium and are 5 to 10 times more powerful than traditional magnets. They can be found in desk toys marketed to adults, magnetic construction sets, magnetic jewelry, and electronics. The US Consumer Product Safety Commission has issued multiple warnings of the dangers of high-powered magnets.[80] The maker of one of the most popular of these desk toys (Buckyballs) has since stopped production,[81] but similar toys are still available at many retailers.

It has been reported that in more than 50% of magnet ingestions the patient has ingested between 2 and 6 magnets.[17] Ingestion of multiple magnets is particularly dangerous, because they can attract each other across bowel walls. This situation leads to pressure necrosis, ulceration, and bowel perforation and fistula formation. Magnets can also cause bowel obstruction, which may lead to volvulus.[82] Peritonitis, pneumoperitoneum, sepsis, and death may follow. Ulceration and indentation of the mucosa may occur in as few as 8 hours.[16] After ingesting multiple magnets, a child may have coughing, gagging, or drooling. Subsequent symptoms may be nonspecific, such as vomiting and diarrhea. Unless many magnets were swallowed, these symptoms may be mild until the patient develops symptoms of bowel obstruction, such as abdominal pain and distension.

Because of the increased risks and ubiquity of these magnets, Hussain and colleagues[16] have developed a new algorithm for management of magnet ingestions. The ingestion should be confirmed by radiograph. Multiple views are necessary to determine whether multiple magnets are involved, because 2 magnets that are stuck

---

Box 4
Risk factors for worse outcomes after button battery ingestion

- Ingestion of a button battery 20 mm or greater
- Age less than 4 years
- Ingestion of more than 1 battery
- Unwitnessed ingestion or unknown time of ingestion
- Misdiagnosis at initial presentation
- Delayed removal of the battery

together across bowel walls may appear to be only a single magnet on a single-view radiograph.[83] A single magnet may be managed conservatively. If the magnet is in the stomach or esophagus, removal should be considered if the patient is at risk for additional ingestions. The magnet should be followed with serial radiographs. Parents should be instructed to remove any magnetic objects from the child's environment, including buckles or buttons on clothing. Laxative solutions such as PEG 3350 can be used to help the magnets pass.

If multiple magnets are noted in the stomach or esophagus, they should be removed promptly by endoscopy. If the ingestion was greater than 12 hours before removal, a pediatric surgeon should be involved as well. If the magnets have moved beyond the stomach and the patient is symptomatic, they should be removed by a pediatric surgeon. If the patient is asymptomatic and there is no sign of obstruction or perforation on radiograph, the magnets should be removed by enteroscopy or colonoscopy. Alternatively, the magnets may be followed with serial radiographs, but symptoms of obstruction and perforation may be subtle. If the magnets do not progress or if the patient becomes symptomatic, the magnets should be removed immediately.[16] Magnet detectors cannot reliably identify magnets because high-powered magnets may be small.[14]

COMPLICATIONS

Of the more than 100,000 foreign bodies ingested each year, approximately 1500 of the patients who ingest them die. It has been previously reported that 80% to 90% of ingested foreign objects pass spontaneously through the GI tract and less than 1% cause severe complications requiring surgical intervention. However, all swallowed foreign bodies should be considered as potential medical emergencies, because of the risk of aspiration and subsequent airway obstruction. Common foreign bodies with a high risk for airway obstruction include balloons, pieces of soft deformable plastic, and food boluses (either cut into large pieces or food which has been poorly chewed).[21] Most foreign bodies pass through the body without causing the patient any discomfort and do not produce any symptoms; however, in some children, significant complications occur. Potential complications from swallowed foreign bodies include airway obstruction, tracheal edema, stenosis, erosion or perforation, abscess formation, bowel obstruction or perforation, mediastinitis, pneumothorax, severe hemorrhage, aortoesophageal fistula, and migration into adjacent structures (Box 5).[19,21,27,42,78,84,85]

Predicting which children with ingested foreign bodies are at risk for complications has been a goal of many of the reports pertaining to ingested foreign objects. The Argentinian foreign body study[19] found that the delayed onset of symptoms (presentation more than 24 hours after ingestion) is associated with an increased risk of complications. Other studies have confirmed that delayed presentation is a significant risk factor and have also identified other potential risk factors for complications after foreign body ingestion, including: objects larger than 3 cm, sharp objects, impaction of the foreign body at the cricopharyngeus or upper esophagus, or a visible foreign body on radiographic examination.[18,27,84]

As discussed earlier, certain foreign bodies, such as magnets and button batteries, carry a high risk of severe complications. Evaluation of these objects is made more difficult because they can be difficult to assess accurately on radiographs. It has been recommended that to prevent morbidity and mortality, in cases of unwitnessed ingestions, coinlike foreign objects should all be presumed to be button batteries until proved otherwise.[86]

Box 5
Potential complications of foreign body ingestion

Esophageal

- Ulceration
- Necrosis
- Arterioesophageal fistula
- Tracheoesophageal fistula
- Esophageal rupture
- Hemorrhage
- Mediastinitis
- Stricture

GI

- Ulceration
- Necrosis
- Bowel obstruction
- Bowel perforation
- Gastric outlet obstruction

SUMMARY

Although most ingested foreign bodies in children pass spontaneously, certain foreign bodies can be harmful. In particular, button batteries, magnets, caustic liquids, and sharp objects pose a significant risk for complications and should have emergent evaluation and removal. Lower-risk foreign bodies, such as coins that have passed into the stomach, may be managed conservatively.

REFERENCES

1. Denney W, Ahmad N, Dillard B, et al. Children will eat the strangest things: a 10-year retrospective analysis of foreign body and caustic ingestions from a single academic center. Pediatr Emerg Care 2012;28(8):731–4.
2. Bronstein AC, Spyker DA, Cantilena LR Jr, et al. 2011 annual report of the American Association of Poison Control Centers' National Poison Data System (NPDS): 29th annual report. Clin Toxicol (Phila) 2012;50(10):911–1164.
3. Paul RI, Christoffel KK, Binns HJ, et al. Foreign body ingestions in children: risk of complication varies with site of initial health care contact. Pediatrics 1993; 91(1):121–7.
4. Conners GP, Chamberlain JM, Weiner PR. Pediatric coin ingestion: a home-based survey. Am J Emerg Med 1995;13(6):638–40.
5. Uyemura MC. Foreign body ingestion in children. Am Fam Physician 2005;72(2): 287–91.
6. Kay M, Wyllie R. Pediatric foreign bodies and their management. Curr Gastroenterol Rep 2005;7(3):212–8.
7. McNeill MB, Sperry SL, Crockett SD, et al. Epidemiology and management of oesophageal coin impaction in children. Dig Liver Dis 2012;44(6):482–6.

8. Timmers M, Snoek KG, Gregori D, et al. Foreign bodies in a pediatric emergency department in South Africa. Pediatr Emerg Care 2012;28(12):1348–52.
9. Waltzman ML. Management of esophageal coins. Curr Opin Pediatr 2006;18(5): 571–4.
10. Eisen GM, Baron TH, Dominitz JA, et al. Guideline for the management of ingested foreign bodies. Gastrointest Endosc 2002;55(7):802.
11. Rempe B, Iskyan K, Aloi M. An evidence-based review of pediatric retained foreign bodies. Pediatr Emerg Med Pract 2009;6(12):1–20.
12. Hesham A-Kader H. Foreign body ingestion: children like to put objects in their mouth. World J Pediatr 2010;6(4):301–10.
13. Wadhera R, Kalra V, Gulati SP, et al. Child abuse: multiple foreign bodies in gastrointestinal tract. Int J Pediatr Otorhinolaryngol 2013;77(2):287–9.
14. McCormick S, Brennan P, Yassa J, et al. Children and mini-magnets: an almost fatal attraction. Emerg Med J 2002;19(1):71–3.
15. Chandra S, Hiremath G, Kim S, et al. Magnet ingestion in children and teen-agers: an emerging health concern for pediatricians and pediatric subspecial-ists. J Pediatr Gastroenterol Nutr 2012;54(6):828.
16. Hussain SZ, Bousvaros A, Gilger M, et al. Management of ingested magnets in children. J Pediatr Gastroenterol Nutr 2012;55(3):239–42.
17. Liu S, Li J, Lv Y. Gastrointestinal damage caused by swallowing multiple mag-nets. Front Med 2012;6(3):280–7.
18. Sung SH, Jeon SW, Son HS, et al. Factors predictive of risk for complications in patients with oesophageal foreign bodies. Dig Liver Dis 2011;43(8):632–5.
19. Chinski A, Foltran F, Gregori D, et al. Foreign bodies in the oesophagus: the experience of the Buenos Aires Paediatric ORL Clinic. Int J Pediatr 2010; 2010:1–6.
20. Goins JL, Evans AK. Retrieval of a penny from the pediatric esophagus: a cost analysis. Int J Pediatr Otorhinolaryngol 2011;75(12):1553–7.
21. Heim SW, Maughan KL. Foreign bodies in the ear, nose, and throat. Am Fam Physician 2007;76(8):1185–9.
22. Arana A, Hauser B, Hachimi-Idrissi S, et al. Management of ingested foreign bodies in childhood and review of the literature. Eur J Pediatr 2001;160(8): 468–72.
23. Diniz LO, Towbin AJ. Causes of esophageal food bolus impaction in the pediat-ric population. Dig Dis Sci 2012;57(3):690–3.
24. Rybojad B, Niedzielska G, Niedzielski A, et al. Esophageal foreign bodies in pe-diatric patients: a thirteen-year retrospective study. ScientificWorldJournal 2012; 2012:102642.
25. Louie MC, Bradin S. Foreign body ingestion and aspiration. Pediatr Rev 2009; 30(8):295–301.
26. Little DC, Shah SR, St Peter SD, et al. Esophageal foreign bodies in the pediatric population: our first 500 cases. J Pediatr Surg 2006;41(5):914–8.
27. Digoy GP. Diagnosis and management of upper aerodigestive tract foreign bodies. Otolaryngol Clin North Am 2008;41(3):485–96.
28. Donnelly L, Frush D, Bisset G. The multiple presentations of foreign bodies in children. Am J Roentgenol 1998;170(2):471–7.
29. Teng M, Doniger SJ. Subungual wooden splinter visualized with bedside sonog-raphy. Pediatr Emerg Care 2012;28(4):392–4.
30. Friedman DI, Forti RJ, Wall SP, et al. The utility of bedside ultrasound and patient perception in detecting soft tissue foreign bodies in children. Pediatr Emerg Care 2005;21(8):487–92.

31. Spina P, Minniti S, Bragheri R. Usefulness of ultrasonography in gastric foreign body retention. Pediatr Radiol 2000;30(12):840–1.
32. Moammar H, Al-Edreesi M, Abdi R. Sonographic diagnosis of gastric-outlet foreign body: case report and review of literature. J Family Community Med 2009;16(1):33–6.
33. Bernstein JM, Burrows SA, Saunders MW. Lodged oesophageal button battery masquerading as a coin: an unusual cause of bilateral vocal cord paralysis. Emerg Med J 2007;24(3):e15.
34. McLarty JD, Krishnan M, Rowe MR. Disk battery aspiration in a young child: a scarcely reported phenomenon. Arch Otolaryngol Head Neck Surg 2012; 138(7):680–2.
35. Conners GP, Hadley JA. Esophageal coin with an unusual radiographic appearance. Pediatr Emerg Care 2005;21(10):667–9.
36. Raney LH, Losek JD. Child with esophageal coin and atypical radiograph. J Emerg Med 2008;34(1):63–6.
37. Schlesinger AE, Crowe JE. Sagittal orientation of ingested coins in the esophagus in children. AJR Am J Roentgenol 2011;196(3):670–2.
38. Lee JB, Ahmad S, Gale CP. Detection of coins ingested by children using a handheld metal detector: a systematic review. Emerg Med J 2005;22(12): 839–44.
39. Seikel K, Primm PA, Elizondo BJ, et al. Handheld metal detector localization of ingested metallic foreign bodies: accurate in any hands? Arch Pediatr Adolesc Med 1999;153(8):853–7.
40. Bassett KE, Schunk JE, Logan L. Localizing ingested coins with a metal detector. Am J Emerg Med 1999;17(4):338–41.
41. Schalamon J, Haxhija EQ, Ainoedhofer H, et al. The use of a hand-held metal detector for localisation of ingested metallic foreign bodies–a critical investigation. Eur J Pediatr 2004;163(4–5):257–9.
42. Wildhaber BE, Le Coultre C, Genin B. Ingestion of magnets: innocent in solitude, harmful in groups. J Pediatr Surg 2005;40(10):e33–5.
43. Conners GP. Esophageal coin ingestion: going low tech. Ann Emerg Med 2008; 51(4):373–4.
44. Macgregor D, Ferguson J. Foreign body ingestion in children: an audit of transit time. J Accid Emerg Med 1998;15(6):371–3.
45. Mandell GA, Rosenberg HK, Schnaufer L. Prolonged retention of foreign bodies in the stomach. Pediatrics 1977;60(4):460–2.
46. Stringer MD, Kiely EM, Drake DP. Gastric retention of swallowed coins after pyloromyotomy. Br J Clin Pract 1991;45(1):66–7.
47. Stanley P, Law BS, Young LW. Down's syndrome, duodenal stenosis/annular pancreas, and a stack of coins. Am J Dis Child 1988;142(4):459–60.
48. Cetinkursun S, Sayan A, Demirbag S, et al. Safe removal of upper esophageal coins by using Magill forceps: two centers' experience. Clin Pediatr (Phila) 2006;45(1):71–3.
49. Arms JL, Mackenberg-Mohn MD, Bowen MV, et al. Safety and efficacy of a protocol using bougienage or endoscopy for the management of coins acutely lodged in the esophagus: a large case series. Ann Emerg Med 2008;51(4): 367–72.
50. Dahshan AH, Kevin Donovan G. Bougienage versus endoscopy for esophageal coin removal in children. J Clin Gastroenterol 2007;41(5):454–6.
51. Morrow SE, Bickler SW, Kennedy AP, et al. Balloon extraction of esophageal foreign bodies in children. J Pediatr Surg 1998;33(2):266–70.

52. Gauderer MW, DeCou JM, Abrams RS, et al. The 'penny pincher': a new technique for fast and safe removal of esophageal coins. J Pediatr Surg 2000; 35(2):276–8.

53. Waltzman ML, Baskin M, Wypij D, et al. A randomized clinical trial of the management of esophageal coins in children. Pediatrics 2005;116(3):614–9.

54. Jona JZ, Glicklich M, Cohen RD. The contraindications for blind esophageal bouginage for coin ingestion in children. J Pediatr Surg 1988;23(4):328–30.

55. Mehta D, Attia M, Quintana E, et al. Glucagon use for esophageal coin dislodgment in children: a prospective, double-blind, placebo-controlled trial. Acad Emerg Med 2001;8(2):200–3.

56. Arora S, Galich P. Myth: glucagon is an effective first-line therapy for esophageal foreign body impaction. CJEM 2009;11(2):169–71.

57. Zhang X, Liu J, Li J, et al. Diagnosis and treatment of 32 cases with aortoesophageal fistula due to esophageal foreign body. Laryngoscope 2011;121(2): 267–72.

58. Wyllie R. Foreign bodies in the gastrointestinal tract. Curr Opin Pediatr 2006; 18(5):563–4.

59. Allotey J, Duncan H, Williams H. Mediastinitis and retropharyngeal abscess following delayed diagnosis of glass ingestion. Emerg Med J 2006;23(2):e12.

60. ASGE Standards of Practice Committee, Ikenberry SO, Jue TL, et al. Management of ingested foreign bodies and food impactions. Gastrointest Endosc 2011;73(6):1085–91.

61. Hurtado CW, Furuta GT, Kramer RE. Etiology of esophageal food impactions in children. J Pediatr Gastroenterol Nutr 2011;52(1):43–6.

62. El-Matary W, El-Hakim H, Popel J. Eosinophilic esophagitis in children needing emergency endoscopy for foreign body and food bolus impaction. Pediatr Emerg Care 2012;28(7):611–3.

63. Lao J, Bostwick HE, Berezin S, et al. Esophageal food impaction in children. Pediatr Emerg Care 2003;19(6):402–7.

64. Lee J, Anderson R. Best evidence topic report. Proteolytic enzymes for oesophageal meat impaction. Emerg Med J 2005;22(2):122–3.

65. Maini S, Rudralingam M, Zeitoun H, et al. Aspiration pneumonitis following papain enzyme treatment for oesophageal meat impaction. J Laryngol Otol 2001;115(7):585–6.

66. Cavo JW Jr, Koops HJ, Gryboski RA. Use of enzymes for meat impactions in the esophagus. Laryngoscope 1977;87(4 Pt 1):630–4.

67. Kay M, Wyllie R. Caustic ingestions in children. Curr Opin Pediatr 2009;21(5): 651–4.

68. Riffat F, Cheng A. Pediatric caustic ingestion: 50 consecutive cases and a review of the literature. Dis Esophagus 2009;22(1):89–94.

69. Aronow SP, Aronow HD, Blanchard T, et al. Hair relaxers: a benign caustic ingestion? J Pediatr Gastroenterol Nutr 2003;36(1):120–5.

70. Harley EH, Collins MD. Liquid household bleach ingestion in children: a retrospective review. Laryngoscope 1997;107(1):122–5.

71. Pelclova D, Navratil T. Do corticosteroids prevent oesophageal stricture after corrosive ingestion? Toxicol Rev 2005;24(2):125–9.

72. Fulton JA, Hoffman RS. Steroids in second degree caustic burns of the esophagus: a systematic pooled analysis of fifty years of human data: 1956-2006. Clin Toxicol (Phila) 2007;45(4):402–8.

73. Litovitz T, Whitaker N, Clark L, et al. Emerging battery-ingestion hazard: clinical implications. Pediatrics 2010;125(6):1168–77.

74. Litovitz T, Whitaker N, Clark L. Preventing battery ingestions: an analysis of 8648 cases. Pediatrics 2010;125(6):1178–83.
75. National Battery Ingestion Hotline. NBIH button battery ingestion triage and treatment guideline. 2011. Available at: http://www.poison.org/battery/guideline.asp. Accessed April 3, 2013.
76. Mallon PT, White JS, Thompson RL. Systemic absorption of lithium following ingestion of a lithium button battery. Hum Exp Toxicol 2004;23(4):193–5.
77. Takagaki K, Perito ER, Jose FA, et al. Gastric mucosal damage from ingestion of 3 button cell batteries. J Pediatr Gastroenterol Nutr 2011;53(2):222–3.
78. Brumbaugh DE, Colson SB, Sandoval JA, et al. Management of button battery-induced hemorrhage in children. J Pediatr Gastroenterol Nutr 2011;52(5):585–9.
79. Honzumi M, Shigemori C, Ito H, et al. An intestinal fistula in a 3-year-old child caused by the ingestion of magnets: report of a case. Surg Today 1995;25(6):552–3.
80. US Consumer Product Safety Commission. Magnets information center. 2013. Magnets Information Center Web site. Available at: http://www.cpsc.gov/en/Safety-Education/Safety-Education-Centers/Magnets/. Accessed April 27, 2013.
81. Martin A. Maker of Buckyball says it will stop selling them. New York Times 2012; 2012:B3.
82. Hernandez Anselmi E, Gutierrez San Roman C, Barrios Fontoba JE, et al. Intestinal perforation caused by magnetic toys. J Pediatr Surg 2007;42(3):E13–6.
83. Butterworth J, Feltis B. Toy magnet ingestion in children: revising the algorithm. J Pediatr Surg 2007;42(12):e3–5.
84. Lai A, Chow T, Lee D, et al. Risk factors predicting the development of complications after foreign body ingestion. Br J Surg 2003;90(12):1531–5.
85. Brown JC, Murray KF, Javid PJ. Hidden attraction: a menacing meal of magnets and batteries. J Emerg Med 2012;43(2):266–9.
86. Soccorso G, Grossman O, Martinelli M, et al. 20 mm lithium button battery causing an oesophageal perforation in a toddler: lessons in diagnosis and treatment. Arch Dis Child 2012;97(8):746–7.

Injury Prevention
Opportunities in the Emergency Department

Marlene D. Melzer-Lange, MD[a,b,]*, Mark R. Zonfrillo, MD, MSCE[c],
Michael A. Gittelman, MD[d,e]

KEYWORDS

- Injury prevention • Emergency department • Safety center • Community advocacy
- Behavioral change • Anticipatory guidance

KEY POINTS

- Injuries continue to plague children in the United States, causing the greatest morbidity and mortality.
- Previous education about injury risk and strategies for prevention has solely rested on the primary care provider (PCP) during well-child care visits.
- Although some success in changing family behavior has been shown in the primary care setting, the emergency department (ED) may be an additional place to provide injury-prevention interventions.
- PCPs, hospital departments and divisions, and hospital advocacy organizations should work together with their ED to better assist ED staff to provide optimal injury prevention.
- Although everyone needs to play their role in combating pediatric injuries, the ED promises to be a very suitable location to start to address the problem.

INTRODUCTION

Injury is the principal cause of morbidity and mortality in children in the United States. In fact, injuries cause more deaths in children and youth than all diseases combined.[1] Unlike cancer, cardiovascular disease, and other chronic illnesses, injuries disproportionately affect children. It is estimated that more than 9000 children aged 0 to 19 years

Financial Disclosure: The authors have no financial conflicts to disclose.
[a] Emergency Department Trauma Center, Children's Hospital of Wisconsin, 9000 West Wisconsin Avenue, Milwaukee, WI 53226, USA; [b] Section of Emergency Medicine, Department of Pediatrics, Children's Corporate Center, Medical College of Wisconsin, C550, 999 North 92nd Street, Milwaukee, WI 53226, USA; [c] Division of Emergency Medicine, Center for Injury Research and Prevention, Children's Hospital of Philadelphia, Perelman School of Medicine, University of Pennsylvania, 34th and Civic Center Boulevard, Philadelphia, PA 19104, USA; [d] Clinical Pediatrics, University of Cincinnati School of Medicine, 231 Albert Sabin Way, Cincinnati, OH 45229, USA; [e] Division of Emergency Medicine, Comprehensive Children's Injury Center, Cincinnati Children's Hospital Medical Center, 3333 Burnet Avenue, ML #2008, Cincinnati, OH 45229, USA
* Corresponding author. Department of Pediatrics, Children's Corporate Center, Medical College of Wisconsin, C550, 999 North 92nd Street, Milwaukee, WI 53226.
E-mail address: mmelzer@mcw.edu

will die from an injury each year.[2] Unfortunately, deaths are only the tip of the injury problem, as more than 8 million nonfatal injured patients will seek care annually at United States emergency departments (EDs).[2] Injuries requiring any medical attention or resulting in restricted activity affect approximately 20 million children and adolescents, and cost roughly $17 billion annually in medical costs.[3] Injury is the result of any intentional or unintentional damage to the body resulting from some type of external force. Thus, most injuries that may result in catastrophic bodily damage are due to mechanisms of great velocity, or can occur rapidly with minimal exposure.[4] It is necessary to identify the best setting and technique for the prevention of injuries to children because they result in such extensive morbidity and death.

HISTORY OF INJURY PREVENTION

The concept that injuries are a public health problem that can be prevented in the same fashion as disease is recent. Most injury-prevention interventions in the past concentrated solely on attempting to have the subject change behavior. Much of the advice offered to parents encouraged them to "be careful." In the early 1920s and 1930s, most home and traffic safety efforts were primarily in the form of pamphlets and posters attempting to persuade individuals to change their actions. However, these interventions showed little effect, and new ideas to change other external factors besides subject behavior, so that force could be minimized, was sought. This concept was first introduced by Hugh DeHaven, a World War I pilot survivor. He showed that pilots who fell hundreds of feet, despite their individual factors, were more likely to survive if the force was distributed and the impact reduced. Dr John Gordon, an epidemiologist at Harvard in the mid-nineteenth century, studied the distribution and causes of injury in the same way as for classic infectious diseases.[5] He concluded that any effect on the environment, the host, or the agent could minimize the injury suffered by the individual. Dr William Haddon, the "grandfather of injury prevention," agreed with controlling different factors to prevent injury, and further described that these variables could be controlled before the injury event occurs (primary prevention), at the time of the event (secondary prevention), or after the injury takes place (tertiary prevention) to minimize morbidity and mortality. Many injury-prevention experts use Haddon's concepts or matrix to determine which interventions can be used at different times, thus to have the greatest impact on reducing injury (**Table 1**).

As a result of the work of injury-prevention experts such as Gordon and Haddon, many experts today concentrate on the "4 Es" when designing injury-prevention interventions: Education, Engineering/technology, Enforcement/legislation, and Environmental modifications. Although the greatest change in reducing injury has been shown in manufacturing new safety products that address specific concerns (eg, booster seats, changing bicycle handlebars) and legislation to encourage specific safety behaviors (eg, drinking and driving laws), education about potential risks that encourage individuals to actively change their behavior continues to be an important aspect in preventing injuries.

SETTING FOR INJURY-PREVENTION EDUCATION: PRIMARY CARE OFFICE VERSUS THE ED

Typically, the task of educating families and children about injury risks has fallen on the pediatrician/primary care provider (PCP) during well-child visits as anticipatory guidance is discussed. Unlike educational efforts in the form of public service announcements, educational interventions in the office setting have been shown to be effective

Table 1
Sample Haddon matrix for the prevention of bicycle-related injuries

	Host	Agent	Physical Environment	Social Environment
Pre-event	Age Riding skill Gender	Bicycle in need of repair (eg, brakes, tires) Poorly sized bicycle for host Reflectors Bicycle stability factors	Weather Separate from traffic (eg, no bicycle trails, narrow roads, no shoulder)	Funding for bike lanes Affordability of appropriate gear Traffic
Event	Helmet wearing	Type of handlebars on bicycle	Type of surface riding on	Affordability of helmets Helmet laws Attitudes
Post-event	Age Physical condition Ability to call for help		Emergency Medical Services (EMS) system Trauma centers	Support for trauma care Training of EMS personnel

for certain injury problems, such as car-seat use, smoke-detector ownership, and adjusting the temperature of hot water from taps.[6] Unfortunately, according to most of the literature, the benefits of educating families and encouraging behavioral change in the office setting have been small and commonly dissipate over time.[7]

The American Academy of Pediatrics TIPP (The Injury Prevention Program) is one of the best known office-based injury-prevention programs, as it helped to integrate the developmental stages of infants and children with the types of injuries to which they are susceptible. A combination of screening for risk, provider education for the specific injury, and brochures are used to educate the family at the appropriate time during a well-child visit.[8] Success for the TIPP program included improving family knowledge of injury-prevention topics within diverse groups.[9] Barriers have been the dissemination of the program to pediatric trainees and the cost of the program to the practicing physicians or clinics. In general, barriers cited for not providing adequate injury prevention in the primary setting include time, choice of topic on which to counsel, lack of pediatrician education on the topic, and competing priorities for anticipatory guidance.[10]

Innovative primary physicians have moved from efforts at education alone to providing more hands-on assistance or providing safety products along with education to increase effectiveness. Quinlan and colleagues[11] discussed car-seat use with families while he developed systems in which the primary care visit is linked to car-seat checks. In this study, through the use of car-seat checks at the primary care clinic, use of in-car restraint systems increased from 17% among infants to 50% among toddlers and to 88% among children who should have been using a booster seat. In addition, in a subset that underwent evaluation, researchers found that there was a significant positive effect on use of in-car restraint systems at follow-up. Another innovative intervention in the primary care setting allowed families to practice "hands-on" safety practices. In a randomized trial, Powell and colleagues[12] showed increased injury-prevention knowledge among a group of families with children younger than 6 years, by offering home safety education using a "safe home" toolkit in a dermatology clinic waiting room. In these interventions where education was linked with written or hands-on injury-prevention products, greater behavioral change was demonstrated in the primary care settings.

Recently, physicians have proposed that ED staff, not solely PCPs in their office, should educate families about injury prevention during ED visits.[13] ED physicians care for the more seriously injured patients, making them well suited to discuss prevention.[14] Furthermore, families of lower socioeconomic status are at increased risk for being more seriously injured, and it is these patients who disproportionately use urgent care or EDs for their medical management.[15] Adolescents, an extremely high-risk group for deaths caused by injury, also often use the ED as their sole source of care.[16-18] If these higher-risk families and patients are seeking care in the ED, they are likely not receiving the appropriate injury-prevention anticipatory guidance from their PCP. The ED has promise as a venue for injury screening and education to occur because it is located in a medical setting that can often meet the needs of the patient, offer resources when appropriate, and even potentially provide safety product(s) if available.[19]

Several investigators have described that families value and use the injury-prevention education they have received in the ED setting.[20] One example of a successful ED primary prevention educational intervention was completed by Quan and colleagues.[21] In this study, parents received computerized discharge instructions regarding 3 drowning-prevention strategies (wear a life vest, swim in safe areas, and do not drink alcohol while swimming and boating). Ninety-seven percent of parents recalled receiving the safety information and 60% found that the information was "very useful" when contacted 1 to 2 weeks later. In addition, 35% of parents reported considering the purchase of life vests for their children. Of note, there were no differences in how parents perceived the information based on their child's illness severity or other demographics. Another research group examined the time needed to screen for injury-prevention practices and the value of educating a group of patients and families arriving at a pediatric trauma center.[22] Screening took just 2 minutes, the injury-prevention intervention took 9 minutes, and most families remembered the injury-prevention messages 3 months after the intervention. The knowledge that families value injury-prevention interventions, that most EDs have resources to provide injury-prevention messages, and that many at-risk patients present to EDs helps to build the case that the ED is an excellent setting within which to provide educational interventions regarding injury prevention.

MODELS FOR EDUCATION ON BEHAVIORAL CHANGE

In focusing on opportunities for the ED staff to provide injury-prevention education, it is important to consider behavioral-change models that may be applicable to addressing the host (patient) described in the Haddon matrix. Several models and theories have been identified to promote injury prevention that can be applied to preventing injuries and other health risks: (1) Health Belief Model, (2) Social Cognitive Theory and Injury, (3) Stages of Change Model, and (4) Teachable Moment.[23]

Health Belief Model

In the Health Belief Model, Rosenstock and colleagues[24] described how persons' own perceived risk, their perceived severity of the condition, their perceived barriers to adopt the promoted behavior, and their perceived benefits if they adopt the behavior would lead them to change their behaviors around a given condition. The Health Belief Model was originally applied to how people accepted screening for tuberculosis, but has since been applied for injury prevention and other health-improvement opportunities. Using this model in ED injury-prevention work is attractive because ED staff members are likely to screen and discuss with their injured patients how they perceive their risk for injury, and probe the patients' future injury-prevention plans. However, this model may be time consuming, and ED staff would need to have a consistent plan to carry out screening of all patient risks, and to develop future plans for all types of injury prevention following ED care.

Social Cognitive Theory

In Social Cognitive Theory, individuals learn healthy strategies by watching what others do and modeling that behavior.[25] An example used in the media is having celebrities wear seat belts in movies or public service announcements. In the ED setting, this theory can be applied through the use of placards with known public figures practicing injury-prevention behaviors. In particular, the use of sports celebrities who are known to youth may be most successful. Although it may be impractical to have ED staff practice injury-prevention strategies in the ED, many ED staff will promote the use of safety equipment through their own personal testimony that they and their families use such practices.

Stages of Change Model

In the Stages of Change Model, individuals are viewed by their readiness to make changes in their health behavior: Precontemplation, Contemplation, Preparation, Action, and Maintenance.[26] In the ED, staff may be primed to discuss the patient's willingness to make a change. The commonly asked question, "Do you own a bicycle helmet?," is a good example of the Preparation stage in this model, and one that takes little time on the part of ED staff. However, it may be challenging to successfully use this model in the ED, as more time may be necessary to fully assess the patient's full readiness and to provide adequate follow-up.

Teachable Moment

The Teachable Moment construct is examined as an event that prompts a person to adopt risk-reducing behaviors.[27] This theory is one that many ED staff use when they care for injured patients. Education regarding the use of bicycle helmets in the ED when a patient presents after a bicycle crash is one example. This construct is very attractive in the ED setting because the injury may represent a call to action to the patient, family, and the ED provider. How often do ED providers hear families mention that their child is not going to be riding a bicycle without a helmet after a crash? The challenge of using this theory in the ED is the time involved and the fact that, for severe injuries requiring a high level of care, it can be practically difficult to provide such guidance.

Whereas many of these models have been applied to health-behavior change such as smoking or drinking cessation, few have been applied or evaluated in injury prevention and within the ED setting. Each offers an application for clinicians to use as they consider their injury-prevention educational efforts while in the ED.

SUCCESSFUL ED INTERVENTIONS

So, how might behavioral change theory be applied to the pediatric patient seen in the pediatric ED? Using the Teachable Moment model, one may suspect that the visit for an injury may prompt patients and their families to take greater action to prevent future injuries, and providers may be interested in discussing these strategies at the time of the ED visit. One study examining children presenting to the ED after ingestion found that only 25% of families received verbal instruction about poisoning prevention, and that this education was more likely to occur in urban academic EDs rather than in rural or suburban hospitals.[28] Another study using the Teachable Moment theory in the ED was a case-control design among children in minor vehicle crashes. This study actually showed no difference between the injured group and the control group in adopting booster seats following the ED intervention. Most importantly, is that both groups of children, whether injured or not, had improved by almost 50% their ownership and use of booster seats following the ED educational intervention.[29] One limitation noted by the investigators was that the children in the intervention group had such minor injuries that their teachable moment may not have been much different to that of the controls. In examining the teachable moment among assault victims at 2 different urban EDs, Johnson and colleagues[30] noted that youth and parents found their ED visit moderately stressful and that using a Teachable Moment Index may help assess which patients would be most amenable to a violence-prevention intervention.

Some EDs have used computerized kiosks to better screen for risk and to minimize the discussion required by staff while in the ED. The idea behind these kiosks is similar to the notion of the TIPP program used by PCPs; however, by being computerized, tailored printouts about behavioral change can be offered. In one ED, psychologists and ED physicians developed a kiosk in which adolescents responded to a mental health screen to identify youth at risk for suicidal thoughts.[31] Providers could then use the screen to direct resources and care to prevent a potential suicide attempt. Gielen and colleagues[32] conducted a randomized controlled trial of using a kiosk in a pediatric ED. The kiosk tested also allowed for both screening of the risk for injury and the provision of tailored information on injury prevention. The investigators found that low-income families in their study were able to use the kiosk and that those who received injury-prevention information were likely to read and share this information with others. Moreover, the kiosk screening was endorsed by families and did not interfere with patient care. These kiosks offer an opportunity for screening and providing injury-prevention information to families who are waiting for care in the ED, with little need for staff interaction during the educational process.

Similar to work done by Quinlan in the primary care setting, EDs have found that providing education in conjunction with offering safety products entices greater behavioral change by families. Posner and colleagues[33] conducted a randomized home-safety intervention within their ED. In this intervention, parents were provided either with comprehensive home-safety education coupled with free safety equipment or focused, ED-specific discharge instructions on injury prevention. Families who received the more comprehensive education and the free safety equipment improved more in pretesting and posttesting of their injury-prevention knowledge, and were also much more likely to report using the free safety equipment following the ED visit. Another study in which products were provided to families in the ED in conjunction with education was done by Gittelman and colleagues[34] in Cincinnati. In this randomized controlled trial, children of booster-seat age who did not use a booster seat were randomly assigned to 1 of 3 groups: (1) received standard discharge instructions (control); (2) received a 5-minute booster-seat training (education only group); or (3) received a 5-minute booster-seat training and a free booster seat (education and product group). At follow-up, only 1% of the control parents and 9% of the education-only parents purchased and used a booster seat after their pediatric ED visit, whereas 98% of parents in the education and product group reported using the booster seat; 75% of these parents reported using the seat 100% of the time. Providing free or reduced-cost safety equipment with education can promote a greater likelihood that the family will practice optimal injury-prevention strategies after their ED visit.

To provide families with safety equipment in the ED setting as education about injuries is offered, some pediatric EDs have opened safety resource centers, located either in the waiting room of their busy ED or in the lobby of the children's hospital.[19] While families are waiting to be brought to an ED room, this allows a special opportunity to provide safety education and products to families. In some sites, brochures and safety products such as bicycle helmets, cabinet locks, and car safety seats are available at discounted prices, or in some cases free to low-income families. Some centers are staffed by injury-prevention specialists who are available to answer questions and dispense safety products with advice on how to use them. At present, 29 children's hospitals have safety centers somewhere in their institution, with varying hours of operation.[35] Although staffing these safety centers is not without cost, the stores who have a staff person available for busy times of the day are more likely to be successful in dispensing both information and safety products.[36]

Although motivational interviewing techniques can be time consuming for the ED staff, several studies have used this model with some success. Initially, successes using this technique were used to alter behavioral risk factors around smoking, diet, and alcohol use, but newer studies have looked at preventing injuries.[37] The patient-centered interview is conducted at a time when the patient may have reasons to change behaviors, "by helping clients to explore and resolve ambivalence."[38] Johnston and colleagues[39] successfully showed that a brief session of behavior-change counseling offered in the ED changed injury-related risk behaviors and the risk of reinjury with regard to the use of bicycle helmets and seat belts. Although training to perform motivational interviewing demands time and staff interest, many hospitals and EDs have been able to train champions who can then serve in that role when a patient is identified. By investing in motivational interviewing resources, EDs have the opportunity to prevent injuries and decrease future injury costs.[40]

LINKING THE ED TO THE COMMUNITY

Another injury-prevention strategy that EDs may use is to direct children and youth at increased risk for injury to resources within their community. Although many understand that counseling families about injury prevention in the ED is important, targeting youth and families who are higher risk through screening, identification, and referral to intervention may be the most effective injury-prevention strategy. For example, many secondary injury-prevention programs target youth who are intentionally injured through an assault. By providing case-management services, referrals to community-based organizations, youth development services, and family support, these intervention programs, initiated in the ED with crisis intervention, offer a real opportunity to serve youth at increased risk of reinjury. Project UJIMA, a program offered in Milwaukee, provides crisis intervention at the time of the ED visit. Community liaisons, employees of the hospital violence intervention team, come to the ED and address the traumatic event with the patient and family, but then also discuss the feelings of revenge and the deleterious effects of seeking revenge before ED discharge. Even after the ED visit, the same community liaison, who has gained rapport with the family, provides home visitation, school advocacy, mental health services, and youth development in the community.[41] Other such programs refer youth to community resources such as mentoring or counseling.[42,43] When ED staff identifies the community resources available to address specific issues that face youth at risk, there are significant opportunities to provide injury-prevention education and to refer at-risk patients to resources in the community for longer-term follow-up.

PREPARING THE ED FOR INJURY-PREVENTION INTERVENTIONS

In each hospital, there is likely a group of professionals who share a common interest in injury prevention. Convening these stakeholders is important, as resources may be more effectively shared and coordinated. Likely stakeholders include professionals from trauma surgery, continuity, or primary care clinics, emergency medicine, the neonatal intensive care unit, adolescent medicine, child protection, and community services. Having an injury resource group, made up of the many professionals within that institution, permits a coordinated approach throughout the hospital. Through regular meetings, the professionals share best practices, new research, resources, and strategies on injury prevention, and can disseminate consistent messages throughout the hospital, clinics, and community settings linked with that hospital. If there are existing hospital/community programs such as Safe Kids or the Injury Free Coalition for Kids in one's local region, these stakeholders, along with hospital professionals, will likely make efforts more effective.[44]

Understanding the type of injuries, age groups, and neighborhoods most affected is paramount to the ED staff for designing targeted injury-prevention strategies. By tailoring electronic medical records to prompt providers to enter injury circumstances, more details about injuries cared for can be captured. With this information, priorities can be determined and partners identified. This type of ED surveillance can help target high-risk patients or areas for better injury-prevention efforts. For example, one could use a template in the medical record to assess the prevalence of bicycle-helmet usage per community and target communities with the most bicycle-related injuries. Once this information is analyzed, helmets could be distributed in high-risk communities to reduce injury risks.

Once the ED staff has designed strategies to combat local injuries, staff should also plan on how to prepare the ED environment. This approach includes identifying staff champions who can sustain injury-prevention efforts and work with others to successfully educate patients and families. In addition, it is important to take advantage of the time and "real estate" available in the ED to promote injury prevention. Placards and patient information signs in waiting and examination rooms can be used to prompt conversations, and these may be changed seasonally to discuss season-sensitive topics such as bicycle safety or winter safety. Safety centers that provide injury-prevention products either at a discounted rate or complimentary to families, along with education on how to fit and use the product, are a consideration. Brochures, Web sites, and information should be available for augmenting verbal discussions. When available, hospital volunteers or trainees can also be used to further relay injury-prevention messages and resources.

HEALTH SYSTEMS AND HOSPITAL PARTNERS
Injury-Prevention Programs

Hospital-based and community-based injury-prevention programs provide an opportunity for research, education, and advocacy to reduce childhood injury. Intradisciplinary groups can include: health care providers (physicians, advanced providers, nurses); epidemiologists and biostatisticians; engineers; behavioral psychologists; public relations and outreach specialists; and trainees including postgraduate, graduate, and undergraduate. The purpose of an intradisciplinary group is to identify a need and target (either at the local, regional, or national level) and a comprehensive approach to obtain injury reduction. A cyclical "Research-to-Action-to-Impact" Paradigm is one such example, which includes injury surveillance, in-depth research, development and dissemination of interventions, measurement of impact, and resurveillance.[45] Similarly, programs such as local Safe Kids[46] and Injury Free Coalitions[47] have hospital-based and community-based programs that provide education and advocacy for road traffic safety, recreational safety, and home safety. All of these programs provide opportunities for health care providers to participate in injury-prevention activities with various approaches and level of involvement. **Table 2** provides a list of injury-prevention organizations that can help to set up injury-prevention programs at any ED site. Recently, the Children's Hospital Association conducted a survey of unintentional injury-prevention services at children's hospitals.[48] This extensive survey provides an understanding of the injury-prevention infrastructure at children's hospitals nationwide, and provides information useful to ED providers as they collaborate with hospital leaders. This information may also be useful to those ED champions who are developing injury-prevention work in their ED.

Trauma Programs

Trauma centers based in the Unites States are required by the American College of Surgeons Committee to have injury-prevention activities integrated into their programs.[49] Although the breadth and depth of these injury prevention activities are variable,[50] they all provide natural opportunities for education and advocacy to patients and families. In addition, trauma programs are uniquely poised to affect groups that may be at higher risk of injury and reinjury.[51] Many trauma centers also maintain trauma registries, which can assist with injury surveillance and be used to customize injury-prevention efforts within the community.[52]

Table 2 Organizations involved in injury-prevention efforts	
Resource	**Description**
American Academy of Pediatrics (AAP) Council on Injury Poisoning and Prevention www.aap.org/sections/ipp	Member-based organization promoting pediatric safety and injury policy, programs, education, and advocacy
The Centers for Disease Control and Prevention (CDC) National Center for Injury Prevention and Control www.cdc.gov/injury	Federal program to reduce injury, disability, death, and costs associated with injuries outside the workplace
Injury Free Coalition for Kids www.injuryfree.org	Hospital-based injury education and advocacy for local communities
Health Resources and Services Administration Maternal and Child Health mchb.hrsa.gov	Government program focused on health of women, children, and infants
National Network for Hospital Based Violence Intervention Programs nnhvip.org	Collaborative organization to promote violence-prevention research and best practices
Safe Kids www.safekids.org	International organization providing resources for children and families
Society for Advancement of Violence and Injury Research (SAVIR) www.savirweb.org	Member-based organization promoting research and advocacy for injury and violence prevention

Primary Care Setting

The primary care setting has long served as a ubiquitous resource of injury-anticipatory guidance for patients and families, and there is evidence for its success.[53] PCPs' injury-prevention efforts commonly include the provision of age-appropriate and developmentally appropriate safety information, from birth through adolescence.[7] There are many competing health-advice topics for primary care providers to discuss,[54,55] although emerging evidence shows that injury-prevention strategies that are based on behavioral theory are more likely to be successful,[56] and that the use of technology in primary care may help facilitate injury-prevention efforts.[57] To most effectively deliver injury-prevention messages, the content and delivery of injury-anticipatory guidance in the primary care setting should take into account measurable and evidence-based outcome standards.[58]

Newborn Nurseries and Care Units

Injury-prevention–based anticipatory guidance for newborns includes safety information for the home, sleep, and transportation. Many hospitals have policies that prohibit newborns from being discharged to their families until certain tasks are completed, including installing a car seat or reading materials on "shaken baby syndrome." First-time and disadvantaged mothers are at higher risk of unsafe practices, and often need more substantial support and education. Some creative methods to increase knowledge include educational baby books that mothers can read to their children, the content of which includes information about development, safety, and other anticipatory guidance.[59] Regardless of the mode of delivery, injury-prevention messaging for parents of newborns should be provided among other "well-baby" health guidance in a standardized manner. Finally, targeting these high-risk mothers in the newborn nursery and neonatal intensive care unit can help to connect them with greater community resources for further support after discharge.

SUMMARY

Injuries continue to plague children in the United States, causing the greatest morbidity and mortality. Unfortunately, in the past, education about injury risk and strategies for prevention has solely rested on the PCP during well-child care visits. Although some success in changing family behavior has been shown in this setting, the ED may be a more appropriate place to provide injury-prevention interventions. Besides the fact that the injury event or even the ED visit itself may serve as a teachable moment, the ED also has the ability to survey injuries in the community, use the hospital setting to screen patients, and provide products and offer resources to assist families within the ED setting to change their risky behaviors. PCPs, hospital departments and divisions, and hospital advocacy organizations should work together with their ED to better assist ED staff to provide optimal injury-prevention care. Although everyone needs to play their role in combating pediatric injuries, the ED would seem to be a most suitable location to address the problem.

REFERENCES

1. Sleet D, Schieber R, Dellinger A. Childhood injuries. In: Breslow L, editor. The encyclopedia of public health, vol. 1. New York: Macmillan Reference; 2002. p. 184–7.
2. Centers for Disease Control and Prevention (CDC), National Centers for Injury Prevention and Control. National action plan for child injury prevention. Available

at: http://www.cdc.gov/safechild/pdf/National_Action_Plan_for_Child_Injury_ Prevention.pdf. Accessed January 8, 2013.

3. Danseco ER, Miller TR, Spicer RS. Incidence and costs of 1987-1994 childhood injuries: demographic breakdowns. Pediatrics 2000;105(2):E27.

4. National Committee for Injury Prevention and Control (U.S.). Injury prevention: meeting the challenge. New York: Oxford University Press; 1989.

5. Christoffel T, Gallagher SS. Conceptual and historical underpinnings of injury and injury prevention. In: Injury prevention and public health: practical knowledge, skills, and strategies. 2nd edition. Sudbury (MA): Jones Publishers and Bartlett; 2006. p. 25–48.

6. The David and Lucille Packard Foundation. The future of children. Available at: http://futureofchildren.org/futureofchildren/publications/docs/10_01_Exec Summary.pdf. Accessed April 2, 2013.

7. Bass JL, Christoffel KK, Widome M, et al. Childhood injury prevention counseling in primary-care settings—a critical review of the literature. Pediatrics 1993;92(4):544–50.

8. American Academy of Pediatrics. TIPP: a guide to safety counseling in office practice. Elk Grove Village (IL): American Academy of Pediatrics; 1994.

9. Powell EC, Tanz RR, Uyeda A, et al. Injury prevention education using pictorial information. Pediatrics 2000;105(1):e16.

10. Kottke TE, Brekke ML, Solberg LI. Making "time" for preventive services. Mayo Clin Proc 1993;68(8):785–91.

11. Quinlan KP, Holden J, Kresnow M. Providing car seat checks with well-child visits at an urban health center: a pilot study. Inj Prev 2007;13(5):352–4.

12. Powell EC, Malanchinski J, Sheehan KM. A randomized trial of a home safety education intervention using a safe home model. J Trauma 2010;69(4): S233–6.

13. Mace SE, Gerardi MJ, Dietrich AM, et al. Injury prevention and control in children. Ann Emerg Med 2001;38(Suppl 4):405–14.

14. Gittelman MA, Durbin DR. Injury prevention: is the pediatric emergency department the appropriate place? Pediatr Emerg Care 2005;21(7):460–7.

15. Marcin JP, Schembri MS, He JS, et al. A population-based analysis of socioeconomic status and insurance status and their relationship with pediatric trauma hospitalization and mortality rates. Am J Public Health 2003;93(3):461–6.

16. Lehmann CU, Barr J, Kelly PJ. Emergency department utilization by adolescents. J Adolesc Health 1994;15(6):485–90.

17. Melzer-Lange M, Lye PS. Adolescent health care in a pediatric emergency department. Ann Emerg Med 1996;27(5):633–7.

18. Wilson KM, Klein JD. Adolescents who use the emergency department as their usual source of care. Arch Pediatr Adolesc Med 2000;154(4):361–5.

19. Gittelman MA, Pomerantz WJ, Frey LK. Use of a safety resource center in a pediatric emergency department. Pediatr Emerg Care 2009;25(7):429–33.

20. Gittelman MA, Pomerantz WJ, Fitzgerald MR, et al. Injury prevention in the emergency department: a caregiver's perspective. Pediatr Emerg Care 2008;24(8): 524–8.

21. Quan L, Bennett E, Cummings P, et al. Do parents value drowning prevention information at discharge from the emergency department? Ann Emerg Med 2001;37(4):382–5.

22. Ehrlich PF, Drongowski A, Swisher-McClure S, et al. The importance of a preclinical trial: a selected injury intervention program for pediatric trauma centers. J Trauma 2008;65(1):189–95.

23. Trifiletti LB, Gielen AC, Sleet DA, et al. Behavioral and social sciences theories and models: are they used in unintentional injury prevention research? Health Educ Res 2005;20(3):298–307.
24. Rosenstock IM, Strecher VJ, Becker MH. Social-learning theory and the health belief model. Health Educ Q 1988;15(2):175–83.
25. Miller NE, Dollard J, Yale University Institute of Human Relations. Social learning and imitation. New Haven (CT): Yale University Press; 1941.
26. Prochaska JO, Diclemente CC. Stages and processes of self-change of smoking—toward an integrative model of change. J Consult Clin Psychol 1983;51(3): 390–5.
27. McBride CM, Emmons KM, Lipkus IM. Understanding the potential of teachable moments: the case of smoking cessation. Health Educ Res 2003;18(2):156–70.
28. Demorest RA, Posner JC, Osterhoudt KC, et al. Poisoning prevention education during emergency department visits for childhood poisoning. Pediatr Emerg Care 2004;20(5):281–4.
29. Gittelman MA, Pomerantz WJ, Ho M, et al. Is an emergency department encounter for a motor vehicle collision truly a teachable moment? J Trauma Acute Care Surg 2012;73(4 Suppl 3):S258–61.
30. Johnson SB, Bradshaw CP, Wright JL, et al. Characterizing the teachable moment: is an emergency department visit a teachable moment for intervention among assault-injured youth and their parents? Pediatr Emerg Care 2007;23(8): 553–9.
31. Pailler ME, Fein JA. Computerized behavioral health screening in the emergency department. Pediatr Ann 2009;38(3):156–60.
32. Gielen AC, McKenzie LB, McDonald EM, et al. Using a computer kiosk to promote child safety: results of a randomized, controlled trial in an urban pediatric emergency department. Pediatrics 2007;120(2):330–9.
33. Posner JC, Hawkins LA, Garcia-Espana F, et al. A randomized, clinical trial of a home safety intervention based in an emergency department setting. Pediatrics 2004;113(6):1603–8.
34. Gittelman MA, Pomerantz WJ, Laurence S. An emergency department intervention to increase booster seat use for lower socioeconomic families. Acad Emerg Med 2006;13(4):396–400.
35. Edmonds S, Gittelman MA, Hill KS, et al. National study of children's hospital safety centers. Pediatric Academic Societies' Annual Meeting. Washington, DC, May 7th, 2013.
36. Gittelman MA, Pomerantz WJ. Starting a pediatric emergency department safety resource center. Pediatr Ann 2009;38(3):149–55.
37. Dunn C, Deroo L, Rivara FP. The use of brief interventions adapted from motivational interviewing across behavioral domains: a systematic review. Addiction 2001;96(12):1725–42.
38. Rollnick S, Miller WR. What is motivational interviewing? Behav Cogn Psychother 1995;23(4):325–34.
39. Johnston BD, Rivara FP, Droesch RM, et al. Behavior change counseling in the emergency department to reduce injury risk: a randomized, controlled trial. Pediatrics 2002;110(2 Pt 1):267–74.
40. Neighbors CJ, Barnett NP, Rohsenow DJ, et al. Cost-effectiveness of a motivational intervention for alcohol-involved youth in a hospital emergency department. J Stud Alcohol Drugs 2010;71(3):384–94.
41. Marcelle DR, Melzer-Lange MD. Project UJIMA: working together to make things right. WMJ 2001;100(2):22–5.

42. Becker MG, Hall JS, Ursic CM, et al. Caught in the crossfire: the effects of a peer-based intervention program for violently injured youth. J Adolesc Health 2004;34(3):177–83.

43. Cunningham RM, Resko SM, Harrison SR, et al. Screening adolescents in the emergency department for weapon carriage. Acad Emerg Med 2010;17(2): 168–76.

44. Tamburro RF, Shorr RI, Bush AJ, et al. Association between the inception of a SAFE KIDS Coalition and changes in pediatric unintentional injury rates. Inj Prev 2002;8(3):242–5.

45. Children's Hospital of Philadelphia Center for Injury Research and Prevention. Research, action, impact. Available at: http://injury.research.chop.edu/about/ research-approach. Accessed March 30, 2013.

46. Safe Kids Worldwide. Available at: http://www.safekids.org. Accessed March 1, 2013.

47. Pressley JC, Barlow B, Durkin M, et al. A national program for injury prevention in children and adolescents: the injury free coalition for kids. J Urban Health 2005;82(3):389–402.

48. Children's Hospital Association. 2011 Survey of Injury Prevention Services at Children's Hospitals. Available at: http://www.childrenshospitals.net/AM/Template. cfm?Section=Injury_Prevention1&Template=/CM/ContentDisplay.cfm& ContentID=61891. Accessed January 10, 2013.

49. American College of Surgeons. Resources for optimal care. Available at: http:// www.facs.org/trauma/optimalcare.pdf. Accessed January 2, 2013.

50. McDonald EM, MacKenzie EJ, Teitelbaum SD, et al. Injury prevention activities in U.S. trauma centres: are we doing enough? Injury 2007;38(5):538–47.

51. Ameratunga SN. Injury prevention and trauma centres: is it an oxymoron? Injury 2007;38(5):550–1.

52. Zehtabchi S, Nishijima DK, McKay MP, et al. Trauma registries: history, logistics, limitations, and contributions to emergency medicine research. Acad Emerg Med 2011;18(6):637–43.

53. Nelson CS, Wissow LS, Cheng TL. Effectiveness of anticipatory guidance: recent developments. Curr Opin Pediatr 2003;15(6):630–5.

54. Barkin SL, Scheindlin B, Brown C, et al. Anticipatory guidance topics: are more better? Ambul Pediatr 2005;5(6):372–6.

55. Belamarich PF, Gandica R, Stein RE, et al. Drowning in a sea of advice: Pediatricians and American Academy of Pediatrics policy statements. Pediatrics 2006;118(4):E964–78.

56. Gielen AC, Sleet D. Application of behavior-change theories and methods to injury prevention. Epidemiol Rev 2003;25:65–76.

57. Williams J, Nansel TR, Weaver NL, et al. Safe n' sound: an evidence-based tool to prioritize injury messages for pediatric health care. Fam Community Health 2012;35(3):212–24.

58. Schor EL. The future pediatrician: promoting children's health and development. J Pediatr 2007;151(5):S11–6.

59. Reich SM, Bickman L, Saville BR, et al. The effectiveness of baby books for providing pediatric anticipatory guidance to new mothers. Pediatrics 2010; 125(5):997–1002.

Index

Note: Page numbers of article titles are in **boldface** type.

A

Abscess(es)
    peritonsillar, ultrasonography for, 1146–1148
    skin. *See* Skin and soft tissue infections.
Abuse, child, altered mental status in, 1097
Acetaminophen poisoning, 1210
Acid ingestions, 1230–1231
Activated charcoal, for poisoning, 1204
Active distraction, for pain management, 1169
Acute Concussion Evaluation, 1108–1109
Adenovirus, in bronchiolitis, 1021
Advanced Trauma Life Support Guidelines, for cervical spine injury, 1126
Aggression, 1191–1195
Airway management
    in ingested foreign body obstruction, 1234
    in office emergencies, 1155–1157
Alar ligament, avulsion of, 1131
ALARA (As Low As Reasonably Achievable) concept, 1141–1142
Albuterol, for asthma, 1037–1039
Alcohols, poisoning from, 1208
Alkali ingestions, 1230–1231
Altered mental status, **1083–1106**
    persistent, 1096–1099, 1102–1103
    transient, 1085–1096, 1099–1102
    types of, 1083–1084
Alveolar pneumocytes, in bronchiolitis, 1020
American Academy of Pediatrics TIPP (The Injury Prevention Program), 1243
American Association of Poison Control Centers, 1221
Aminophylline, for asthma, 1042
Analgesia. *See* Pain management.
Anterior cord syndrome, 1127
Antibiotics
    for bronchiolitis, 1027
    for skin and soft tissue infections, 1070–1074
Anticholinergic drugs, abuse of, 1214
Antidepressants, for suicidal ideation and attempts, 1189
Anti-inflammatory agents, for bronchiolitis, 1026–1027
Antipsychotics, for aggressive and violent persons, 1193–1195
Antiviral agents, for bronchiolitis, 1027
Anxiety, in procedures, 1166–1168
Anxiolytics, for procedures, 1170–1172
Aortoesophageal fistula, from button battery ingestion, 1233

Pediatr Clin N Am 60 (2013) 1255–1271
http://dx.doi.org/10.1016/S0031-3955(13)00152-1
0031-3955/13/$ – see front matter © 2013 Elsevier Inc. All rights reserved.

pediatric.theclinics.com

Confidentiality, in suicidal situations, 1187
Confusional migraine, 1094–1095
Congestive heart failure, versus bronchiolitis, 1023
Conversion disorder, 1095–1096
Coronary artery anomalies, 1090
Corticosteroids
    for asthma, 1040
    for bronchiolitis, 1026–1027
Cough
    in bronchiolitis, 1021
    in retained foreign body, 1222
C-reactive protein, for fever without source, 1053–1054, 1056
Culture, viral, for bronchiolitis, 1025
Cultures, viral
    for bronchiolitis, 1022
    for fever without source, 1054, 1057

D

Daptomycin, for skin and soft tissue infections, 1073
Debridement, pain management for, 1175–1176
Decolonization, of methicillin-resistant *Staphylococcus aureus,* 1075
Decontamination, gastrointestinal, for poisoning, 1204–1207
DeHaven, Hugh, injury prevention concept of, 1242
Dehydration, altered mental status in, 1098
Dens, fractures of, 1131
Designer drugs, 1211–1214
Developmental disorders, 1195–1197
Dexamethasone, for asthma, 1040
Dextromethorphan abuse, 1214
Diabetic ketoacidosis, altered mental status in, 1098
Digital blocks, 1176–1177
Dimenhydrinate, abuse of, 1214
Diphenhydramine, for aggressive and violent persons, 1194
Disaster preparedness, 1159
Distraction
    for autism spectrum disorders, 1196
    for developmental disorders, 1196
    for pain management, 1169
Documentation, of office emergency response, 1155
Doxycycline, for skin and soft tissue infections, 1073
Drainage, for abscess, 1067–1069
Drooling, in retained foreign body, 1222
Dysphagia
    in caustic ingestions, 1230–1231
    in retained foreign body, 1222
Dysplasia, arrhythmogenic right ventricular, 1092

E

Echocardiography, 1146
Education

United States Postal Service

Statement of Ownership, Management, and Circulation
(All Periodicals Publications Except Requestor Publications)

1. Publication Title	2. Publication Number	3. Filing Date
Pediatric Clinics of North America	4 2 4 - 6 6 0 0	9/14/13

4. Issue Frequency	5. Number of Issues Published Annually	6. Annual Subscription Price
Feb, Apr, Jun, Aug, Oct, Dec	6	$191.00

7. Complete Mailing Address of Known Office of Publication *(Not printer) (Street, city, county, state, and ZIP+4®)*

Elsevier Inc.
360 Park Avenue South
New York, NY 10010-1710

Contact Person
Stephen R. Bushing
Telephone *(Include area code)*
215-239-3688

8. Complete Mailing Address of Headquarters or General Business Office of Publisher *(Not printer)*

Elsevier Inc., 360 Park Avenue South, New York, NY 10010-1710

9. Full Names and Complete Mailing Addresses of Publisher, Editor, and Managing Editor *(Do not leave blank)*

Publisher *(Name and complete mailing address)*

Linda Belfus, Elsevier, Inc., 1600 John F. Kennedy Blvd. Suite 1800, Philadelphia, PA 19103-2899

Editor *(Name and complete mailing address)*

Kerry Holland, Elsevier, Inc., 1600 John F. Kennedy Blvd. Suite 1800, Philadelphia, PA 19103-2899

Managing Editor *(Name and complete mailing address)*

Adrianne Brigido, Elsevier, Inc., 1600 John F. Kennedy Blvd. Suite 1800, Philadelphia, PA 19103-2899

10. Owner *(Do not leave blank. If the publication is owned by a corporation, give the name and address of the corporation immediately followed by the names and addresses of all stockholders owning or holding 1 percent or more of the total amount of stock. If not owned by a corporation, give the names and addresses of the individual owners. If owned by a partnership or other unincorporated firm, give its name and address as well as those of each individual owner. If the publication is published by a nonprofit organization, give its name and address.)*

Full Name	Complete Mailing Address
Wholly owned subsidiary of	1600 John F. Kennedy Blvd., Ste. 1800
Reed/Elsevier, US holdings	Philadelphia, PA 19103-2899

11. Known Bondholders, Mortgagees, and Other Security Holders Owning or Holding 1 Percent or More of Total Amount of Bonds, Mortgages, or Other Securities. If none, check box ☐ None

Full Name	Complete Mailing Address
N/A	

12. Tax Status *(For completion by nonprofit organizations authorized to mail at nonprofit rates) (Check one)*
The purpose, function, and nonprofit status of this organization and the exempt status for federal income tax purposes:
☐ Has Not Changed During Preceding 12 Months
☐ Has Changed During Preceding 12 Months *(Publisher must submit explanation of change with this statement)*

PS Form **3526**, September 2007 (Page 1 of 3 (Instructions Page 3)) PSN 7530-01-000-9931 **PRIVACY NOTICE:** See our Privacy policy in www.usps.com

---

13. Publication Title	14. Issue Date for Circulation Data Below
Pediatric Clinics of North America	June 2013

15. Extent and Nature of Circulation		Average No. Copies Each Issue During Preceding 12 Months	No. Copies of Single Issue Published Nearest to Filing Date
a. Total Number of Copies *(Net press run)*		2309	2075
b. Paid Circulation (By Mail and Outside the Mail)	(1) Mailed Outside-County Paid Subscriptions Stated on PS Form 3541. *(Include paid distribution above nominal rate, advertiser's proof copies, and exchange copies)*	1111	988
	(2) Mailed In-County Paid Subscriptions Stated on PS Form 3541 *(Include paid distribution above nominal rate, advertiser's proof copies, and exchange copies)*		
	(3) Paid Distribution Outside the Mails Including Sales Through Dealers and Carriers, Street Vendors, Counter Sales, and Other Paid Distribution Outside USPS®	690	570
	(4) Paid Distribution by Other Classes Mailed Through the USPS (e.g. First-Class Mail®)		
c. Total Paid Distribution *(Sum of 15b (1), (2), (3), and (4))*		1801	1558
d. Free or Nominal Rate Distribution (By Mail and Outside the Mail)	(1) Free or Nominal Rate Outside-County Copies Included on PS Form 3541	78	99
	(2) Free or Nominal Rate In-County Copies Included on PS Form 3541		
	(3) Free or Nominal Rate Copies Mailed at Other Classes Through the USPS (e.g. First-Class Mail)		
	(4) Free or Nominal Rate Distribution Outside the Mail (Carriers or other means)		
e. Total Free or Nominal Rate Distribution (Sum of 15d (1), (2), (3) and (4))		78	99
f. Total Distribution (Sum of 15c and 15e)		1879	1657
g. Copies not Distributed (See instructions to publishers #4 (page #3))		430	418
h. Total (Sum of 15f and g)		2309	2075
i. Percent Paid (15c divided by 15f times 100)		95.85%	94.03%

16. Publication of Statement of Ownership
☐ If the publication is a general publication, publication of this statement is required. Will be printed ☐ Publication not required
in the October 2013 issue of this publication.

17. Signature and Title of Editor, Publisher, Business Manager, or Owner

[signature]

Stephen R. Bushing – Inventory Distribution Coordinator

Date
September 14, 2013

I certify that all information furnished on this form is true and complete. I understand that anyone who furnishes false or misleading information on this form or who omits material or information requested on the form may be subject to criminal sanctions (including fines and imprisonment) and/or civil sanctions (including civil penalties).

PS Form **3526**, September 2007 (Page 2 of 3)

Moving?

Make sure your subscription moves with you!

To notify us of your new address, find your **Clinics Account Number** (located on your mailing label above your name), and contact customer service at:

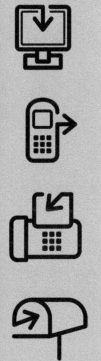

Email: journalscustomerservice-usa@elsevier.com

800-654-2452 (subscribers in the U.S. & Canada)
314-447-8871 (subscribers outside of the U.S. & Canada)

Fax number: 314-447-8029

Elsevier Health Sciences Division
Subscription Customer Service
3251 Riverport Lane
Maryland Heights, MO 63043

*To ensure uninterrupted delivery of your subscription, please notify us at least 4 weeks in advance of move.

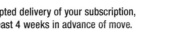

Printed and bound by CPI Group (UK) Ltd, Croydon, CR0 4YY

03/10/2024

01040412-0004